Robotic Surgery

Editor

JULIO TEIXEIRA

SURGICAL CLINICS
OF NORTH AMERICA

www.surgical.theclinics.com

Consulting Editor
RONALD F. MARTIN

April 2020 • Volume 100 • Number 2

ELSEVIER

1600 John F. Kennedy Boulevard • Suite 1800 • Philadelphia, Pennsylvania, 19103-2899

http://www.surgical.theclinics.com

SURGICAL CLINICS OF NORTH AMERICA Volume 100, Number 2
April 2020 ISSN 0039–6109, ISBN-13: 978-0-323-70847-0

Editor: John Vassallo, j.vassallo@elsevier.com
Developmental Editor: Casey Potter

Surgical Clinics of North America (ISSN 0039–6109) is published bimonthly by Elsevier Inc., 360 Park Avenue South, New York, NY 10010-1710. Months of publication are February, April, June, August, October, and December. Business and Editorial Offices: 1600 John F. Kennedy Blvd., Suite 1800, Philadelphia, PA 19103-2899. Periodicals postage paid at New York, NY and additional mailing offices. Subscription prices are $430.00 per year for US individuals, $891.00 per year for US institutions, $100.00 per year for US & Canadian students and residents, $507.00 per year for Canadian individuals, $1130.00 per year for Canadian institutions, $536.00 for international individuals, $1130.00 per year for international institutions and $250.00 per year for foreign students/residents. To receive student/resident rate, orders must be accompanied by name of affiliated institution, date of term, and the *signature* of program/residency coordinator on institution letterhead. Orders will be billed at individual rate until proof of status is received. Foreign air speed delivery is included in all *Clinics* subscription prices. All prices are subject to change without notice. POSTMASTER: Send address changes to *Surgical Clinics*, Elsevier Health Sciences Division, Subscription Customer Service, 3251 Riverport Lane, Maryland Heights, MO 63043. **Customer Service (orders, claims, online, change of address): Telephone: 1-800-654-2452 (U.S. and Canada); 314-447-8871 (outside U.S. and Canada). Fax: 314-447-8029. E-mail: journalscustomerservice-usa@elsevier.com (for print support); journalsonlinesupport-usa@elsevier.com (for online support)**.

Reprints. For copies of 100 or more, of articles in this publication, please contact the Commercial Reprints Department, Elsevier Inc., 360 Park Avenue South, New York, New York 10010-1710. Tel. 212-633-3874; Fax: 212-633-3820, E-mail: reprints@elsevier.com.

The Surgical Clinics of North America is also published in Spanish by McGraw-Hill Interamericana Editores S.A., P.O. Box 5-237 06500 Mexico D.F. Mexico; and in Portuguese by Interlivros Edicoes Ltda., Rua Comandante Coelho 1085, CEP 21250, Rio de Janeiro, Brazil; and in Greek by Paschalidis Medical Publications, Athens Greece.

The Surgical Clinics of North America is covered in *MEDLINE/PubMed (Index Medicus)*, *EMBASE/Excerpta Medica*, *Current Contents/Clinical Medicine*, *Current Contents/Life Sciences*, *Science Citation Index*, and *ISI/BIOMED*.

Contributors

CONSULTING EDITOR

RONALD F. MARTIN, MD, FACS
Colonel (Retired), United States Army Reserve, Executive Vice President, Kalispell Regional Healthcare, Chief Physician Executive, Kalispell Regional Medical Group, Division of HPB Surgery and Surgical Oncology, Kalispell, Montana, USA

EDITOR

JULIO TEIXEIRA, MD, FACS
Associate Professor of Surgery, Donald and Barbara Zucker School of Medicine at Hofstra/Northwell, Northwell Health Hofstra University, Chief of Minimally Invasive Surgery, System Director of the Northwell Bariatric Surgery Collaborative, Lenox Hill Hospital–Northwell Health Surgery, New York, New York, USA

AUTHORS

POPPY ADDISON, MD
Surgical Resident, Department of Surgery, Lenox Hill Hospital, New York, New York, USA

JENNIFER L. AGNEW, MD
Attending Surgeon, Lenox Hill Hospital, Assistant Professor of Surgery, Donald and Barbara Zucker School of Medicine at Hofstra/Northwell, New York, New York, USA

KULVINDER S. BAJWA, MD
Division of Minimally Invasive and Elective General Surgery, Department of Surgery, McGovern Medical School, The University of Texas Health Science Center at Houston, Houston, Texas, USA

GARTH BALLANTYNE, MD
Clinical Professor of Surgery, NYU Grossman School of Medicine, New York, New York, USA

JUSTIN BLASBERG, MD, MPH, FACS
Director of Robotic Thoracic Surgery, Associate Professor of Surgery, Yale School of Medicine, New Haven, Connecticut, USA

HARRISON BROWNING, MD
Digestive Health Institute, AdventHealth Tampa, Tampa, Florida, USA

KAREN CHANG, MD
Good Samaritan Medical Center, Tufts University School of Medicine, SMG Surgical Specialties, Brockton, Massachusetts, USA

LINUS CHUANG, MD
Department of Obstetrics, Gynecology and Reproductive Biology, Nuvance Health, Danbury, Connecticut, USA

TANUJA DAMANI, MD
Surgical Director, Center for Esophageal Health, NYU Langone Health, Clinical Assistant Professor of Surgery, NYU Grossman School of Medicine, New York, New York, USA

NAOMI-LIZA DENNING, MD
Department of Surgery, Donald and Barbara Zucker School of Medicine at Hofstra/Northwell, Manhasset, New York, USA; Cohen Children's Medical Center at Northwell Health, New Hyde Park, New York, USA

DAVID EARLE, MD, FACS
Director, New England Hernia Center, North Chelmsford, Massachusetts, USA; Associate Professor of Surgery, Tufts University School of Medicine, Boston, Massachusetts, USA

MELISSA M. FELINSKI, DO
Division of Minimally Invasive and Elective General Surgery, Department of Surgery, McGovern Medical School, The University of Texas Health Science Center at Houston, Houston, Texas, USA

ABIGAIL FONG, MD
Department of Surgery, City of Hope National Medical Center, Duarte, California, USA; Department of Surgery, Cedars-Sinai Medical Center, Los Angeles, California, USA

YUMAN FONG, MD
Sangiacomo Chair and Chairman, Department of Surgery, City of Hope National Medical Center, Duarte, California, USA

JOHN GAROFALO, MD
Department of Obstetrics, Gynecology and Reproductive Biology, Nuvance Health, Norwalk, Connecticut, USA

FAHRI GOKCAL, MD
Good Samaritan Medical Center, Tufts University School of Medicine, Brockton, Massachusetts, USA

ALFREDO D. GUERRÓN, MD, FACS
Division of Metabolic and Weight Loss Surgery, Assistant Professor, Department of Surgery, Duke University Health System, Durham, North Carolina, USA

JONATHAN M. HEMLI, MD, MSc, FRACS
Surgical Director, Clinical Research, Department of Cardiovascular and Thoracic Surgery, Lenox Hill Hospital–Northwell Health, New York, New York, USA; Associate Professor, Cardiovascular and Thoracic Surgery, Donald and Barbara Zucker School of Medicine at Hofstra/Northwell, Hempstead, New York, USA

POUYA IRANMANESH, MD
Division of Minimally Invasive and Elective General Surgery, Department of Surgery, McGovern Medical School, The University of Texas Health Science Center at Houston, Houston, Texas, USA

RAMÓN DÍAZ JARA, MD
Research Fellow, Division of Metabolic and Weight Loss Surgery, Department of Surgery, Duke University Health System, Durham, North Carolina, USA

MICHELLE P. KALLIS, MD
Department of Surgery, Donald and Barbara Zucker School of Medicine at Hofstra/
Northwell, Manhasset, New York, USA; Cohen Children's Medical Center at Northwell
Health, New Hyde Park, New York, USA

PRATISTHA KOIRALA, MD, PhD
Department of Obstetrics, Gynecology and Reproductive Biology, Nuvance Health,
Danbury, Connecticut, USA

OMAR YUSEF KUDSI, MD, MBA, FACS
Good Samaritan Medical Center, Tufts University School of Medicine, Brockton,
Massachusetts, USA

KELLY J. LAFARO, MD, MPH
Department of Surgery, Johns Hopkins University School of Medicine, Baltimore,
Maryland, USA

KENNETH LUBERICE, MD
Digestive Health Institute, AdventHealth Tampa, Tampa, Florida, USA

JOSEPH MARTZ, MD
Chief, Division of Colon and Rectal Surgery, Western Region Northwell/Lenox Hill
Hospital, Vice Chairman, Associate Professor, Department of Surgery, Lenox Hill
Hospital, Donald and Barbara Zucker School of Medicine at Hofstra/Northwell, New York,
New York, USA

MINA MEKHAIL, BSc (Hons)
Medical Student, St. George's University, School of Medicine, St George's, Grenada,
West Indies

DAVID MIKHAIL, MD, FRCSC
Endourology Fellow, The Smith Institute for Urology (Northwell Health), New Hyde Park,
New York, USA

ASHLEY S. MOON, MD
Department of Obstetrics, Gynecology and Reproductive Biology, Nuvance Health,
Danbury, Connecticut, USA

YURI NOVITSKY, MD, FACS
Professor of Surgery, Columbia University Irving Medical Center, Director,
Comprehensive Hernia Center, Department of Surgery, New York, New York,
USA

NIRAV C. PATEL, MD, FRCS
Vice Chairman, Department of Cardiovascular and Thoracic Surgery, Lenox Hill Hospital–
Northwell Health, Director, Robotic Cardiac Surgery, Northwell Health, New York,
New York, USA; Professor, Cardiovascular and Thoracic Surgery, Donald and Barbara
Zucker School of Medicine at Hofstra/Northwell, Hempstead, New York, USA

DINA PODOLSKY, MD
Assistant Professor of Surgery, Columbia University Irving Medical Center,
Comprehensive Hernia Center, Department of Surgery, New York, New York, USA

DANA PORTENIER, MD, FACS
Division of Metabolic and Weight Loss Surgery, Assistant Professor, Department of
Surgery, Duke University Health System, Durham, North Carolina, USA

JOSE M. PRINCE, MD
Vice Chair, Department of Surgery, Donald and Barbara Zucker School of Medicine at Hofstra/Northwell, Manhasset, New York, USA; Associate Professor of Surgery and Pediatrics, Donald and Barbara Zucker School of Medicine at Hofstra/Northwell, Hempstead, New York, USA; Chief, Division of Pediatric Surgery, Cohen Children's Medical Center at Northwell Health, New Hyde Park, NY, USA

DIMITAR RANEV, MD
Department of Surgery, Lenox Hill Hospital–Northwell Health, New York, New York, USA

LEE RICHSTONE, MD
Chairman of Urology, Lennox Hill Hospital–Northwell Health, New York, New York, USA

ALEXANDER S. ROSEMURGY, MD
Digestive Health Institute, AdventHealth Tampa, Tampa, Florida, USA

SHARONA ROSS, MD
Digestive Health Institute, AdventHealth Tampa, Tampa, Florida, USA

MANU SANCHETI, MD, FACS
Director of Robotic Thoracic Surgery, Assistant Professor of Surgery, Emory Saint Joseph's Hospital, Emory Healthcare, Atlanta, Georgia, USA

JOSEPH SARCONA, MD
Urology Resident Physician, Lennox Hill Hospital–Northwell Health, New York, New York, USA

GARY SCHWARTZ, MD, FACS
Department of Thoracic Surgery and Lung Transplantation, Baylor University Medical Center, Clinical Assistant Professor of Surgery, Texas A&M Health Science Center, Dallas, Texas, USA

SHINIL K. SHAH, DO
Division of Minimally Invasive and Elective General Surgery, Department of Surgery, McGovern Medical School, The University of Texas Health Science Center at Houston, Houston, Texas, USA; Michael E Debakey Institute for Comparative Cardiovascular Science and Biomedical Devices, Texas A&M University, College Station, Texas, USA

CAMILLE STEWART, MD
Department of Surgery, City of Hope National Medical Center, Duarte, California, USA

ISWANTO SUCANDY, MD
Digestive Health Institute, AdventHealth Tampa, Tampa, Florida, USA

JULIO TEIXEIRA, MD, FACS
Associate Professor of Surgery, Donald and Barbara Zucker School of Medicine at Hofstra/Northwell, Northwell Health Hofstra University, Chief of Minimally Invasive Surgery, System Director of the Northwell Bariatric Surgery Collaborative, Lenox Hill Hospital–Northwell Health Surgery, New York, New York, USA

MAI-LINH T. VU, MD
Complete Women Care, Long Beach, California, USA

ERIK B. WILSON, MD
Division of Minimally Invasive and Elective General Surgery, Department of Surgery, McGovern Medical School, The University of Texas Health Science Center at Houston, Houston, Texas, USA

Contents

Foreword: Robotic Surgery   xiii

Ronald F. Martin

Preface: One Hundred Years of Evolution in Surgery: From Asepsis to Artificial Intelligence   xv

Julio Teixeira

History of Computer-Assisted Surgery   209

Dimitar Ranev and Julio Teixeira

Robotic surgery is growing rapidly, with more than 5000 units in operation worldwide. The most widely used robotic surgery system originated from the concept of telepresence, which led to government-sponsored research and development. The resulting work was taken over by private industry, which led to Food and Drug Administration clearance of the first systems in 2000 to 2001. Robotic surgery offers significant advantages over open surgery; its most important feature is the introduction of a computer into the operating room, with the resulting potential for data collection and analysis that will shape surgical practice in the future.

Robotic Cardiac Surgery   219

Jonathan M. Hemli and Nirav C. Patel

 Video content accompanies this article at http://www.surgical. theclinics.com.

Robotic minimally invasive direct coronary artery bypass is the most common robotic coronary procedure performed worldwide. It can be used to treat isolated left anterior descending (LAD) stenosis or can be coupled with percutaneous coronary intervention to diseased non-LAD targets in patients with multivessel disease. Virtually all types of mitral valve repair can be performed using the robot; valve replacement can also be undertaken. The robot can be used to repair atrial septal defects and resect cardiac myxoma. Increased cost of the robotic procedure may be offset by fewer perioperative complications, shorter hospital stay, and faster postoperative recovery.

Robotic Thoracic Surgery   237

Gary Schwartz, Manu Sancheti, and Justin Blasberg

Minimally invasive surgery for diseases of the chest offsets the morbidity of painful thoracic Incisions while allowing for meticulous dissection of major anatomic structures. This benefit translates to improved outcomes and recovery following the surgical management of benign and malignant esophageal pathologic condition, mediastinal tumors, and lung resections. This anatomic region is particularly amenable to a robotic approach given the fixed space and need for complex intracorporeal dissection. As robotic platforms continue to evolve, more complex thoracic surgical interventions will be facilitated, translating to improved outcomes for our patients.

Robotic Foregut Surgery   249

Tanuja Damani and Garth Ballantyne

Robotic-assisted surgery for benign esophageal disease is described for treatment of achalasia, gastroesophageal reflux, paraesophageal hernias, epiphrenic diverticula, and benign esophageal masses. Robotic Heller myotomy has operative times, relief of dysphagia, and conversion rates comparable to laparoscopic approach, with lower incidence of intraoperative esophageal perforation. The use of robotic platform for primary antireflux surgery is under evaluation, due to prolonged operative time and increased operative costs, with no differences in postoperative outcomes or hospital stay. Studies have shown benefits of robotic surgery in complex reoperative foregut surgery with respect to decreased conversion rates, lower readmission rates, and improved functional outcomes.

Robotic Liver Resection   265

Kelly J. Lafaro, Camille Stewart, Abigail Fong, and Yuman Fong

Robotic surgery has rapidly evolved. It is particularly attractive as an alternative minimally invasive approach in liver surgery because of improvements in visualization and articulated instruments. Limitations include increased operative times and lack of tactile feedback, but these have not been shown in studies. Considerations unique to robotic surgery, including safety protocols, must be put in place and be reviewed at the beginning of every procedure to ensure safety in the event of an emergent conversion. Despite the lack of early adoption by many hepatobiliary surgeons, robotic liver surgery continues to evolve and find its place within hepatobiliary surgery.

Robotic Biliary Surgery   283

Karen Chang, Fahri Gokcal, and Omar Yusef Kudsi

Robotic cholecystectomy is safe and feasible approach and can be combined with common bile duct exploration to address complicated pathology in a single setting. This article summarizes reported outcomes after robotic biliary surgery. A technical overview of robotic multiport and single port cholecystectomy is provided. Last, the approach to benign bile duct disease during robotic cholecystectomy, including reconstruction of the biliary tree, is described.

Robotic Pancreatic Surgery for Solid, Cystic, and Mixed Lesions   303

Alexander S. Rosemurgy, Sharona Ross, Kenneth Luberice, Harrison Browning, and Iswanto Sucandy

Robotic surgery is flourishing worldwide. Pancreatic cancer is the fourth leading cause of cancer death in the United States. Most pancreatic operations are undertaken for the management of pancreatic adenocarcinoma. Therefore, it is essential for all physicians caring for patients with cancer to understand the role and importance of molecular tumor markers. This article details our technique and application of the robotic platform to robotic pancreatectomy. The use of the robot does not change the nature of pancreatic operations, but it is our belief that it will improve patient outcomes and, possibly, survival by reducing perioperative complications.

Robotic Colorectal Surgery   337

Poppy Addison, Jennifer L. Agnew, and Joseph Martz

The role of robotics in colon and rectal surgery has been established as an important and effective tool for the surgeon. Its inherent technologies have provided for increased visualization and ease of dissection in the minimally invasive approach to surgery. The value of the robot is apparent in the more challenging aspects of colon and rectal procedures, including the intracorporeal anastomosis for right colectomies and the low pelvic dissection for benign and malignant diseases.

Urologic Robotic Surgery   361

David Mikhail, Joseph Sarcona, Mina Mekhail, and Lee Richstone

Urologists have always been leaders in advancing surgical technology and were the first to utilize modern robotic surgery for robotic-assisted laparoscopic radical proctectomy. Surgeon ergonomics, instrument precision, operative time, and postoperative recovery were all objectively improved. In urology, robotic surgery is now used for all intra-abdominal, retroperitoneal, and pelvic procedures and has been expanded to renal transplants and pediatric use. Modern robotic surgery has become an essential part of treating complex urologic disease in the developed world. Urologists continue to lead the way with the latest robotic surgical systems, including the newly approved single port systems.

Robotic-Assisted Laparoscopic Ventral Hernia Repair   379

David Earle

Robotic-assisted laparoscopic ventral hernia repair (RA-LVHR) has many options. Before applying these techniques, it is important to identify the patient's goals for hernia repair, align yourself with those goals, and apply a technique appropriate for the clinical scenario, and most likely to meet the goals. Fundamental principles of hernia repair must be maintained: avoiding thermal injury to hollow viscera, adequate dissection of abdominal wall, appropriate mesh:defect ratio, stronger fixation where overlap is limited, and more overlap where fixation points are weak. This manuscript will detail available techniques for RA-LVHR along with their their advantages and disadvantages.

Robotic Inguinal Hernia Repair   409

Dina Podolsky and Yuri Novitsky

Robotic inguinal hernia repair represents the natural progression of minimally invasive inguinal hernia surgery. This article highlights all aspects of a robotic transabdominal preperitoneal (rTAPP) inguinal hernia repair with mesh, starting with preoperative planning and patient selection, key technical steps, and common postoperative complications and recovery. The most recent published data on robotic inguinal hernia repair are comprehensively reviewed, confirming that rTAPP is a safe and effective option for the repair of unilateral and bilateral inguinal hernias.

Robotic Primary and Revisional Bariatric Surgery 417

Pouya Iranmanesh, Kulvinder S. Bajwa, Melissa M. Felinski, Shinil K. Shah, and Erik B. Wilson

In this article, we review the role of robotics in bariatric surgery. After a brief overview of the evolution of minimally invasive bariatric surgery, we discuss possible advantages of robotic systems and subsequently go into more details about each procedure, including adjustable gastric bands, sleeve gastrectomy, Roux-en-Y gastric bypass, and biliopancreatic diversion with duodenal switch. We also discuss outcomes of robotics in reoperative bariatric surgery. Considerations about training are presented as well.

Pediatric Robotic Surgery 431

Naomi-Liza Denning, Michelle P. Kallis, and Jose M. Prince

Pediatric robotic-assisted surgery is quickly gaining traction in pediatric surgical disciplines but presents unique challenges as compared to adult robotic surgery. Small abdominal and thoracic cavities limit working space and operative indications differ from the adult population. This article describes the development of pediatric robotic-assisted surgery, discusses technical limitations and benefits, and reviews training considerations particular to robotic surgery. Applications and published outcomes of common procedures in urology, general and thoracic surgery, otolaryngology, and pediatric surgical oncology are described. Finally, costs and the anticipated future direction of pediatric robotic-assisted surgery are discussed.

Robotic Surgery in Gynecology 445

Ashley S. Moon, John Garofalo, Pratistha Koirala, Mai-Linh T. Vu, and Linus Chuang

 Video content accompanies this article at http://www.surgical.theclinics.com.

The robotic-assisted laparoscopic surgical approach has improved complex gynecologic surgeries. It has the advantages of excellent visualization through the high-resolution 3-dimensional view, a wrist-like motion of the robotic arms and improved ergonomics. Similar to conventional laparoscopic surgeries, it is associated with a decrease in long-term surgical morbidity, early recovery and return to work, and improved esthetics. We discuss preoperative planning, surgical techniques, and some of the latest clinical results of robotic-assisted laparoscopic gynecologic surgery.

Complications of Robotic Surgery 461

Ramón Díaz Jara, Alfredo D. Guerrón, and Dana Portenier

Robotic-assisted surgery has represented a revolution for surgical practice and minimally invasive surgery. The case volume is increasing exponentially and the numbers continue to grow particularly owing to urology and general surgery subspecialties. Nonetheless, robotic surgery is not exempt from complications, which can occur during the preoperative, intraoperative, and postoperative periods, and in particular with issues related to patient preparation, team dynamics, equipment failure, complications related to the surgical act, and surgical outcomes.

SURGICAL CLINICS
OF NORTH AMERICA

FORTHCOMING ISSUES

June 2020
Surgical Oncology for the General Surgeon
Randall Zuckerman and Neal Wilkinson,
Editors

August 2020
Wound Management
Michael D. Caldwell and Michael J. Harl,
Editors

October 2020
Rural Surgery
Tyler G. Hughes, *Editor*

RECENT ISSUES

February 2020
Contemporary Melanoma Management:
A Surgical Perspective
Rohit Sharma, *Editor*

December 2019
Inflammatory Bowel Disease
Sean J. Langenfeld, *Editor*

October 2019
Practicing Primary Palliative Care
Pringl Miller, *Editor*

SERIES OF RELATED INTEREST

Advances in Surgery
https://www.advancessurgery.com/
Surgical Oncology Clinics
https://www.surgonc.theclinics.com/
Thoracic Surgery Clinics
http://www.thoracic.theclinics.com/

THE CLINICS ARE AVAILABLE ONLINE!
Access your subscription at:
www.theclinics.com

Foreword
Robotic Surgery

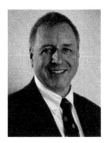

Ronald F. Martin, MD, FACS
Consulting Editor

Throughout the history of surgery, we surgeons have had to wrestle with how to incorporate new ideas and technology. As our understanding of the human condition has evolved, that task has become sometimes easier and sometimes less easy. For the first 6000 years or so of recorded surgical history, everything we could do didn't really make that much of an impact on overall longevity or societal cost. Of course, there were some large gains here and there, but much of what improved health and longevity was outside of the traditional confines of surgery. During the twentieth century, especially the latter half of the century, the discipline of surgery really started to make an impact on public health. Advances in our ability to control physiology (both in and out of the operating room) and advances in operative skill and techniques in the areas of cardiac, pulmonary, general, orthopedic, and neurological surgery all led to dramatic changes to our ability to improve health and increase longevity. These advances accompanied their own technological growths but also brought us an unparalleled increase in cost to society. It also led us to a new era in which the main question shifted, or should have shifted, from what *can* we do to what *should* we do? As the century came to a close, the advances in minimally invasive surgery brought even more focus to the question of capability and feasibility as opposed to necessity or prudence.

From a surgical standpoint, the twenty-first century has been largely marked by the advance of robotic surgery. As the reader of this issue will note, *robotic surgery* is probably better described as *computer-assisted operating*. Robotic devices serve as a computer interface between the operator and the instruments. In some cases, that allows for some surgeons who struggle with "straight" videoscopic operations to mitigate some technical challenges. In other cases, it allows videoscopic operations to be done that otherwise may not be possible by other means. The use of the robotic interface very much influences what we can do.

However, there are some potential downsides to computer-assisted operating: cost of equipment (purchase and service) and operative time probably being chief among them at present. The counterargument can be made that since the operative word in

Surg Clin N Am 100 (2020) xiii–xiv
https://doi.org/10.1016/j.suc.2020.02.001
0039-6109/20/© 2020 Published by Elsevier Inc.

"computer-assisted operating" is "computer," it is likely that the cost curve will deflect to some degree in a favorable manner over time. Perhaps, operative efficiency will improve as well as the human part of the equation develops the human-computer interface. What computer-assisted operating will not likely help us with is the process of identifying the correct diagnosis and understanding the correct solution, those will remain in the cognitive arena of our surgical discipline. Of course, artificial intelligence is always nipping at that heel as well.

How and when we incorporate computer-assisted surgery should be guided by 1 question: what problem are we trying to solve? It should not necessarily reflect surgeon preference or be a marketing tool (though both of those may factor in). Our discipline and our industry need to take a good long look in the mirror and ask ourselves if we are motivated by what is good for our patients, their families, and our communities or are we motivated by other factors?

As with any such challenge, we must first educate ourselves on what computer-assisted surgery is and what it can offer us. Dr Teixiera and his colleagues have produced an outstanding collection of articles that will inform and educate the reader about computer-assisted surgery from its inception through the current day as well as yield additional insight as to where things may go. These articles will be invaluable not only as a review of our current capability but also as to how we can incorporate the technology as it exists. We are indebted to them for their phenomenal work.

Of note, the *Surgical Clinics of North America* enters its 100th year this year. That is quite an achievement for any publication. Somewhat coincidentally, the December issue of this year will be my 100th issue as Consulting Editor for the series. It has been a tremendous honor to be part of this series and to watch it also develop through its digital transformation in addition to our print media. We have been fortunate to have worked with so many talented and brilliant people along the way.

In the few weeks leading up to this issue being completed, we lost a very great friend and contributor to this series, Dr Stanley J. Dudrick. I first met Stan when I was a resident in general surgery. He had come to a meeting in our town, and I gave him a ride back to his hotel on a rainy night. I was awestruck by meeting the man who pioneered parenteral nutrition. Conversely, he was the most unassuming and kind human being one could ever wish to meet. Over the years, we developed a close friendship. A few years back, Stan was kind enough to work on a 2-volume issue on surgical nutrition that still stands as a landmark contribution to this series and to the literature in general. Working with Stan on those 2 volumes was one of the highlights of my surgical career. Our thoughts go out to Stan's family. We are so sorry for their loss and so grateful that they shared Stan and his talents with us. Stan was a true giant who never thought of himself as anything other than a proud member of the surgical community. He will be missed.

Ronald F. Martin, MD, FACS
Colonel (retired), United States Army Reserve
Kalispell Regional Healthcare
Kalispell Regional Medical Group
Division of HPB Surgery and
Surgical Oncology
310 Sunnyview Lane
Kalispell, MT 59901, USA

E-mail address:
rfmcescna@gmail.com

Preface

One Hundred Years of Evolution in Surgery: From Asepsis to Artificial Intelligence

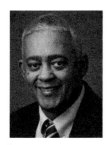

Julio Teixeira, MD, FACS
Editor

The twentieth century witnessed a dramatic evolution in the field of surgery. The introduction of aseptic technique, improvements in anesthesia and perioperative care, and the standardization of hospital care by the American College of Surgeons unleashed an era of creativity and scientific experimentation that led to explosive growth in surgery.

Major historical political events, including the major world wars and the expansion of the industrial revolution, provided the environment for the science of surgery to rapidly evolve in the areas of trauma, critical care, and vascular surgery.

In the 1950s, we witnessed major developments in the fields of cardiothoracic surgery, the introduction of cardiopulmonary bypass, and eventually, transplantation surgery.

The *Surgical Clinics of North America* was a witness to these events in the evolution of surgery and provided a trusted source to document these advances in the science and art of surgery.

In the last 50 years, we have continued to witness rapid growth of the science of surgery determined to meet the needs of our society. Expansion and sophistication in plastic surgery, transplantation, trauma, and critical care continue to transform the field of surgery.

New developments in cameras and imaging and new diagnostic tools have led to dramatic shifts in paradigm in how we approach disease. The introduction of flexible endoscopy and later laparoscopy was a major revolution. Minimal access surgery has impacted all disciplines in surgery universally, leading to lower complications, less pain, and a shift from inpatient to outpatient surgery.

Typically, major paradigm shifts in surgery have lagged behind major changes in technology. Although robotic surgery was first introduced 20 years ago, it struggled

Surg Clin N Am 100 (2020) xv–xvi
https://doi.org/10.1016/j.suc.2020.01.001
0039-6109/20/© 2020 Published by Elsevier Inc.

to demonstrate significant advantages over laparoscopic surgery. The initial systems offered the advantages of 3D visualization and wristed instrumentation but found the surgeons well adjusted to the limitations of "straight stick" laparoscopy. In addition, other factors, such as cost, access, and increased operative time, further limited its adoption, and consequently, the ability to find legitimate indications in most fields in surgery with the exception of urology.

We are currently witnessing the fourth industrial revolution. The coalescence of major technological forces, including Big Data Science, machine learning, and advanced robotic systems, is transforming every aspect of human life, and surgery is no exception.

The evolution of simple laparoscopic surgery to robotic surgery is fundamentally the exchange of a video camera for a computer as the primary interface between the surgeon and the patient. Robotics as we understand it today is the mechanical interface that allows for a digital interventional platform.

This basic, fundamental exchange allows for an infinite number of opportunities that will transform both the surgeon's and the patient's experience.

The applications being developed include data harvesting and assessment of surgeon performance to the introduction of deep learning techniques in computer vision that will assist the surgeon in interpreting anatomy. Other more sophisticated systems will track the surgeon's movements and patient data and synchronize with outcomes data to provide us with early warning systems for complications.

The most provocative aspect is how these systems will participate in the surgical decision-making process in real time. Already we are gathering data on tissue perfusion, helping us decide on the appropriate location for an anastomosis. Molecular markers are determining resection margins, and smart staplers are automatically stopping the stapling process to allow for increased compression or to advise us on making a better choice of staple heights.

These complex systems are based on recurrent convolutional neural networks that are constantly learning and updating from every staple firing and becoming increasingly efficient. Even more evolved systems based on differential programming will gather structured and unstructured data in real time from many sources, including electronic health records, anesthesia monitoring systems, video images, and surgeon's data to arrive at decisions that we will increasingly rely on.

We are at a dawn of a new age in surgery, as we witness the dramatic growth in robotic surgery. The proliferation and commercialization of new robotic surgical systems over the next few years will drive competition, lower cost, and accelerate the adoption of these technologies. The 100th edition of the *Surgical Clinics of North America* recognizes this historical moment and provides a review of the state-of-the-art.

Julio Teixeira, MD, FACS
Zucker School of Medicine Surgery
Northwell Health Hofstra University
Lenox Hill Hospital–Northwell Health
Surgery
186 East 76th Street, 1st Floor
New York, NY 10021, USA

E-mail address:
Jteixeira@northwell.edu

History of Computer-Assisted Surgery

Dimitar Ranev, MD[a],*, Julio Teixeira, MD[b]

KEYWORDS

- History • Robot • Robotic • Surgery • Computer-assisted

KEY POINTS

- Computer-assisted robotic surgery is a rapidly growing field affecting multiple surgical specialties.
- The most widely used robotic platform today originated from the collaboration among researchers, government agencies (NASA and the Department of Defense), and the private industry during the 1980s and 1990s.
- Intuitive Surgical's da Vinci system was cleared by the Food and Drug Administration in 2000 and Computer Motion's ZEUS system in 2001. The 2 companies merged in 2003.
- Robotic surgery places a computer between the surgeon and patient, opening the door to data collection and analysis that is the prerequisite for future automated, artificial intelligence–driven surgery.

INTRODUCTION

Computer assistance, robotics, virtual reality, automation, and artificial intelligence (AI) are concepts that when applied to surgery, would have seemed like science fiction to our surgical predecessors, even less than half a century ago. Technology is transforming not only our daily lives, but our surgical practice at an astonishing pace. The number of articles on robotic surgery indexed on PubMed has increased from 2 to 8 per year before the year 2000, to more than 700 per year in 2017 to 2018 (**Fig. 1**). By reviewing the history, one can better understand, and hopefully join, this ongoing technological revolution.

DEFINITION OF ROBOTIC SURGERY

"Robotic surgery" is commonly used to refer to the da Vinci surgical system and other similar platforms, whereas "computer-assisted surgery" usually implies surgical planning, navigation, and image-guidance. The precise definition is complicated because

[a] Department of Surgery, Long Island Jewish Forest Hills - Northwell Health, 102-01 66th Road, Forest Hills, NY 11375, USA; [b] Zucker School of Medicine at Hofstra/Northwell, Lenox Hill Hospital – Northwell Health, 186 East 76th Street, New York, NY 10021, USA
* Corresponding author.
E-mail address: dranev@northwell.edu

Surg Clin N Am 100 (2020) 209–218
https://doi.org/10.1016/j.suc.2019.11.001
0039-6109/20/© 2019 Elsevier Inc. All rights reserved.

surgical.theclinics.com

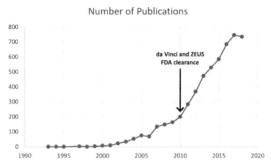

Fig. 1. Number of "robotic surgery" publications indexed on PubMed per year.

terms that are introduced for marketing purposes do not necessarily reflect the technology being used. For example, "robotic surgery" may suggest a degree of autonomous operation, which is currently not the case. There are many technical terms related to this subject that are used throughout the text (**Table 1**). The definition and understanding of these terms will become increasingly important as surgical technology progresses. In this text, the authors use "robotic surgery" in the widest sense, not limited to specific commercial products and applications.

Mechanical automated machines have been present since antiquity. The ancient Greek philosopher Archytas designed a steam-powered flying pigeon in 350 B.C. In

Table 1	
Definition of robotic surgery technical terms	
Term	**Definition**
Robot	Moves independently and performs a physical task
Mini-, micro-, nano-robot	Robots of decreasing sizes
Bot	Software, program designed to behave like a human on a network (ie, the Internet)
Cobot	Collaborative robot, physically interacts with humans in a shared workspace (unlike most industrial robots)
Android	Humanoid, manlike in appearance
Gynoid	Also "fembot," humanoid, resembling a woman
Cyborg	Cybernetic organism, with upgraded mechanical parts (prosthetics)
Automaton	Independently performs pre-programed task(s)
Drone	Unmanned remotely controlled vehicle
Augmented reality	Interposing a computer-generated image over a view of the real world
Virtual reality	Transporting one's awareness to a computer-generated, simulated environment
Telepresence	Transporting one's awareness to a different (remote) location
Machine learning	Software that uses mathematical models to analyze data, allowing it to make predictions and decisions
Artificial intelligence	"Cognitive" functions displayed by machines, like learning and decision making
Quantum computing	Computers that use quantum theory principles making them massively faster and more powerful than current silicone chip computers

the fifteenth century, Leonardo da Vinci designed his famous *robot:* a mechanical knight, moved by pulleys and cables, based on knowledge from his anatomic dissections. Although these devices can be seen as early "robots," today's perception of a robot was shaped by science fiction during the twentieth century.

The origin of the term "robot" is the Old Church Slavonic word for labor (rabota/работа). The term was written by Czech science fiction writer Karel Čapek (and coined by his brother, Josef Čapek) in the 1920 play *R.U.R. (Rossum's Universal Robots)*. There, a race of artificial beings created for work, rebel against and eventually wipe out humanity. The play became popular internationally, and in 1938 its adaptation became the first piece of science fiction broadcasted on television. By the 1940s, Isaac Asimov had further popularized robots, adding the word "robotic" and defining the "Three Laws of Robotics." Curiously, Isaac Asimov was offered collaboration with the Defense Advanced Research Projects Agency (DARPA) during the cold war, the same agency that was instrumental in developing the technology behind today's surgical robots.[1] An example of robotics in trauma, vascular, and hand surgery was seen on the big screen in 1980, when a robot performed Luke Skywalker's prosthetic hand replantation with an excellent outcome.[2]

A contemporary definition of "robot" is found in the Merriam-Webster Dictionary: "a machine that resembles a living creature in being capable of *moving independently* (as by walking or rolling on wheels) and *performing complex actions* (such as grasping and moving objects)."[3] Robots became reality in 1961, as the first industrial robot, named Unimate, began operation at a General Motors assembly plant in Ewing Township, New Jersey, performing automated tasks dangerous to humans.[4]

The first robotic surgical procedure, a stereotactic brain biopsy, was performed in 1985 by Kwoh and colleagues.[5] The device was called PUMA: an adapted industrial robotic arm that was used to position the biopsy needle, eliminating tremor and improving precision. This evolved into multiple subsequent devices that gained approval from the Food and Drug Administration (FDA) and are in widespread use today. PUMA was the basis of developing the PROBOT (Integrated Surgical Supplies Ltd., Mesa, AZ), which was used successfully for TURP. Another device, ROBODOC, was a related system used in hip replacement, allowing for precise coring of the femur head to allow placement of the prosthesis. PAKY was a platform designed for percutaneous approach to the kidney.[6] All of these devices were designed to serve a single purpose, for a specific procedure and specialty. Their development was driven by the pursuit of precision, usually with the use of radiological guidance. The development of today's most widely used robotic surgery platform, however, originated from a different concept: telepresence.

ORIGIN OF ROBOTIC SURGERY

Today's most widely adopted robotic surgical technology is the product of a collaboration among researchers at the Stanford Research Institute (SRI), government agencies (National Aeronautics and Space Administration [NASA] and the Department of Defense [DOD]), and private companies.

The concept of telepresence would allow a surgeon to begin a life-saving procedure soon after the moment of injury, from a remote and safe location, while the patient is still being transported from the hostile environment. The term telepresence first emerged as NASA scientists developed a heavy helmet-mounted and ceiling-suspended displays, initially with the goal of reviewing data from the Voyager mission.[7] In 1984, former Atari employee Jaron Lanier founded VLP Research and designed a head-mounted display and gloves (DataGlove) that allowed data manipulation on the screen and included haptic feedback. Lanier coined the term virtual reality.

STANFORD RESEARCH INSTITUTE

In 1986, Phil Green, PhD, at SRI began federally funded research on a remote surgical manipulator capable of performing microsurgery. The head-mounted display and gloves, however, proved inadequate for the task and were subsequently replaced by a stereoscopic monitor and a workstation using instrument handles. In 1987, US Army Colonel (COL) Richard Satava, MD, joined SRI and construction of the first prototype began. The device, named "telepresence surgical system" by Dr Green, consisted of 2 separate parts: a telepresence surgeon's workstation and a remote surgical unit. The workstation included a 3-dimensional (3D) monitor requiring the surgeon to wear polarized glasses, included a speaker and was designed ergonomically to achieve an immersive virtual reality experience for the operator. The remote surgical unit included a stereoscopic camera and 2 manipulators with exchangeable tips. The instruments allowed 4 degrees of freedom and provided force-feedback. In 1989, COL Satava viewed Dr Jacques Perrisat's video of a laparoscopic cholecystectomy at the Society of American Gastrointestinal and Endoscopic Surgeons Meeting in Louisville, Kentucky. Realizing their telepresence system's multiple advantages in laparoscopy (elimination of fulcrum effect, tremor reduction, improved dexterity, stereoscopic vision), COL Satava helped redirect the focus of the project from microsurgery to laparoscopic surgery. In 1992, COL Satava was assigned to the Advanced Biomedical Technologies program of DARPA.[8,9]

At DARPA, SRI's prototype was the centerpiece of a larger concept: medical forward surgical treatment (MEDFAST). The surgeon would perform the life-saving procedure remotely, with the patient-side unit located at an armored vehicle used for patient transport. This concept integrated the platform with the vehicle and other medical technologies developed by DARPA, like digital radiography and robotic scrub nurse capable of exchanging instruments and dispensing medications. MEDFAST was a complete mobile operating room with anesthesia equipment, suction, and electrosurgery, and future plans to add a computed tomography scanner. Because the platform was intended for a moving vehicle, tremor reduction was added to the surgeon workstation, and the camera system was improved by increasing magnification and resolution and providing stability: the camera's position could adjust to external motion, keeping a stable view for the surgeon.

SRI was then tasked with building and installing the telepresence system at the Uniformed Services University of the Health Sciences in Bethesda, MD. In addition, a training simulator was requested. The prototype was shown in 1993 during field exercises in Augusta, Georgia, and the following year at the Association of the US Army Annual Convention. At that time, the 2 components still required a cable connection.

SRI, funded by DARPA, then began testing the system in animal models. When COL Satava left SRI for DARPA, he was replaced by vascular surgeon Jon Bowersox, MD, PhD. Dr Bowersox successfully performed various vascular surgical tasks.[10] The system required bedside assistance for suture placement and cutting. Keeping the focus on trauma surgery, the platform was then used to treat visceral injuries in the in vivo porcine models, followed by urologic procedures like nephrectomy and bladder repair. In all cases, the procedures were successful, but lasted significantly longer than the open counterpart. Degrees of freedom limited to 4, fixed camera position, and inability to clutch the controllers contributed to the prolonged operative time. Interestingly, the operative time was shorter for laparoscopic and microsurgical applications. With the latest version, microwave communication between the components was possible, and the prototype allowed 6 degrees of freedom. Although the device provided force-feedback, suture breakage was common and, surprisingly, surgeons performed better with the force-feedback turned off. Force is just one of many sensations necessary to perform a fine motor task. In 1998, scientists at MIT confirmed this observation while working on another DARPA-supported, force-feedback–enabled robotic surgical system: the Black Falcon.[11] This observation, that a high-resolution 3D image allows the surgeon to judge tissue tension and compensate for the lack of tactile feedback, is the reason today's most popular robotic platform does not offer haptics. In 1995, Intuitive Surgical acquired SRI's intellectual property.

COMPUTER MOTION

The first FDA-cleared robotic surgical system was developed by a private company, Computer Motion, founded by Dr Yulun Wang in 1990. The work was supported by grants from NASA and DARPA. The Automated Endoscopic System for Optimal Positioning (AESOP) was designed to hold and guide a laparoscope under the control of the surgeon. To achieve that, AESOP used a voice-controlled robotic arm. The system was FDA-cleared in 1994 using the faster 510k process setting a precedent for future robotic systems. In 1996, Computer Motion introduced HERMES, an integrated system for the operating room, allowing voice-control of various functions like lighting and insufflation. The same year, they introduced ZEUS: a complete robotic surgery system including AESOP and 2 laparoscopic instruments with 6 and later 7 degrees of freedom, tremor elimination, and motion scaling. The robotic arms were mounted to the operating table and the 3D display required the surgeon to wear polarized glasses. In 1998, ZEUS was used for the first time in a human, performing tubal re-anastomosis, and in 1999 it was used in coronary artery bypass grafting. ZEUS received FDA approval in 2001. The same year, ZEUS was used to perform the first telesurgical procedure, a laparoscopic cholecystectomy, with the patient located in Strasbourg, France, and the surgeon, Dr Jacques Marescaux, located in New York City.[12] The process required a dedicated high-speed transatlantic cable connection. In 2001, Computer Motion's SOCRATES received FDA approval. The system was designed for tele-mentoring and was successfully used for multiple procedures at remote areas in Canada by Dr Mehran Anvari, MBBS, PhD, and his team.[13] In 2003, Computer Motion merged with Intuitive Surgical.

INTUITIVE SURGICAL

Intuitive Surgical was founded in 1995 by Fred Moll, MD; John Freund, MD; and engineer Robert Younge. Building on SRI's designs, their first prototype was named Lenny, short for Leonardo, and included 3 robotic arms: 1 for the laparoscope, and 2 non-interchangeable instruments with 7 degrees of freedom. SRI's polarized 3D system was replaced by active shutter video display and glasses. The second prototype, Mona, named after Leonardo's *Mona Lisa*, added interchangeable instruments, but lacked a camera-holding arm, requiring a bedside assistant to hold the laparoscope. Mona became the first surgical robot to begin human trials in 1997, a year before ZEUS. The first operation, a laparoscopic cholecystectomy, was performed by Dr Jacques Himpens, a bariatric surgeon in Dendermonde, Belgium. The report of this first robotic surgery was declined by both *The New England Journal of Medicine* and *The Lancet*, being judged "inappropriate" or "very unlikely to have actually happened," but was published in *Surgical Endoscopy* as a letter to the editor. A year later, Dr Guy-Bernard Cadière, known for performing the first laparoscopic adjustable gastric banding in 1992, performed the first procedure to include suturing: a Nissen fundoplication, using the improved system to include a laparoscope-holding arm. Dr Cadière also reported the first robotic bariatric surgery, an adjustable gastric banding, in 1998, highlighting the benefits of robotics in this patient population. Of note, all of these reports used the term telepresence laparoscopic surgery.[14]

Intuitive Surgical's next generation system, the da Vinci, improved significantly on the previous prototype. All robotic arms originated from a single patient cart, which obviated the need to mount each arm to the operating table and solved issues with table positioning. Visualization was improved by a new 3D laparoscope and a system providing separate video feeds to the left and right eye of the surgeon. The instrument-arm interface was improved and as a result less prone to failures, and the controllers were upgraded. Human trials began in 1998, and over the next few years the da Vinci was used for various minimally invasive procedures across different surgical specialties. It received FDA clearance in 2000, using the same 510k process as Computer Motion, allowing rapid introduction into the market. Like ZEUS, da Vinci was initially targeted at cardiothoracic surgery, but found better success in urology. Laparoscopic prostatectomy is very technically challenging, requiring fine suturing in an inverted direction to perform the bladder-to-urethra anastomosis. The da Vinci allowed urologic surgeons a smooth transition from an open to a minimally invasive approach, leading to improved patient outcomes, that became evident in trials.[15]

Over the next few years, Computer Motion and Intuitive Surgical's products competed as the adoption of robotic surgery grew. A patent war ensued between the 2 companies, which concluded with a merger in 2003. ZEUS was discontinued in favor of da Vinci, whereas Computer Motion's technology was used to improve the next generation of systems.

Multiple generations of the platform followed: the Da Vinci S, Si, Si HD, X, and Xi. Although the concept remained the same, significant improvements in technology and instrumentation allowed the increasing adoption across surgical specialties: dual surgeon consoles, smaller profile instruments, rotating boom, multi-quadrant capability, table motion, advanced energy devices, and surgical staplers. Initially, gynecology and urology dominated robotic surgery, but since 2016, general surgery has become the fastest growing and most common application of the Da Vinci. As of June 2019, more than 5000 da Vinci systems were deployed around the world, more than half of which are located in the United States. More than 6 million robotic procedures have been performed.[16] In 2019, 2 new systems were introduced, the da Vinci SP, a flexible, single port platform for transoral surgery, and Ion, a percutaneous lung biopsy system.

OTHER ROBOTIC SYSTEMS

In 2017, TransEnterix's Senhance system became the first to gain FDA clearance since da Vinci and ZEUS in 2000 and 2001. The company calls the system "digital laparoscopy" as opposed to robotic surgery. The system introduced different technology, like eye-tracking for camera control, separate carts for each arm, no docking to trocars, and pressure/force sensors. The system is FDA approved for adult colorectal, gynecologic, and hernia surgery and cholecystectomy. CMR Surgical's Versius system is another platform pending FDA clearance. Similar to Senhance, the robotic arms are mounted on separate carts and do not dock to the trocars. The company emphasizes cost-effectiveness, connectivity, and easy software updates. Medicaroid is a joint venture between Japanese companies Kawasaki Heavy Industries and Sysmex, currently developing a surgical robot. In October 2018, Medicaroid announced partnership with Karl Storz Endoscopy. Medtronic, already on the market with the Mazor X Robotic Guidance System for Spinal Surgery, is also partnered with Karl Storz Endoscopy and in development of a surgical robot. The company has the major advantage of having existing surgical energy and stapling technology that can be integrated into its future system from its launch. Verb Surgical, a joint venture announced in 2015 between Johnson & Johnson and Google, aims to bring robotics and AI into the operating room.

Critics of robotic surgery quote higher cost and longer operative time with minimal to no measurable clinical benefits. Although robotic assistance allows easier transition from open to minimally invasive surgical practice, with all of the associated benefits, comparison of robotic to laparoscopic surgery is more complicated. Some of the major advantages of robotic surgery, like wristed instruments and 3D vision, have become available in laparoscopic systems (**Table 2**). Improved ergonomics, an issue not usually addressed in clinical outcome studies, is an important factor to consider, as surgeons are prone to posture-related musculoskeletal injuries and lower extremity venous disease. The final and most significant advantage of robotic surgery is beyond what can be measured in a clinical trial. It is the introduction of a computer between the surgeon and patient.

FUTURE

The evolution of robotic technology will include improved hardware and, more importantly, software. The most obvious future developments will improve on the current systems to address some limitations: smaller size of instruments, arms, and carts, allowing for faster docking and reducing instrument collisions and clutter; automatic instrument exchanges; and elimination of energy cords, haptics, and tissue-sensing technology. Improved surgeon interface will allow for control of other operating room functions and integration of radiological images with the surgical video feed, which in real-time will achieve an augmented reality experience. Finally, the cost of robotic equipment will need to decrease to allow for wider adoption. All of these developments will be accelerated by what is soon to become a very competitive market for manufacturers.

Another stage in hardware will involve different concepts like flexible and mini-robotics. In 2006 and 2007, the first reports of transoral appendectomy and

Table 2 Advantages and disadvantages of the da Vinci system compared with standard laparoscopy	
Advantages	**Disadvantages**
Immersive 3-dimensional view of the operating field	Higher cost
Wristed instruments (7 degrees of freedom)	Longer operative time
Surgeon-controlled assistant instrument	Bulky equipment
Surgeon-controlled, stable camera image	No haptic feedback
Motion scaling up to 3:1, tremor filtering, fulcrum and torque elimination	Robotic arm collision leading to limited range of motion
Improved adjustable ergonomics	Proprietary system: software and hardware modifications not possible
Improved mentoring with dual console, pointers, and touchscreen	
Shorter learning curve	
Single company, centralized control of training and certification	

transvaginal cholecystectomy[17,18] caused excitement about Natural Orifice Translu-minal Endoscopic Surgery (NOTES). Thirteen years later, NOTES has failed to replace laparoscopy. As a transition to NOTES, laparoscopic single-site surgery was intro-duced, but has not achieved wide adoption because of the limited workspace and lack of triangulation. Experts have pushed the limits of flexible endoscopy in proced-ures like endoscopic submucosal dissection, peroral endoscopic myotomy, full-thickness resection, and suturing. However, there are major limitations, as the flexible endoscope is a 70-year-old design, created for visual inspection, not for performing surgery. Achieving a stable operative field and tissue retraction is challenging, adding to the long learning curve of these procedures. Flexible robotic platforms will greatly facilitate these techniques and allow for a shorter learning curve and wider adoption. Surgical mini-robots are another future development and multiple prototypes are already in existence.[19]

Although bringing new high-tech hardware to the operating room is exciting, the true revolution in surgery will come from how we use software and data. In today's robotic systems, the computer functions solely to translate the surgeon's hand motions into the robotic arms. Future platforms will capture these interactions in addition to the sur-gical video feed, generating enormous amounts of data ("big data"). Analysis of this data will allow machine learning and AI to become part of surgical practice. The pos-sibilities are limitless: quality improvement, real-time feedback, and early warning to prevent complications, and, eventually, automation. Researchers are already "training" software to "understand" surgical videos.[20] Real-time processing of intrao-perative video, possibly in combination with radiological imaging, will allow true, inde-pendent, automatic robotic surgery. Data sharing will enable collaboration between surgeons around the world. The amount of surgical data will also transform surgical training. Complicated simulations will become possible, including different surgical approaches, anatomic variants, and intraoperative complications. These intelligent simulators will change the way surgeons are trained and evaluated. Software ad-vances will be facilitated by new technology already on the horizon, like quantum computing and 5G wireless connectivity.

SUMMARY

There are considerable challenges facing the field of robotic surgery. New technology translates to higher cost, which remains a major limitation to wider adoption of ro-botics. In addition, tele-surgery and medicine require transmission of data over net-works, which causes privacy and security concerns. Safety of both patients and staff remains an issue when working with complicated, heavy, automated equipment. Similar to industrial robots, as technology becomes more advanced and cost-effective, it will start to replace human health care workers. Mass adoption in hospitals may result in technological unemployment, as hospitals are among the largest em-ployers in many major cities. Last, the problems associated with autonomous surgical robots and true AI, while still in the realm of science fiction, could become real in the future.

On the other hand, computer-assisted and robotic surgery has many benefits. A ro-botic arm offers improved strength, endurance, and precision. Remote operation and expendability make the robots suitable for distant and/or hostile environments like deep sea, space, and war. Robots pose no ethical concerns related to work hours, compensation, or working conditions. Reprogramming and remote software updates could allow the expansion of a single device's scope to multiple different procedures, subspecialties, and subjects. Surgical data processing and sharing will allow for worldwide, real-time collaboration between surgeons, next-level quality improvement, and simulation training. Image-guided, flexible, and miniature robots will allow remote, incisionless, painless, awake surgery: the ultimate minimally invasive procedures. Most importantly, the robot translates the art of surgery into a digital language that a computer can understand. This opens the door to a future of artificial surgical intelligence.

DISCLOSURE

The authors have nothing to disclose.

REFERENCES

1. The write stuff: Asimov's secret Cold War mission | The Times. Available at: https://www.thetimes.co.uk/article/the-write-stuff-asimovs-secret-cold-war-mission-jc8k5w9pb7b. Accessed August 20, 2019.
2. 2-1B Droid. StarWars.com. Available at: https://www.starwars.com/databank/2-1b-droid. Accessed July 7, 2019.
3. Definition of ROBOT. Available at: https://www.merriam-webster.com/dictionary/robot. Accessed August 12, 2019.
4. Unimateâ€"The first industrial robot. Robotics online. Available at: https://www.robotics.org/joseph-engelberger/unimate.cfm. Accessed August 12, 2019.
5. Kwoh YS, Hou J, Jonckheere EA, et al. A robot with improved absolute positioning accuracy for CT guided stereotactic brain surgery. IEEE Trans Biomed Eng 1988;35(2):153–61.
6. Shah J, Vyas A, Vyas D. The history of robotics in surgical specialties. Am J Robot Surg 2014;1(1):12–20.
7. George EI, Brand TC, LaPorta A, et al. Origins of robotic surgery: from skepticism to standard of care. JSLS 2018;22(4). https://doi.org/10.4293/JSLS.2018.00039.
8. Satava RM. Robotic surgery: from past to future–a personal journey. Surg Clin North Am 2003;83(6):1491–500, xii.
9. Satava RM. Surgical robotics: the early chronicles: a personal historical perspective. Surg Laparosc Endosc Percutan Tech 2002;12(1):6–16.
10. Bowersox JC, Shah A, Jensen J, et al. Vascular applications of telepresence surgery: initial feasibility studies in swine. J Vasc Surg 1996;23(2):281–7.
11. Madhani AJ, Niemeyer G, Salisbury JK. The black falcon: a teleoperated surgical instrument for minimally invasive surgery. In: Proceedings. 1998 IEEE/RSJ International Conference on Intelligent Robots and Systems. Innovations in Theory, Practice and Applications (Cat. No. 98CH36190) 1998; Vol 2; 936–41, vol.2. doi:10.1109/IROS.1998.727320
12. Marescaux J, Leroy J, Rubino F, et al. Transcontinental robot-assisted remote telesurgery: feasibility and potential applications. Ann Surg 2002;235(4):487–92.
13. Anvari M. Remote telepresence surgery: the Canadian experience. Surg Endosc 2007;21(4):537–41.
14. My experience performing the first telesurgical procedure in the world: Bariatric Times. Available at: http://bariatrictimes.com/my-experience-performing-the-first-telesurgical-procedure-in-the-world/. Accessed August 17, 2019.
15. Tewari A, Srivasatava A, Menon M, Members of the VIP Team. A prospective comparison of radical retropubic and robot-assisted prostatectomy: experience in one institution. BJU Int 2003;92(3):205–10.
16. Investor Relations. Intuitive surgical. Available at: https://isrg.gcs-web.com/investors. Accessed August 20, 2019.

17. Rao GV, Reddy DN, Banerjee R. NOTES: human experience. Gastrointest Endosc Clin N Am 2008;18(2):361–70.
18. Zorrón R, Filgueiras M, Maggioni LC, et al. NOTES. Transvaginal cholecystectomy: report of the first case. Surg Innov 2007;14(4):279–83.
19. Zygomalas A, Kehagias I, Giokas K, et al. Miniature surgical robots in the era of NOTES and LESS: dream or reality? Surg Innov 2015;22(1):97–107.
20. Padoy N. Machine and deep learning for workflow recognition during surgery. Minim Invasive Ther Allied Technol 2019;28(2):82–90.

Robotic Cardiac Surgery

Jonathan M. Hemli, MD, MSc, FRACS[a,b], Nirav C. Patel, MD, FRCS[a,b,c],*

KEYWORDS

- Robotic • CABG • MIDCAB • TECAB • Mitral valve

KEY POINTS

- One-half of all robotic cardiac cases are coronary artery bypass procedures, the remainder being comprised almost entirely of mitral valve and concomitant procedures.
- Minimally invasive direct coronary artery bypass (MIDCAB) is the most common robotic coronary procedure. The left internal mammary artery (LIMA) is harvested using the robotic instruments, followed by an off-pump LIMA-left anterior descending (LAD) anastomosis performed through a small left thoracotomy.
- MIDCAB can be used to treat isolated LAD stenosis, or it can be a component of hybrid coronary revascularization, coupled with percutaneous coronary intervention to diseased non-LAD targets in multivessel disease.
- Robotic total endoscopic coronary artery bypass is technically more challenging, although also has favorable results.
- The robot can be used for all types of mitral valve repair, irrespective of complexity. Valve replacement can be undertaken for those patients deemed not suitable for repair.

 Video content accompanies this article at http://www.surgical.theclinics.com.

INTRODUCTION

The evolution of robotic-assisted cardiac surgery has been relentless ever since the first coronary and mitral valve procedures were performed in the late 1990s. Iterative advancements in technology have resulted in enhanced 3-dimensional stereoscopic visual systems, improved ergonomic instruments with greater flexibility, dexterity and multiple degrees of freedom of movement, programmable instrument carts with integrated energy sources, and the ability for the surgeon to continually hone their skills on a training simulator.

The da Vinci system (Intuitive Surgical, Inc, Sunnyvale, CA, USA) is the commercial robot most commonly used in cardiac surgery. In addition to providing all of the

[a] Department of Cardiovascular & Thoracic Surgery, Lenox Hill Hospital, Northwell Health, 130 East 77th Street, 4th Floor, New York, NY 10075, USA; [b] Cardiovascular & Thoracic Surgery, Zucker School of Medicine at Hofstra/Northwell, Hempstead, NY, USA; [c] Robotic Cardiac Surgery, Northwell Health, 130 East 77th Street, 4th Floor, New York, NY 10075, USA
* Corresponding author. Department of Cardiovascular & Thoracic Surgery, Lenox Hill Hospital, Northwell Health, 130 East 77th Street, 4th Floor, New York, NY 10075.
E-mail address: nipatel@northwell.edu

Surg Clin N Am 100 (2020) 219–236
https://doi.org/10.1016/j.suc.2019.12.005
0039-6109/20/© 2019 Elsevier Inc. All rights reserved.

surgical.theclinics.com

advantages of a robotic platform, the current da Vinci systems are able to seamlessly integrate more than 1 video console, aptly facilitating the training of the next generation of robotic cardiac surgeons.

Recognizing the benefits inherent in a robotic approach, between 2007 and 2009, there was a 75% increase in the number of da Vinci systems purchased in the United States alone.[1] Similarly, over a 4-year period, robotic-assisted cardiac surgery increased 6-fold.[2]

Yanagawa and associates[2] analyzed the outcomes of 5199 patients who underwent a robotic cardiac surgical procedure between 2008 and 2011, who were propensity matched with individuals who had more traditional, nonrobotic, cardiac operations. The investigators found that, when compared with the nonrobotic procedures, those patients who underwent robotic surgery had significantly lower mortality, shorter length of hospital stay, and fewer perioperative complications overall.

Of all robotic cardiac surgical procedures performed worldwide, approximately one-half are robotic coronary artery bypass operations. Robotic mitral valve surgery constitutes almost the entirety of the remainder, although these operations not uncommonly include concomitant tricuspid valve repair and/or antiarrhythmia maze procedures. Robotic-assisted atrial septal defect (ASD) repair and resection of intracardiac tumors comprise less than 1% of all robotic cardiac cases.[3]

ROBOTIC CORONARY SURGERY

Robotic techniques for coronary artery bypass grafting (CABG) have now been consistently used for more than 2 decades. The term "robotic-assisted coronary surgery," however, can refer to several different procedures (**Fig. 1**).

Robotic Minimally Invasive Direct Coronary Artery Bypass

Minimally invasive direct coronary artery bypass (MIDCAB) is, today, by far, the robotic-assisted CABG procedure most commonly performed worldwide. This operation entails harvesting of the left internal mammary artery (LIMA) using robotic instruments, with a subsequent open anastomosis to the left anterior descending (LAD) being fashioned, off-pump, via a small left minithoracotomy.

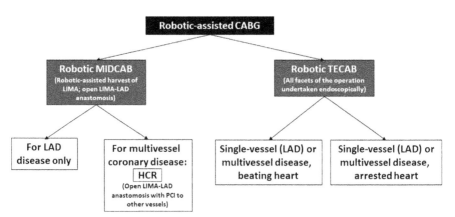

Fig. 1. Robotic-assisted coronary artery surgery encompasses a spectrum of possible procedures.

Indications
Robotic MIDCAB can be offered to patients with isolated disease of the LAD, or, alternately, it can be used in patients with multivessel coronary stenoses, coupled with percutaneous techniques to all diseased non-LAD vessels; this latter approach constitutes a hybrid coronary revascularization (HCR) strategy.

The 2012 American College of Cardiology Foundation/American Heart Association (AHA)/American College of Physicians/American Association for Thoracic Surgery/Preventive Cardiovascular Nurses Association/Society for Cardiovascular Angiography and Interventions/Society of Thoracic Surgeons ((STS) Guideline for the Diagnosis and Management of Patients with Stable Ischemic Heart Disease offers a class IIb recommendation for HCR, stating that it may be a reasonable alternative to CABG or multivessel percutaneous coronary intervention (PCI), so as to improve the risk-benefit ratio of the procedures.[4] The 2014 European Society of Cardiology/European Association for Cardio-Thoracic Surgery Guidelines on Myocardial Revascularization mention HCR as an option when multivessel PCI is deemed to be unsuitable, or when CABG is considered to be at prohibitive risk.[5]

Hemodynamically unstable patients are not suitable candidates for a robotic MIDCAB, nor is robotic MIDCAB an appropriate technique to use in an emergency setting. Patients with limited pulmonary reserve who are unable to tolerate single-lung ventilation are also not ideal for an MIDCAB operation. Significantly impaired left ventricular systolic function has been regarded by some as a relative contraindication to a robotic procedure, although favorable results in this setting have been reported.[6] A robotic MIDCAB is technically more challenging in the obese patient and has been associated with longer operative times.[7] However, there is no inherent reason a higher body mass index should preclude a robotic approach, and, indeed, satisfactory outcomes have been described in this patient cohort.[8] Patients who have had previous cardiac surgery can also potentially be offered a reoperative robotic MIDCAB.[9]

Surgical technique
After deflation of the left lung, 3 ports are introduced into the left pleural cavity, under vision, typically in the second, fourth, and sixth interspaces (**Fig. 2**). The pleural cavity is insufflated with carbon dioxide.

The LIMA is harvested as a skeletonized vessel, in its entire length, using the robotic instruments only (Video 1). The pericardium is opened using the robotic instruments, typically over the right ventricular outflow tract, and the LAD is identified (Video 2).

After removal of the robot, the patient is systemically heparinized, and a left anterior muscle-sparing minithoracotomy is performed, most commonly by extending the middle (robot camera) port incision. Rib trauma is minimized, and a soft tissue wound protector is used to provide circumferential, atraumatic exposure (Applied Medical, Rancho Santa Margarita, CA, USA).

The LIMA-LAD anastomosis is undertaken under direct-vision, using standard off-pump coronary grafting techniques (Video 3).[10] Graft flow and patency are assessed using a transit-time flow measurement system (Medistim VeriQ, Medistim USA Inc, Plymouth, MN, USA) before wound closure.

For patients undergoing robotic MIDCAB as part of an HCR management algorithm, an MIDCAB-first approach is typically adopted, followed by interval PCI, typically within 4 to 6 weeks of surgery. A MIDCAB-first strategy allows the surgical revascularization to be performed without concern for the potential bleeding that may be associated with the dual antiplatelet therapy that is mandatory after PCI with drug-eluting stents. MIDCAB procedures have, in fact, been undertaken in patients taking dual antiplatelet agents without undue bleeding,[11] although these findings have not

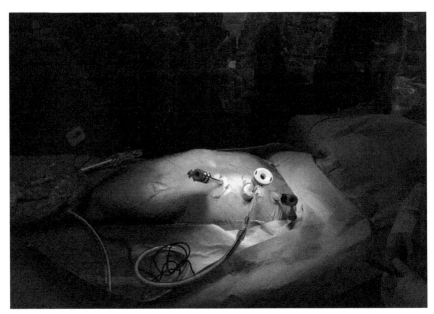

Fig. 2. Three ports have been placed into the left pleural cavity in preparation for docking of the da Vinci robot.

necessarily been consistent among all surgical groups.[12] More importantly, the MIDCAB-first approach allows the patency of the LIMA-to-LAD bypass graft to be interrogated during the subsequent PCI procedure. A PCI-first strategy is typically pursued in those patients who present with an acute coronary syndrome in which the culprit vessel is not the LAD, or in those individuals in whom the angiographic severity of at least one of the non-LAD stenoses is greater than that of the disease within the LAD itself. In these patients, subsequent LIMA-to-LAD grafting is undertaken on uninterrupted dual antiplatelet therapy. Alternately, simultaneous MIDCAB and PCI have been adopted by some centers.[13,14]

Results

There is a plethora of data now available that affirms the advantages of robotic MIDCAB, both as a stand-alone procedure for patients with isolated LAD disease and as part of a more global HCR strategy for patients with multivessel disease. Numerous studies detail the excellent results of a robotic-assisted LIMA-to-LAD graft, with or without PCI to non-LAD vessels, reporting low perioperative mortality and morbidity as well as excellent mid- to longer-term graft patency.[15] Moreover, when compared with sternotomy CABG, robotic MIDCAB procedures (and HCR overall) have been consistently associated with shorter intensive care and hospital stays, a reduced perioperative transfusion requirement, less postoperative pain, and faster recovery.[16-27] Of course, a sternal-sparing robotic MIDCAB completely negates the risk of sternal wound infection that is otherwise inherent to all sternotomy procedures.

Despite the advantages of robotic MIDCAB (and HCR), an analysis from the STS Adult Cardiac Surgery Database revealed that HCR represented only 0.48% of all CABG volume in the United States between 2011 and 2013.[28]

Numerous investigators have described the learning curve inherent to robotic MIDCAB. Oehlinger and colleagues[29] noted a marked decrease in LIMA harvest time over the course of 100 consecutive procedures. Bonatti and associates[30] similarly described significant improvements in LIMA harvest times after 38 cases, whereas Kappert and coworkers[31] noted better operative times after 35 cases. In their experience of 77 consecutive cases, Hemli and colleagues[32] not only found that LIMA harvest times decreased with increasing surgical experience but also noted that other components of the operation became faster as well, including port-placement time, and total robotic-use time (**Fig. 3**). The investigators found that a 10% decrease in operating times could be expected for each doubling of the number of cases performed, although they noted that the greatest improvements occurred within the first 20 cases. The learning curve for robotic MIDCAB may, in fact, be shorter than would be otherwise expected, particularly for those surgeons who are already comfortable with off-pump surgical techniques.

Robotic Total Endoscopic Coronary Artery Bypass

The first robotic total endoscopic coronary artery bypass (TECAB) was performed by Loulmet and associates in 1998.[33] In some respects, robotic TECAB represents the ultimate in minimally invasive CABG, because the entire operation is performed through port access, within the closed chest. Not only is the internal mammary harvested endoscopically but also the coronary anastomoses themselves are constructed wholly within the chest using robotic instruments.

In contrast to robotic MIDCAB, which only revascularizes the LAD, a TECAB procedure can facilitate grafting to multiple arterial territories. Moreover, unlike a robotic MIDCAB operation, which is almost invariably completed off-pump, TECAB procedures can be performed either on the beating heart or on the arrested heart.

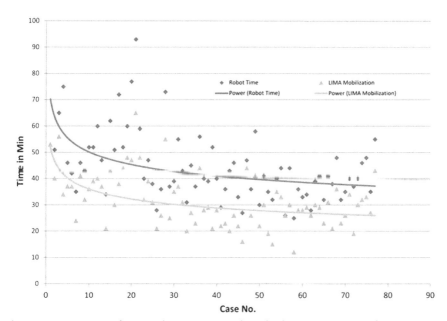

Fig. 3. Learning curves for LIMA harvest time and total robotic-use time in robotic MIDCAB. (*From* Hemli JM, Henn LW, Panetta CR, et al. Defining the learning curve for robotic-assisted endoscopic harvesting of the left internal mammary artery. Innovations (Phila) 2013; 8: 353-8; *with permission*).

Arrested-heart TECAB incorporates peripheral cannulation to establish cardiopulmonary bypass and the use of endoscopic techniques to cross-clamp the aorta and administer cardioplegia.

The adoption of robotic TECAB by the cardiac surgical community has been significantly slower than that of MIDCAB, in large part because of the technical complexity of the procedure, the challenges inherent in working entirely within the closed chest, and the longer learning curves associated with the operation. Although it is not widely practiced, robotic TECAB is nevertheless carried out on a routine basis in a limited number of dedicated centers worldwide.

In a recent review of the literature, Gobolos and colleagues[34] analyzed the outcomes of 2397 TECAB cases and reported a perioperative mortality of 0.8% (slightly higher in beating-heart cases than in arrested-heart cases), a stroke rate of 1.0%, and an incidence of new renal failure of 1.6%. These favorable results tend to be achieved at the expense of longer operative times, a not insignificant conversion rate to larger incisions, a 4.2% reexploration rate for bleeding, and a longer learning curve for the procedure.

Leonard and coworkers[35] conducted a metaanalysis of all TECAB reports from 2000 to 2017. They also report encouraging results, with low operative mortality (0.8%), infrequent stroke (1.5%), an incidence of perioperative myocardial infarction of 2.28%, and 94.8% graft patency at a mean follow-up of just more than 10 months.

Bonaros and associates[36] reported a multicenter experience of 500 TECAB cases, performed between 2001 and 2011. Intraoperative conversions to larger incisions were required in 10% of patients. Median operative time was, once again, on the longer side. The investigators found that independent predictors of procedural success included a less-technically challenging operation (such as a single-vessel or an arrested-heart TECAB) and a non–learning curve case.

ROBOTIC VALVE SURGERY

Robotic-assisted valve surgery is primarily focused on the mitral valve, such that this is now a routine technique used in a multitude of centers around the world.

Mitral Valve

The first robotic-assisted mitral valve repair, using an early prototype of the da Vinci system, was performed by Carpentier and associates[37] in 1998, followed rapidly thereafter by Mohr and colleagues.[38] The first complete robotic-assisted mitral valve repair in the United States was performed by Chitwood and coworkers[39] under a Food and Drug Administration (FDA) safety and efficacy trial in 2000. In 2002, after a multicenter phase 2 trial, the FDA approved the da Vinci system for generalized use in mitral valve surgery.[40]

Indications

Any patient requiring mitral valve surgery is, at least theoretically, a potential candidate for a robotic-assisted approach. The indications for mitral valve intervention in these individuals are no different than they would be for a patient undergoing a traditional median sternotomy; these are summarized in the AHA/American College of Cardiology and European guidelines for the management of patients with valvular heart disease.[41,42] Robotic mitral repair techniques can be applied to both degenerative and functional valve pathologic condition; valve replacement can be performed for those patients not deemed candidates for repair. Patients with a history of atrial fibrillation requiring a concomitant ablation or antiarrhythmia maze procedure are good candidates for a robotic-assisted strategy, as are those who need concurrent intervention on the tricuspid valve.

Patients with poor left ventricular function, a heavily calcified mitral annulus, severe pulmonary hypertension, limited pulmonary reserve, significant aortic insufficiency, peripheral arterial disease, and/or moderate to severe pectus excavatum are not ideal candidates for a robotic approach. Patients who require concomitant CABG, an aortic valve procedure, and/or surgery of the ascending aorta or arch, cannot be adequately treated via minimal-access robotic surgery and should be managed via a median sternotomy. Contraindications to a robotic mitral valve procedure are summarized in **Box 1**.

Perioperative assessment

Robotic mitral valve surgery necessitates peripheral cannulation to establish cardiopulmonary bypass. Patients must therefore be assessed for the presence of aortoiliofemoral atherosclerotic disease; significant peripheral vascular disease may preclude femoral arterial cannulation. A preoperative computed tomographic (CT) angiogram of the chest/abdomen/pelvis is useful to quantify the burden of calcium in the descending aorta and in the pelvic vessels,[43,44] and the intraoperative transesophageal echocardiogram (TEE) adds further information about any atheromatous plaque that may be present in the arch. If there is undue concern regarding an elevated stroke risk secondary to retrograde arterial flow via the femoral artery, an alternate surgical strategy should be used. The surgeon may still elect to pursue a robotic-assisted approach, but use the right axillary artery for perfusion, rather than the femoral artery, reducing the risk of an adverse neurologic outcome[45]; alternatively, the operation can be completed via a minimal-access right thoracotomy (without the robot), either cannulating the right axillary artery or the ascending aorta directly. Finally, a right-chest approach may be abandoned altogether in favor of sternotomy.

A preoperative coronary angiogram is typically required to screen for coronary artery disease, although, in the younger population, particularly in those with degenerative valve pathologic condition, a CT coronary angiogram may be sufficient.[46] If isolated coronary disease is identified that is amenable to percutaneous intervention, it may be possible to stent this lesion, to be followed by an interval robotic mitral valve procedure 4 to 6 weeks later, constituting a "hybrid coronary-valve approach."[47]

Box 1
Contraindications to robotic-assisted mitral valve surgery

Absolute contraindications

Concomitant requirement for:
  CABG
  Aortic valve surgery
  Ascending aorta/arch procedure

Relative contraindications

Depressed LV function

Poor pulmonary function

Pulmonary hypertension

Aortic insufficiency

Peripheral arterial disease

Pectus excavatum

Abbreviation: LV, left ventricular.

The importance of the intraoperative TEE in accurately defining the mitral valve pathologic condition to be addressed cannot be overstated. If the surgeon does not think that a minimal-access approach can facilitate a quality outcome, for whatever reason, based on the pathologic condition of the valve, or otherwise, then the surgery should proceed via sternotomy.

Surgical technique

After the patient is appropriately positioned (**Fig. 4**), the right lung is deflated; a 3- to 4-cm slightly curvilinear incision is made in the right inframammary crease, lateral to the nipple, and the pleural cavity is entered through the fourth intercostal space. The inframammary thoracotomy becomes the primary means of access into the chest for the bedside surgical assistant. A soft tissue wound retractor is used to improve exposure; a rib-spreading retractor is usually not required (**Fig. 5**).

Trocars for the left- and right-arm robotic instruments are inserted through the third and fifth interspaces, respectively, anterior to the midaxillary line. An additional port site is used for the left atrial retractor (**Fig. 6**). Carbon dioxide is insufflated into the right pleural space.

The patient is heparinized. Femoral arterial and venous cannulation is typically used to establish cardiopulmonary bypass. Although not mandatory, a second venous drainage cannula, inserted percutaneously into the superior vena cava via the right internal jugular vein, is helpful.

After cardiopulmonary bypass has been established, the pericardium is opened using the robotic instruments, anterior to the right phrenic nerve, which is specifically identified and protected.

A long cross-clamp is passed through a separate incision in the chest wall, usually through the second or third interspace, as posteriorly and cephalad as possible, so as

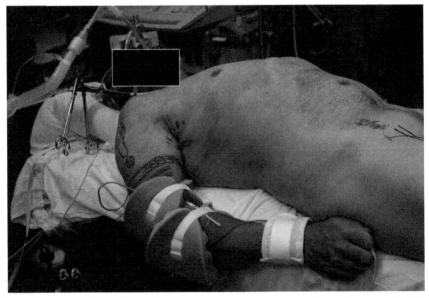

Fig. 4. The patient is positioned for robotic mitral valve surgery. The patient's right side is elevated by 30°, and the entire operating table has been tilted to the left to further expose the right chest. Note the presence of a venous drainage cannula in the superior vena cava (inserted percutaneously via the right internal jugular vein).

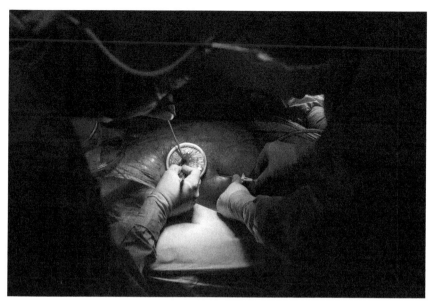

Fig. 5. The working port is created in the right inframammary crease and a soft tissue retractor is used to improve exposure. Avoidance of a rib-spreading retractor helps to reduce postoperative pain.

to avoid conflict with the left robotic-arm trocar, and applied to the aorta (Video 4). Rather than use a cross-clamp, some prefer to use an intraaortic balloon in order to achieve endoaortic occlusion.[48–50]

The robotic instruments are used to dissect out the interatrial groove and open the left atrium. The actual valve repair (or replacement) should proceed in an identical

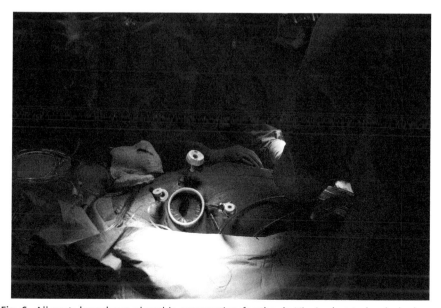

Fig. 6. All ports have been placed in preparation for the da Vinci robot to be docked.

fashion as if the surgeon was operating through a sternotomy. The magnification, flexibility, and excellent exposure afforded by the robotic system facilitate all types of mitral valve repair, irrespective of complexity Video 5.

If an endocardial ablation or maze procedure needs to be undertaken to treat concurrent atrial fibrillation, this can be done at any time while the left atrium is open. Similarly, the orifice of the left atrial appendage can be closed, if required.

Results

There remains little, if any, doubt as to the benefits of a robotic-assisted approach in mitral valve surgery. Numerous reports confirm low perioperative complication rates, reduced transfusion requirements, shorter ventilation times, reduced intensive care and overall lengths of stay, diminished postoperative pain, faster return to normal activities, and greater overall patient satisfaction.[51–53]

A metaanalysis of 6 studies comparing robotic and conventional mitral valve surgery by Cao and colleagues[54] demonstrated that robotic mitral surgery is safe, with low perioperative complication rates, despite somewhat longer cardiopulmonary bypass and cross-clamp times, particularly if performed by experienced surgeons in designated centers of excellence.

Gillinov and coworkers[55] reported the results of the first 1000 cases of robotically assisted mitral surgery performed at the Cleveland Clinic. They found that, of the 992 patients who underwent valve repair for regurgitation, 99.7% left the operating room with, at most, mild residual regurgitation, and 97.9% of patients had less than mild regurgitation by the time of hospital discharge. Mortality was low (0.1%), and perioperative stroke was uncommon (1.4%). The investigators described a definite learning curve to the procedure, confirming that, over the longitudinal course of their review, bypass and cross-clamp times decreased, stroke rates diminished, transfusion rates improved, and intensive care and hospital lengths of stay shortened.

In an analysis of the STS Adult Cardiac Surgery Database, Wang and associates[56] reported the results of 503 patients who underwent robotic mitral valve repair, propensity-matched with a concurrent cohort who had valve repair via sternotomy. The robotic approach was associated with less postoperative atrial fibrillation, reduced rates of transfusion, and shorter lengths of stay, with equivalent mortality at 3 years. Importantly, there was no significant difference in the need for valve reintervention in the midterm, a finding that has been replicated by others.[57] Once again, however, bypass and cross-clamp times were longer in the robotic group than in the sternotomy cohort.

Potential concerns of the robotic technique include the longer bypass and myocardial ischemic times that are replicated in almost all studies, although, as demonstrated by the group at the Cleveland Clinic, and by others,[58] these do seem to improve over time, as surgeons become defter with the procedure. Moreover, the longer perfusion times do not appear to directly correlate with increased perioperative morbidity.[59,60] Concerns regarding an increased risk of perioperative stroke associated with femoral arterial cannulation have largely been mitigated by appropriate preoperative screening for atheroocclusive disease, by judicious patient selection, and by the use of alternate cannulation sites as needed.

Reoperations

Patients who have had prior cardiac surgery may be particularly suited to a minimal-access right chest approach. Peripheral cannulation, avoiding a redo sternotomy, and attaining surgical exposure from the right side serve to minimize dissection around the heart, reducing the risks of injury to the heart or to any patent bypass grafts, should they be present, while concomitantly decreasing the incidence and extent of periop-erative bleeding.

If the risk of using a transthoracic aortic cross-clamp is thought to be prohibitive in a reoperative surgical field, hypothermic fibrillatory arrest represents an attractive alternative.[61]

OTHER ROBOTIC CARDIAC SURGERY
Tricuspid Valve

Virtually any tricuspid valve pathologic condition can be tackled using a robotic-assisted approach, although the most commonly performed procedure is implant of an annuloplasty band to correct functional tricuspid regurgitation in a patient undergo-ing a robotic mitral valve operation.[62] A robotic tricuspid valve operation can, of course, be completed as a stand-alone procedure, in which case its setup and execu-tion essentially mimics that of mitral valve surgery in almost all respects.

Ablation for Atrial Fibrillation and Occlusion of the Left Atrial Appendage

An endocardial cryoablation maze procedure to address coexistent atrial fibrillation is not uncommonly incorporated as part of a robotic mitral valve operation. The cryoa-blation catheters are introduced into the left atrium through the port sites, manipulated with the robotic instruments, and the lesion set can be constructed at any time while the left atrium is open. If the maze procedure is efficiently executed while the surgeon is performing another component of the mitral operation, it should not unduly add to overall cross-clamp or cardiopulmonary bypass times. The safety and longer-term ef-ficacy of endoscopic, robotic-assisted ablation of atrial fibrillation, with or without a simultaneous mitral valve procedure, have been affirmed by numerous investigators.[63,64]

Occlusion of the left atrial appendage can, similarly, be safely and effectively carried out using robotic techniques from within the left atrium,[65] often as part of a more com-plete cryoablation maze procedure, typically in conjunction with mitral valve surgery. Alternatively, it can be undertaken as a dedicated procedure in its own right, approaching the left atrial appendage entirely from its pericardial aspect.[66]

Atrial Septal Defects and Intracardiac Tumors

ASDs of virtually all types have been successfully repaired using robotic instruments, including secundum defects,[67,68] sinus venosus defects with partial anomalous venous return,[69–71] and coronary sinus defects.[72] The procedural setup and conduct are analogous to that of a robotic mitral valve operation.

There have also been reports of successful robotic repair of atrioventricular canal defects,[73,74] ventricular septal defects,[75] as well as an ASD associated with cor tria-triatum sinister.[76]

The most common intracardiac tumor to have been successfully excised using ro-botic technology has been the left atrial myxoma, once again using an operative tech-nique that essentially mimics that of a mitral valve procedure.[77–79] The advantages of the robotic approach include improved surgical exposure, shorter hospital length of stay, reduced postoperative pain, and more rapid functional recovery.[80,81] Myxomas have also been successfully removed from other cardiac chambers, including the right atrium and the left ventricle.[82,83]

Aortic Valve

Although robotic mitral valve surgery is now commonplace, the use of robotics to operate on the aortic valve has, thus far, been sparse and somewhat limited. There are isolated case reports and small case series of successful robotic-assisted aortic valve replacements (AVR),[84,85] and the robot has also been used to successfully excise aortic valve papillary fibroelastoma.[86–88]

In a recent review, Balkhy and colleagues[88] demonstrated the feasibility and safety of a robotic-assisted AVR, although the role of this procedure in the current era of burgeoning transcatheter AVR still remains uncertain.

There have also been case reports of using the robot to perform an apicoaortic conduit for aortic stenosis[89] and to fashion a thoracic aortic anastomosis in an ovine model.[90]

OTHER CONSIDERATIONS

One of the main concerns that still plague robotic surgery is its cost. Most studies have demonstrated that the financial cost of a robotic procedure exceeds that of a nonrobotic one, a phenomenon that is multifactorial in cause.[2] Purchasing the robotic unit, by itself, is expensive. The fixed usage life of the robotic instruments (and the use of single-use consumable items) necessitates continually purchasing more, a cost that is unavoidable. Moreover, the longer operative times reported with some robotic procedures reduce the overall efficiency of the operating suite and come at an opportune cost of being able to perform other cases.

There remains the potential for the cost of the procedure to fall. As surgeons become more comfortable with the procedure, and as case volume increases, operative time would be expected to consistently decrease, and the surgeon should also become defter at minimizing and managing perioperative complications. In addition, the higher in-hospital costs of the robotic operation may be somewhat offset by the patient's shorter hospital stay, faster postoperative recovery, fewer perioperative complications, and earlier return to work.

In a systematic review of the literature, Seco and associates[91] summarized the results of 27 studies that assessed the perioperative outcomes of robotic mitral valve surgery. The investigators concluded that, although cardiopulmonary bypass and cross-clamp times tend to be somewhat on the longer side, the overall short-term mortality and morbidity are low, and that the increased expense of the procedure (accrued by the use of the robot) is more than offset by the patients' shorter hospital stay and faster return to work.

Other limitations of the robotic approach to date have included the lack of proprioception and the absence of tactile feedback provided by the robotic instruments. Further advances in robotic technology may address some of these issues.

SUMMARY

Robotic cardiac surgery will only continue to improve over time. Higher-resolution optics, smaller instruments with lower profiles allowing for finer motor control and coordination, and the incorporation of a "haptic" or tactile feedback system into the robotic arms, will combine to facilitate faster, smoother operations, with consistently reproducible results.

To date, the surgeon operating at the console has always been physically colocated in the same operating suite as the patient and the bedside assistant; this may not always be the case, because one can imagine the potential for remote tele-surgery using robotic technology.

Continued innovation in robotics will undoubtedly translate into even broader application in cardiac surgery, with potential for its use in thoracic aortic procedures, pediatric cases, and even in conjunction with transcatheter valve therapies. Indeed, it may be said that the future of robotic cardiac surgery may very well be limitless.

DISCLOSURE

The authors have nothing to disclose.

SUPPLEMENTARY DATA

Supplementary data related to this article can be found online at https://doi.org/10.1016/j.suc.2019.12.005.

REFERENCES

1. Barbash GI, Glied SA. New technology and health care costs–the case of robot-assisted surgery. N Engl J Med 2010;363:701–4.
2. Yanagawa F, Perez M, Bell T, et al. Critical outcomes in nonrobotic vs robotic-assisted cardiac surgery. JAMA 2015;150:771–7.
3. Doulamis IP, Spartalis E, Machairas N, et al. The role of robotics in cardiac surgery: a systematic review. J Robot Surg 2019;13:51–2.
4. Fihn SD, Gardin JM, Abrams J, et al. 2012 ACCF/AHA/ACP/AATS/PCNA/SCAI/STS guideline for the diagnosis and management of patients with stable ischemic heart disease: a report of the American College of Cardiology Foundation/American Heart Association Task Force on practice guidelines, and the American College of Physicians, American Association for Thoracic Surgery, Preventive Cardiovascular Nurses Association, Society for Cardiovascular Angiography and Interventions, and Society of Thoracic Surgeons. Circulation 2012;126: e354–471.
5. Kolh P, Windecker S, Alfonso F, et al. 2014 ESC/EACTS guidelines on myocardial revascularization: the Task Force on Myocardial Revascularization of the European Society of Cardiology (ESC) and the European Association for Cardio-Thoracic Surgery (EACTS). Developed with the special contribution of the European Association of Percutaneous Cardiovascular Interventions (EAPCI). Eur J Cardiothorac Surg 2014;46:517–92.
6. Gorki H, Patel NC, Balacumaraswami L, et al. Long-term survival after minimal invasive direct coronary artery bypass (MIDCAB) surgery in patients with low ejection fraction. Innovations (Phila) 2010;5:400–6.
7. Vassiliades TA, Nielsen JL, Lonquist JL. Effects of obesity on outcomes in endoscopically assisted coronary artery bypass operations. Heart Surg Forum 2003;6: 99–101.
8. Hemli JM, Darla LS, Panetta CR, et al. Does body mass index affect outcomes in robotic assisted coronary artery bypass procedures? Innovations (Phila) 2012;7: 350–3.
9. Balacumaraswami L, Patel NC, Gorki H, et al. Minimally invasive direct coronary artery bypass as a primary strategy for reoperative myocardial revascularization. Innovations (Phila) 2010;5:22–7.
10. Hemli JM, Patel NC, Subramanian VA. Increasing surgical experience with off-pump coronary surgery does not mitigate the morbidity of emergency conversion to cardiopulmonary bypass. Innovations (Phila) 2012;7:259–65.
11. Hemli JM, Darla LS, Panetta CR, et al. Does dual antiplatelet therapy affect blood loss and transfusion requirements in robotic-assisted coronary artery surgery? Innovations (Phila) 2012;7:399–402.
12. Daniel WT, Liberman HA, Kilgo P, et al. The impact of clopidogrel therapy on postoperative bleeding after robotic-assisted coronary artery bypass surgery. Eur J Cardiothorac Surg 2014;46:e8–13.

13. Bonatti J, Schachner T, Bonaros N, et al. Simultaneous hybrid coronary revascularization using totally endoscopic left internal mammary artery bypass grafting and placement of rapamycin eluting stents in the same interventional session. The COMBINATION pilot study. Cardiology 2008;110:92–5.

14. Kon ZN, Brown EN, Tran R, et al. Simultaneous hybrid coronary revascularization reduces postoperative morbidity compared with results from conventional off-pump coronary artery bypass. J Thorac Cardiovasc Surg 2008;135:367–75.

15. Gaudino M, Bakaeen F, Davierwala P, et al. New strategies for surgical myocardial revascularization. Circulation 2018;138:2160–8.

16. Patel NC, Hemli JM, Kim MC, et al. Short and intermediate-term outcomes of hybrid coronary revascularization for double-vessel disease. J Thorac Cardiovasc Surg 2018;156:1799–807.

17. Sardar P, Kundu A, Bischoff M, et al. Hybrid coronary revascularization versus coronary artery bypass grafting in patients with multivessel coronary artery disease: a meta-analysis. Catheter Cardiovasc Interv 2018;91:203–12.

18. Zhu P, Zhou P, Sun Y, et al. Hybrid coronary revascularization versus coronary artery bypass grafting for multivessel coronary artery disease: systematic review and meta-analysis. J Cardiothorac Surg 2015;10:63.

19. Yang M, Wu Y, Wang G, et al. Robotic total arterial off-pump coronary artery bypass grafting: seven-year single-center experience and long-term follow-up of graft patency. Ann Thorac Surg 2015;100:1367–73.

20. Harskamp RE, Williams JB, Halkos ME, et al. Meta-analysis of minimally invasive coronary artery bypass versus drug-eluting stents for isolated left anterior descending coronary artery disease. J Thorac Cardiovasc Surg 2014;148:1837–42.

21. Halkos ME, Walker PF, Vassiliades TA, et al. Clinical and angiographic results after hybrid coronary revascularization. Ann Thorac Surg 2014;97:484–90.

22. Halkos ME, Liberman HA, Devireddy C, et al. Early clinical and angiographic outcomes after robotic-assisted coronary artery bypass surgery. J Thorac Cardiovasc Surg 2014;147:179–85.

23. Harskamp RE, Puskas JD, Tijssen JG, et al. Comparison of hybrid coronary revascularization versus coronary artery bypass grafting in patients ≥ 65 years with multivessel coronary artery disease. Am J Cardiol 2014;114:224–9.

24. Harskamp RE, Bagai A, Halkos ME, et al. Clinical outcomes after hybrid coronary revascularization versus coronary artery bypass surgery: a meta-analysis of 1,190 patients. Am Heart J 2014;167:585–92.

25. Shen L, Hu S, Wang H, et al. One-stop hybrid coronary revascularization versus coronary artery bypass grafting and percutaneous coronary intervention for the treatment of multivessel coronary artery disease: 3-year follow-up results from a single institution. J Am Coll Cardiol 2013;61:2525–33.

26. Repossini A, Tespili M, Saino A, et al. Hybrid revascularization in multivessel coronary artery disease. Eur J Cardiothorac Surg 2013;44:288–93.

27. Poston RS, Tran R, Collins M, et al. Comparison of economic and patient outcomes with minimally-invasive versus traditional off-pump coronary artery bypass grafting techniques. Ann Surg 2008;248:638–46.

28. Harskamp RE, Brennan JM, Xian Y, et al. Practice patterns and clinical outcomes after hybrid coronary revascularization in the United States: an analysis from the Society of Thoracic Surgeons adult cardiac database. Circulation 2014;130:872–9.

29. Oehlinger A, Bonaros N, Schachner T, et al. Robotic endoscopic left internal mammary artery harvesting: what have we learned after 100 cases? Ann Thorac Surg 2007;83:1030–4.

30. Bonatti J, Schachner T, Bernecker O, et al. Robotic totally endoscopic coronary artery bypass: program development and learning curve issues. J Thorac Cardiovasc Surg 2004;127:504–10.

31. Kappert U, Cichon R, Schneider J, et al. Robotic coronary artery surgery–the evolution of a new minimally-invasive approach in coronary artery surgery. Thorac Cardiovasc Surg 2000;48:193–7.

32. Hemli JM, Henn LW, Panetta CR, et al. Defining the learning curve for robotic-assisted endoscopic harvesting of the left internal mammary artery. Innovations (Phila) 2013;8:353–8.

33. Loulmet D, Carpentier A, d'Attellis N, et al. Endoscopic coronary artery bypass grafting with the aid of robotic-assisted instruments. J Thorac Cardiovasc Surg 1999;118:4–10.

34. Gobolos L, Ramahi J, Obeso A, et al. Robotic totally endoscopic coronary artery bypass grafting: systematic review of clinical outcomes from the past two decades. Innovations (Phila) 2019;14:5–16.

35. Leonard JR, Rahouma M, Abouarab AA, et al. Totally endoscopic coronary artery bypass surgery: a meta-analysis of the current evidence. Int J Cardiol 2018; 261:42–6.

36. Bonaros N, Schachner T, Lehr E, et al. Five hundred cases of robotic totally endoscopic coronary artery bypass grafting: predictors of success and safety. Ann Thorac Surg 2013;95:803–12.

37. Carpentier A, Loulmet D, Aupecle B, et al. Computer assisted open heart surgery. First case operated on with success. C R Acad Sci III 1998;321:437–42.

38. Mohr FW, Falk V, Diegeler A, et al. Computer-enhanced coronary artery bypass surgery. J Thorac Cardiovasc Surg 1999;117:1212–4.

39. Chitwood WR Jr, Nifong LW, Elbeery JE, et al. Robotic mitral valve repair: trapezoidal resection and prosthetic annuloplasty with the da vinci surgical system. J Thorac Cardiovasc Surg 2000;120:1171–2.

40. Nifong LW, Chitwood WR, Pappas PS, et al. Robotic mitral valve surgery: a United States multicenter trial. J Thorac Cardiovasc Surg 2005;129:1395–404.

41. Nishimura RA, Otto CM, Bonow RO, et al. 2014 AHA/ACC guideline for the management of patients with valvular heart disease: executive summary: a report of the American College of Cardiology/American Heart Association Task Force on practice guidelines. J Am Coll Cardiol 2014;63:2438–88.

42. Vahanian A, Alfieri O, Andreotti F, et al. Guidelines on the management of valvular heart disease (version 2012): the Joint Task Force on the Management of Valvular Heart Disease of the European Society of Cardiology (ESC) and the European Association for Cardio-Thoracic Surgery (EACTS). Eur J Cardiothorac Surg 2012;42: S1–44.

43. Leonard JR, Henry M, Rahouma M, et al. Systematic preoperative CT scan is associated with reduced risk of stroke in minimally invasive mitral valve surgery: a meta-analysis. Int J Cardiol 2019;278:300–6.

44. Moodley S, Schoenhagen P, Gillinov AM, et al. Preoperative multidetector computed tomography angiography for planning of minimally invasive robotic mitral valve surgery: impact on decision making. J Thorac Cardiovasc Surg 2013;146:262–8.

45. Bedeir K, Reardon M, Ramchandani M, et al. Elevated stroke risk associated with femoral artery cannulation during mitral valve surgery. Semin Thorac Cardiovasc Surg 2015;27:97–103.

46. Morris MF, Suri RM, Akhtar NJ, et al. Computed tomography as an alternative to catheter angiography prior to robotic mitral valve repair. Ann Thorac Surg 2013; 95:1354–9.

47. Ford RB, Rodriguez E, Nifong LW, et al. Robotic mitral valve repair or replacement. In: KL Franco KL, Thourani VH, editors. Cardiothoracic surgery review. Philadelphia: Lippincott Williams & Wilkins; 2012. p. 410–4.

48. Breves SL, Hong I, McCarthy J, et al. Ascending aortic endoballoon occlusion feasible despite moderately enlarged aorta to facilitate robotic mitral valve surgery. Innovations (Phila) 2016;11:355–9.

49. Yaffee DW, Loulmet DF, Fakiha AG, et al. Fluorescence-guided placement of an endoaortic balloon occlusion device for totally endoscopic robotic mitral valve repair. J Thorac Cardiovasc Surg 2015;149:1456–8.

50. Ward AF, Loulmet DF, Neuburger PJ, et al. Outcomes of peripheral perfusion with balloon aortic clamping for totally endoscopic robotic mitral valve repair. J Thorac Cardiovasc Surg 2014;148:2769–72.

51. Murphy DA, Moss E, Binongo J, et al. The expanding role of endoscopic robotics in mitral valve surgery: 1257 consecutive procedures. J Thorac Cardiovasc Surg 2015;100:1675–82.

52. Mihaljevic T, Jarrett CM, Gillinov AM, et al. Robotic repair of posterior mitral valve prolapse versus conventional approaches: potential realized. J Thorac Cardiovasc Surg 2011;141:72–80.

53. Ramzy D, Trento A, Cheng W, et al. Three hundred robotic-assisted mitral valve repairs: the Cedars-Sinai experience. J Thorac Cardiovasc Surg 2014;147: 228–35.

54. Cao C, Wolfenden H, Liou K, et al. A meta-analysis of robotic vs. conventional mitral valve surgery. Ann Cardiothorac Surg 2015;4:305–14.

55. Gillinov AM, Mihaljevic T, Javadikasgari H, et al. Early results of robotically assisted mitral valve surgery: analysis of the first 1000 cases. J Thorac Cardiovasc Surg 2018;155:82–91.

56. Wang A, Brennan JM, Zhang S, et al. Robotic mitral valve repair in older individuals: an analysis of the Society of Thoracic Surgeons Database. Ann Thorac Surg 2018;106:1388–93.

57. Liu G, Zhang H, Yang M, et al. Robotic mitral valve repair: 7-year surgical experience and mid-term follow-up results. J Cardiovasc Surg (Torino) 2019;60: 406–12.

58. Yaffee DW, Loulmet DF, Kelly LA, et al. Can the learning curve of totally endoscopic robotic mitral valve repair be short-circuited? Innovations (Phila) 2014; 9:43–8.

59. Suri RM, Burkhart HM, Daly RC, et al. Robotic mitral valve repair for all prolapse subsets using techniques identical to open valvuloplasty: establishing the benchmark against which percutaneous interventions should be judged. J Thorac Cardiovasc Surg 2011;142:970–9.

60. Hawkins RB, Mehaffey JH, Mullen MM, et al. A propensity matched analysis of robotic, minimally invasive, and conventional mitral valve surgery. Heart 2018; 104:1970–5.

61. Hollatz A, Balkhy HH, Chaney MA, et al. Robotic mitral valve repair with right ventricular pacing-induced ventricular fibrillatory arrest. J Cardiothorac Vasc Anesth 2017;31:345–53.

62. Lewis CT, Stephens RL, Tyndal CM, et al. Concomitant robotic mitral and tricuspid valve repair: technique and early experience. Ann Thorac Surg 2014; 97:782–7.

63. Ju MH, Huh JH, Lee CH, et al. Robotic-assisted surgical ablation of atrial fibrillation combined with mitral valve surgery. Ann Thorac Surg 2019;107:762–8.
64. Rillig A, Schmidt B, Di Biase L, et al. Manual versus robotic catheter ablation for the treatment of atrial fibrillation: the man and machine trial. JACC Clin Electrophysiol 2017;3:875–83.
65. Ward AF, Applebaum RM, Toyoda N, et al. Totally endoscopic robotic left atrial appendage closure demonstrates high success rate. Innovations (Phila) 2017; 12:46–9.
66. Lewis CT, Stephens RL, Horst VD, et al. Application of an epicardial left atrial appendage occlusion device by a robotic-assisted, right-chest approach. Ann Thorac Surg 2016;101:e177–8.
67. Gao C, Yang M, Wang G, et al. Totally robotic resection of myxoma and atrial septal defect repair. Interact Cardiovasc Thorac Surg 2008;7:947–50.
68. Xiao C, Gao C, Yang M, et al. Totally robotic atrial septal defect closure: 7-year single-institution experience and follow-up. Interact Cardiovasc Thorac Surg 2014;19:933–7.
69. Onan B, Aydin U, Kadirogullari E, et al. Robotic repair of partial anomalous pulmonary venous connection: the initial experience and technical details. J Robot Surg 2019. https://doi.org/10.1007/s11701-019-00943-0.
70. Onan B, Aydin U, Turkvatan A, et al. Robot-assisted repair of right partial anomalous pulmonary venous return. J Card Surg 2016;31:394–7.
71. Lewis CT, Bethencourt DM, Stephens RL, et al. Robotic repair of sinus venosus atrial septal defect with partial anomalous pulmonary venous return and persistent left superior vena cava. Innovations (Phila) 2014;9:388–90.
72. Onan B, Aydin U, Basgoze S, et al. Totally endoscopic robotic repair of coronary sinus atrial septal defect. Interact Cardiovasc Thorac Surg 2016;23:662–4.
73. Bakir I, Onan B, Kadirogullari E. Robotically assisted repair of partial atrioventricular canal defect. Artif Organs 2016;40:917–8.
74. Mandal K, Srivastava AR, Nifong LW, et al. Robot-assisted partial atrioventricular canal defect repair and cryo-maze procedure. Ann Thorac Surg 2016;101:756–8.
75. Gao C, Yang M, Wang G, et al. Totally endoscopic robotic ventricular septal defect repair. Innovations (Phila) 2010;5:278–80.
76. Gao C, Yang M, Xiao C, et al. Totally endoscopic robotic correction of cor triatriatum sinister coexisting with atrial septal defect. Innovations (Phila) 2016;11: 451–2.
77. Schilling J, Engel AM, Hassan M, et al. Robotic excision of atrial myxoma. J Card Surg 2012;27:423–6.
78. Murphy DA, Miller JS, Langford DA. Robot-assisted endoscopic excision of left atrial myxomas. J Thorac Cardiovasc Surg 2005;130:596–7.
79. Tarui T, Ishikawa N, Ohtake H, et al. Totally endoscopic robotic resection of left atrial myxoma with persistent left superior vena cava. Interact Cardiovasc Thorac Surg 2016;23:174–5.
80. Yang M, Yao M, Wang G, et al. Comparison of postoperative quality of life for patients who undergo atrial myxoma excision with robotically assisted versus conventional surgery. J Thorac Cardiovasc Surg 2015;150:152–7.
81. Kesavuori R, Raivio P, Jokinen JJ, et al. Quality of life after robotically assisted atrial myxoma excision. J Robot Surg 2015;9:235–41.
82. Gao C, Yang M, Wang G, et al. Excision of atrial myxoma using robotic technology. J Thorac Cardiovasc Surg 2010;139:1282–5.
83. Onan B, Kahraman Z, Erturk M, et al. Robotic resection of giant left ventricular myxoma causing outflow tract obstruction. J Card Surg 2017;32:281–4.

84. Folliguet TA, Vanhuyse F, Magnano D, et al. Robotic aortic valve replacement: case report. Heart Surg Forum 2004;7:E551–3.

85. Folliguet TA, Vanhuyse F, Konstantinos Z, et al. Early experience with robotic aortic valve replacement. Eur J Cardiothorac Surg 2005;28:172–3.

86. Murphy ET. Robotic excision of aortic valve papillary fibroelastoma and concomitant maze procedure. Glob Cardiol Sci Pract 2013;2012:93–100.

87. Woo YJ, Grand TJ, Weiss SJ. Robotic resection of an aortic valve papillary fibroelastoma. Ann Thorac Surg 2005;80:1100–2.

88. Balkhy HH, Lewis CT, Kitahara H. Robot-assisted aortic valve surgery: state of the art and challenges for the future. Int J Med Robot 2018;14:e1913.

89. Gammie JS, Lehr E, Griffith BP, et al. Robotic-assisted aortic valve bypass (apicoaortic conduit) for aortic stenosis. Ann Thorac Surg 2011;92:726–8.

90. Malhotra SP, Le D, Thelitz S, et al. Robotic-assisted endoscopic thoracic aortic anastomosis in juvenile lambs. Heart Surg Forum 2002;6:38–42.

91. Seco M, Cao C, Modi P, et al. Systematic review of robotic minimally invasive mitral valve surgery. Ann Cardiothorac Surg 2013;2:704–16.

Robotic Thoracic Surgery

Gary Schwartz, MD[a],*, Manu Sancheti, MD[b], Justin Blasberg, MD, MPH[c]

KEYWORDS

- Thoracic surgery • Esophagectomy • Mediastinal mass • Pulmonary lobectomy

KEY POINTS

- A minimally invasive approach is particularly important in thoracic surgery, whereby postoperative pain plays a major role in recovery and outcome.
- Thoracic surgery entails meticulous dissection of major vascular structures in confined spaces, making a robotic approach particularly beneficial.
- A robotic platform can be used for pulmonary resection, benign and malignant esophageal surgery, mediastinal tumors, and diaphragm surgery, all with excellent outcomes.

INTRODUCTION

Surgery of the chest poses significant challenges because of the presence of major vascular structures, consideration of intraoperative ventilation, and marked postoperative pain and associated risk of atelectasis and pneumonia. Minimally invasive surgery has curtailed the pain associated with thoracic incisions, and a robotic platform has enabled increasing proficiency with dissection and reconstruction of delicate structures. Using robotic assistance in thoracic surgery in a thoughtful manner can help optimize outcomes and maximize patient benefit.

ROBOTIC ESOPHAGEAL SURGERY
Introduction

Esophageal surgery is particularly amenable to a minimally invasive approach because of its location in multiple anatomic fields and the subsequent need for several incisions in open surgery. The proximity to significant adjacent structures in the neck, chest, and abdomen makes a robotic approach particularly appealing. Robotic-assisted surgery of the esophagus has been described in both benign and malignant esophageal diseases with excellent outcomes.

[a] Department of Thoracic Surgery & Lung Transplantation, Baylor University Medical Center, Texas A&M Health Science Center, 3410 Worth Street, Suite 545, Dallas, TX 75246, USA; [b] Emory Saint Joseph's Hospital, Emory Healthcare, 5665 Peachtree Dunwoody Road #200, Atlanta, GA 30342, USA; [c] Yale School of Medicine, Lauder Hall, 310 Cedar Street, New Haven, CT 06510, USA
* Corresponding author.
E-mail address: Gary.Schwartz@BSWHealth.org

Surg Clin N Am 100 (2020) 237–248
https://doi.org/10.1016/j.suc.2019.12.001
0039-6109/20/© 2019 Elsevier Inc. All rights reserved.

surgical.theclinics.com

Disease-Specific Applications

Benign esophageal conditions can occur at any level of the esophagus. In the cervical region, Zenker diverticulum is the most prominent. Given the success of the open transcervical and endoscopic transoral approaches, a robotic repair has not been widely adopted, although it has been described via a transaxillary route.[1] In the thorax, benign conditions include leiomyoma and epiphrenic diverticuli. Robotic enucleation of esophageal leiomyoma has been well described even with quite large masses.[2,3] Epiphrenic diverticulectomy can be safely performed via a robotic-assisted transthoracic or transabdominal approach.[4,5]

Benign conditions of the gastroesophageal junction, including refractory gastroesophageal reflux disease and achalasia, are approached transabdominally, although endoscopic approaches are gaining popularity.[6] Further discussion of a robotic-assisted transabdominal approach to these conditions can be found later in the Tanuja Damani and Garth Ballantyne's article, "Robotic Foregut Surgery," in this issue.

Management of malignant disease of the esophagus requires a multidisciplinary team. In general, trimodality therapy using induction chemoradiotherapy followed by surgical resection is the gold standard for early-stage disease. Surgical approach varies based on tumor location, patient surgical history, and surgeon preference. Commonly performed approaches include transabdominal transhiatal, Ivor-Lewis, and McKeown esophagectomies. A left thoracoabdominal approach is rarely used and does not translate well to minimally invasive surgery. Recent reports of esophagectomy via a limited transcervical approach alone highlight the evolving application of robotic technology.[7]

The open transabdominal transhiatal approach to esophagectomy has been well described as comparable to a transthoracic approach in terms of oncologic outcomes and complications.[8] Initial application of robotic assistance to esophagectomy was via this approach, with more recent and larger series demonstrating equivalent outcomes.[9–12] Cervical reconstruction of the esophagus can be performed in a hand-sewn or stapled manner, with a variety of surgeon-specific preferences and no clear gold standard.

Advantages of a transhiatal approach include no entry into the pleural spaces and therefore decreased pulmonary complications and potential pain. Augmentation with a transverse abdominis block can further improve postoperative analgesia.[13] Disadvantages include suboptimal visualization high into the mediastinum and dissection out of the reach of robotic instrumentation, with potential for mediastinal bleeding and airway complications, although reported rates are similar to other surgical approaches. In addition, as compared with an Ivor-Lewis esophagectomy, a cervical neck dissection has potential for injury to vascular structures, the trachea, and the left recurrent laryngeal nerve, as well as a higher incidence of anastomotic leak; fortunately, this increased leak rate is associated with a lower morbidity than an intrathoracic leak.[14]

Generally, based on surgeon preference and training, and owing to the perceived improved mediastinal lymphadenectomy, a "3-field" or McKeown esophagectomy involves surgery of the cervical, thoracic, and abdominal esophagus. The McKeown technique was adopted early by a robotic approach[15,16] and is quite appealing to most thoracic surgeons because the oncologic benefits of wide margins and extended lymphadenectomy are paired with minimal invasiveness.[17] Disadvantages include entry into the pleural space and the need to turn and reprepare the patient, adding operative time to the procedure, as well as a cervical dissection with added morbidity as in a transhiatal esophagectomy. Cervical reconstruction is similarly performed in the same manner as via a transhiatal approach.

Ivor-Lewis esophagectomy entails transabdominal gastric dissection, lymphade-nectomy, and conduit preparation, followed by closure and turning of the patient and repreparing for a right transthoracic approach, including esophageal dissection, specimen transection and extraction, and reconstruction. This approach has been widely adopted by minimally invasive surgeons because both fields can be approached robotically, with the benefits of an extended mediastinal lympha-denectomy and an intrathoracic anastomosis with a lower leak rate.[14,18,19] Intratho-racic esophagogastric reconstruction can be performed in a variety of manners, including running hand-sewn, linear stapled, and end-to-end circular stapled anastomoses.[19–21]

Delayed esophageal reconstruction is occasionally necessary, most often because of esophageal perforation with a contaminated mediastinum precluding immediate reconstruction. Available conduit is chosen on a case-by-case basis and may include the standard gastric conduit, colon interposition, small bowel (with or without "super-charging"), or rarely, a free myocutaneous graft, with results comparable to 1-stage esophagectomy.[22–25] The substernal tunnel is the most common route of reconstruc-tion, and although experience is limited, robotic reconstruction via this route has been described.[26]

Ultimately, the surgical approach to malignancies of the esophagus is patient and surgeon specific. Each technique has advantages and disadvantages, requiring a thoughtful analysis of each individual patient. Excellent oncologic outcomes as well as quality of life can be achieved using a robotic platform to aid in surgical resection and reconstruction of the esophagus.[27–29]

ROBOTIC MEDIASTINAL SURGERY
Introduction

Historically, the mediastinum has been a difficult location for surgeons to access given the proximity of the heart and great vessels to adjacent structures. Surgeries were traditionally performed via sternotomy, posterolateral thoracotomy, or anterolateral thoracotomy with or without transverse sternotomy (clamshell), incurring prolonged hospital stay and recovery. With video-assisted thoracoscopic surgery (VATS), mini-mally invasive techniques for mediastinal procedures allow for smaller incisions, shorter hospital stay, and quicker recovery.[30] The advent of robotic technology has further pushed the envelope of what is possible in the mediastinum, allowing the sur-geon to perform complex maneuvers that mimic traditional open techniques. Robotics specifically adds the benefits of articulating instruments, 3-dimensional visualization, and stabilized operative movements, which are critical advantages in the mediastinum.

Mediastinal pathologic condition is conventionally described based on specific anatomic landmarks and separated into the anterior, middle, and posterior compart-ment. The differential diagnoses for anterior mediastinal pathologic conditions include thymoma/thymic carcinoma, germ cell tumors, thyroid masses, and ectopic parathy-roid glands. Middle mediastinal masses include lymph nodes, bronchogenic cysts, pericardial cysts, and rarely, solid ectopic tumors. Finally, posterior mediastinal masses include duplication cysts of foregut origin or solid tumors of neurogenic origin.

Preoperative Evaluation

Standard preoperative evaluation is performed for all patients, independent of the platform for resection, with an additional few details specific to robotic-assisted pro-cedures. Computed tomography (CT) with intravenous (IV) contrast is helpful in deter-mining the relationship of a mass to surrounding great vessels and vital structures. As is common with thoracoscopic and robotic procedures, the association of the lesion with surrounding rib spaces is important for port location. Pulmonary function testing is recommended because poor lung reserve may preclude single-lung ventilation. Lung isolation is routinely supplemented with carbon dioxide insufflation at 8 to 10 mm Hg to improve visualization and for cases whereby single-lung ventilation is poorly tolerated.

Preoperative imaging is vital for surgical planning. Port placement and positioning of the robot/patient is a key aspect of all successful robotic operations. In general, port sites are triangulated at least 10 cm away from the target lesion. Port sites and associated robot arms should be separated by at least 8 cm to avoid collisions. In addition, if an assistant port is used, it should ideally be 5 to 7 cm posterior from the robotic ports to minimize assistant to robot arm collisions. The port placement and robot/patient positioning are uniform for anterior mediastinal access but are variable for middle and posterior mediastinal lesions and therefore subjective based on preoperative imaging.

Anterior Mediastinum

The anterior mediastinum is the space in the chest between the anterior border of the pericardium and the sternum. Robotic-assisted surgery has been used for the following anterior mediastinal pathologic conditions: thymectomy for myasthenia gravis, thymoma/thymic carcinomas, lymphoma, germ cell tumors, parathyroid, and thyroid tissues. Cross-sectional imaging is helpful to determine the relationship of an anterior mediastinal mass to surrounding structures. In all cases, obtaining an R0 resection is very important. Hence, thymomas enclosed within the thymic capsule, or Masaoka stage I tumors, have been found to be acceptable for minimally invasive techniques.[31] Minimally invasive resections for Masaoka stage II tumors have been found to acceptable as well, but the use of robotic assistance in this case has not fully been studied.[32] The treatment of anterior mediastinal mature teratomas and dermoid cysts is primarily surgical resection of which robotic assistance is appropriate. Seminomas and nonseminomatous tumors are treated primarily with radiation and chemotherapy, respectively. If persistent after treatment, further robotic-assisted resection may be indicated. Robotic anterior mediastinal procedures for lymphoma are primarily related to excisional biopsies.

Surgical Considerations

Anterior mediastinal masses may be approached from either side of the chest. The patient is placed in the supine position with a rolled sheet along the posterior midclavicular line to elevate the operative side. The arms are tucked with the ipsilateral arm below the operative table.

The port sites are positioned along the midanterior axillary line. Generally, ports are placed in the third, fifth, and seventh interspaces. The pleural space is insufflated with carbon dioxide via the assistant port, which is 5 cm, centered posteriorly between the camera and inferior port. The robot is driven into the operative field from the contralateral side preferably, although the robot boom can be rotated if approaching ipsilaterally. A 0° camera is preferable, but the 30° scope may be needed when visualization is challenging. Instruments used include a grasping device in the nondominant hand (ie, Cadiére forceps) and an energy device in the dominant hand (ie, monopolar, bipolar, or vessel sealer).

Aspects of this operation specific to the robotic platform include the use of rolled gauze (cigars), which can be inserted through the assistant port to absorb minor bleeding and assist with retraction. The identification of key anatomy for this procedure is similar to other open and minimally invasive resections. Defining the phrenic nerve is critical, which helps in the dissection of the mediastinal pleura extending caudad to the inferior pole of the thymic tissue above the diaphragm. Ligation and division of the thymic veins at the superior aspect of the dissection bed are facilitated by use of the robotic vessel sealer or clips, which provide appropriate hemostasis. The contralateral pleura should be opened to allow for identification of the contralateral phrenic nerve. Visualization of the contralateral pleural space can be aided by transition to a 30° camera and traction on the dissected thymus. In addition, a thoracoscope can be placed via a 5-mm trocar in the contralateral space by the assistant. Robotic consoles equipped with appropriate video inputs allow for visualization of the contralateral VATS view from within the robot console, which helps the operating surgeon identify and avoid injury to the contralateral phrenic nerve.

Middle Mediastinum

The middle mediastinum is the space in the chest between the anterior border of the pericardium and the posterior border of the pericardium. Pathologic conditions of the middle mediastinum commonly include the mediastinal lymph nodes often accessed via mediastinoscopy and congenital bronchogenic cysts and pericardial cysts.[33] The use of robotic technology for resection of bronchogenic cysts and pericardial cysts is well published in the literature.[34]

Robotic mediastinal lymphadenopathy may be best accessed via a transthoracic approach as opposed to endobronchial ultrasound or mediastinoscopy in cases of prior neck surgery, radiation treatment, or access to the aortopulmonary window lymph nodes. Congenital mediastinal cysts may be symptomatic because of the mass effect on surrounding tissues. In addition, these cysts can get infected, complicating resection.[35] Resection is often indicated for symptomatic or easily accessible cysts with low operative risk to prevent long-term complications secondary to growth and mass effect. In cases with prior cyst infection or significant scarring, articulating instruments and use of bipolar cautery along with ×10 magnified optics help to define planes of dissection and reduce the risk of injury to surrounding structures.

Surgical Considerations

The location of the tumor and preoperative imaging is vital to determine port and patient positioning for middle mediastinal surgeries. In most cases, a right or left lateral decubitus position will be appropriate for resection. Slight reverse Trendelenburg and anterior tilt of the bed will assist in moving the lung out of the operative field.

Most commonly, a 3-arm approach is appropriate to triangulate toward the target tissue with ports as far away as possible. The camera is placed in the eighth intercostal space just anterior to the posterior axillary line. The other 2 robotic ports are placed anterior and posterior to the camera approximately 8 cm away in the same interspace. If used, an assistant port is placed 5 cm inferior and anterior to the camera trocar. Similar to the anterior mediastinal robotic procedure, carbon dioxide insufflation is used.

The operative steps for a robotic-assisted middle mediastinal procedure is dictated by the specific pathologic condition treated. A 30° camera is helpful for these procedures. In general, vital structures present near the middle mediastinum to be aware of include the aorta, trachea, esophagus, vagus nerve, recurrent laryngeal nerve, and phrenic nerve. Dissection is usually carried out with a bipolar instrument along with a grasping instrument.

Posterior Mediastinum

The posterior mediastinum is the space in the chest between the posterior border of the pericardium and the vertebrae. Procedures related to the foregut and neurogenic pathologic condition are most common, including robotic resection of neurofibromas, schwannoma, neuroganglioma, ganglioneuroblastoma, paraganglioma, and foregut duplication cysts/tumors.

Similar to middle mediastinal tumors, tumors of the posterior mediastinum, specifically neurogenic tumors, may be symptomatic because of the mass effect.[4] Robotic surgical resection in these patients does require careful preoperative planning and preparation. MRI of the spine is critical to define involvement of the intravertebral foramen.[4] If identified, a combined procedure with neurosurgery may be necessary. A functional paraganglioma is a possible diagnosis for a posterior mediastinal tumor. Therefore, a thorough endocrine evaluation for catecholamine levels is important to avoid an intraoperative hypertensive crisis.[4] In the setting of foregut pathologic condition, upper endoscopy or contrast esophagram is recommended before robotic repair.

Surgical Considerations

The location of the tumor on preoperative imaging is helpful to determine port and patient positioning for posterior mediastinal surgeries. In most cases, right or left lateral decubitus positioning will be appropriate for resection. Moderate reverse Trendelenburg and anterior tilt of the bed will assist in retracting the lung out of the operative field.

A 3-arm approach is preferred with triangulation on the target tissue with ports as far away as possible. The camera is placed in the ninth intercostal space just anterior to the posterior axillary line. The other 2 robotic ports are placed anterior and posterior to the camera approximately 8 cm away in the same interspace. If used, an assistant port is placed 5 cm inferior and anterior to the camera trocar. Similar to the anterior and middle mediastinal robotic procedures, carbon dioxide insufflation is used.

The operative steps for a robotic-assisted posterior mediastinal procedure is dictated by the specific pathologic condition treated. Vital structures present near the posterior mediastinum to be cognizant of include the aorta, spine, esophagus, azygous vein, and thoracic duct. A 30° camera is helpful in these procedures for better visualization. Dissection is usually carried out with a bipolar instrument along with a grasping instrument.

ROBOTIC LUNG SURGERY
Introduction

Surgical resection for early-stage non–small cell lung cancer is associated with optimal 5-year survival and the lowest risk of local and distant recurrence compared with other treatment modalities.[36] Although thoracotomy for lung resection has evolved over time with muscle-sparing incisions and improved pain control with catheter delivery systems and long-acting analgesics,[37] open surgery continues to be associated with variable hospital length of stay and risk for perioperative morbidity and mortality. The adoption of minimally invasive lung resection has dramatically changed the management of these patients, reducing hospital length of stay, expediting return to baseline performance status, and shortening the interval of recovery need for patients that might require adjuvant therapy.[38]

Although minimally invasive lung resection is historically performed in a "video-assisted" fashion with 2-dimensional optics and nonarticulating instruments, the incorporation of robotic technology in the lung cancer space has also meant significant technical advantages to the surgeon. Accordingly, an increased robotic adoption and an improved opportunity for patients to realize the benefits of minimally invasive lung resection regardless of hospital size or geography. Increased utilization also provides an opportunity to retrospectively evaluate outcomes associated with this platform as well as specific ways to improve clinical practice for the lung surgery population. The most current robotic system represents a useful tool from which wedge, anatomic resection (segment, lobectomy, pneumonectomy), mediastinal lymphadenectomy, and advanced procedures, including bronchovascular sleeve resections,[39] can be performed. Although the merits of VATS versus robotic resection continue to be debated, overall utilization of minimally invasive surgery to manage both benign and malignant lung conditions remains a significant advantage to the patient.

Preoperative Evaluation

Appropriate selection of patients for robotic lung resection is similar to other minimally invasive techniques. These procedures are best performed with single-lung ventilation; however, unlike VATS, insufflation with carbon dioxide to a pressure of 8 to 10 mm Hg is used in almost all cases and significantly improves visualization. A significant advantage of robotic resection compared to traditional VATS is the visualization provided by insufflation, which is particularly useful in patient whose lung function cannot tolerate single-lung ventilation for the entire procedure. Almost any patient eligible for minimally invasive resection can undergo a robotic procedure, including cases with small or nonpalpable nodules. The incorporation of preoperative localization in the form of either CT-guided dye marking or intraoperative navigational bronchoscopy has helped augment preoperative imaging and improved the efficiency of these cases.[40] Tumor location to central structures that require complex bronchovascular resection and reconstruction may be a contraindication to all but the most advanced surgeon. In addition, invasion of the chest wall may mandate a hybrid approach (robotic lobectomy followed by en bloc chest wall resection through a limited incision overlying the area of interest) or should be considered only after significant experience with less complex cases has been achieved. Significant hilar lymphadenopathy surrounding central structures, particularly in cases where granulomatous disease is prevalent, also represents a potential technical challenge. However, these cases are still more easily accomplished robotically compared with VATS given the technical advantages associated with articulating instruments and bipolar or vessel sealing energy. Patient size would intuitively seem to be a contraindication to robotic lung resection; however, these cases are actually more easily performed robotically rather than with VATS. In select cases, patient habitus may impact precise placement of robotic ports, which has more significant implications compared with VATS.

The workup and preoperative management of patients for lung resection are similar to VATS and have been discussed in previous sections. Preoperative chest CT scan with IV contrast is recommended to assess pulmonary artery branches or other complex anatomy based on tumor location that can assist with surgical planning. Similar to robotic mediastinal and esophageal surgery, precise identification of where the diaphragm inserts helps to define the appropriate rib space for entry. This information is also useful to optimize patient positioning. Staging and cardiopulmonary risk stratification are similar to other robotic and nonrobotic procedures described based on consensus recommendations.[41]

Surgical Considerations

A significant advantage of robotic lobectomy is that port position is essentially independent of the lobe to be resected. The reproducibility of port position allows for improved efficiency for the operating staff as well as for the surgeon. The conduct of robotic lobectomy is similar to open and VATS procedures, including the use of a double lumen endotracheal tube and patient positioning. Bed flexion is more critical in robotic cases compared with VATS; a high riding anterior superior iliac spine (ASIS) can restrict robotic instrument movement and make a straightforward lobectomy significantly more challenging. In cases where a high-riding ASIS limits the ability to achieve a horizontal plane from the axilla down to the 10th rib and the ASIS, a gel roll or folded sheet may be placed under the patient's flank to prop up the inferior aspect of the thorax and achieve this necessary alignment.

The classic description of placing all 4 ports in the either the eighth or ninth interspace, starting at the posterior axillary line, spaced approximately 1 handsbreath apart with additional ports in the anterior axillary, infrascapular, and paraspinous positions, can be modified based on the patient's body habitus and location of the diaphragm. Modification of port position provides the recommended 10-cm distance from the resection target regardless of the location of the pathologic condition, including lower-lobe resection. The first port can be placed in several different ways, although these investigators recommend vision during entry using either an OPTIVIEW style trocar with camera or a Hassan style cut down into the pleural space with S retractors or similar. In either case, avoiding blind insertion helps reduce the risk of inadvertent lung injury, particularly for cases whereby pleural adhesions are suspected. The robotic stapler, a significant advantage of the newer robotic systems, can only be used via a 12-mm port; therefore, placing these larger ports in both the anterior axillary and the infrascapular positions provides significant versatility when performing anatomic resection, particularly for upper lobe tumors. Although not mandatory, an assistant port placed 1 to 2 interspaces between this line, either between the anterior 2 ports or between the posterior axillary and infrascapular ports, allows for retraction, for an access point to feed sponges (cigars), or for removal of specimen without removing instruments and undocking the robotic arms. Consideration for where the assistant port is located relative to the positioning of the robotic arms will help determine whether an anterior or posterior assistant port is optimal. Both 0° and 30° cameras can be used for robotic lung resection, each with specific advantages. In general, a 30° scope is advantageous to see around corners or over the top of structures when visualization may be limited. These recommendations for port positioning and camera are highly reproducible with little variability.

The conduct of lung resection is similar to open and VATS procedures. Although different surgeons advocate for different starting points (fissure vs hilum, artery vs vein, and so forth), the fundamentals of lung resection is the same regardless of the surgical platform. At ×10 magnification, planes are easier to see, and blood loss from lymph node dissection is more easily avoided, particularly with robotic bipolar energy devices that have little thermal spread. In cases where malignancy is either known or suspected, complete hilar and mediastinal lymphadenectomy is recommended before ligation and division of vascular or airway structures, because this significantly improves the ability to see around tubular structures, making division safer. Given the delicate nature of the pulmonary artery and lung parenchyma, careful dissection includes avoiding directly grabbing either structure with an instrument, but rather using cigar-assisted retraction for blunt dissection or exposure. These techniques help facilitate the operation and reduce the risk of parenchymal injury with subsequent air leak.

These technical attributes have led to increased utilization of robotic lung resection over the past decade, with institutional and large database outcomes demonstrating similar rates of margin positivity and risk for morbidity and mortality when compared with open and VATS procedures.[38,42,43] Reported advantages of robotic lung resection include improved lymph node dissection, a greater number of nodes procured, and reduced blood loss compared with either open or VATS procedures.[44,45] Whether there are advantages with regard to hospital length of stay or postoperative pain control remains controversial and is institution dependent. Similar to VATS procedures, the proficiency of robotic lung resection is realized with increased surgeon experience.[46,47] In addition, hospital volume is directly correlated with length of stay and mortality; therefore, incorporating robotic lung resection into one's practice should be more structured than just an occasional attempt at using the system.[48] In the future, improved adoption by open surgeons will likely lead to opportunities for patients managed at nonacademic or rural centers to realize the benefits of minimally invasive resection whereby they might not currently be available.

The major challenges in thoracic surgery stem from the tight working space and proximity of major vital structures. Specific advantages in this space provided by robotic assistance include improved 3-dimensional, high-definition visualization along a wide array of wristed, dexterous instrumentation to facilitate surgical resection. Increased adoption of robotic surgery will facilitate a broader range of patients being offered minimally invasive thoracic surgery, which should translate to improved outcomes and decreased morbidity.

SUMMARY

Robotic surgery has many applications within the chest, including benign and malignant esophageal surgery, mediastinal masses, and pulmonary lobectomy. Less common procedures include diaphragm plication and reconstruction as well as pleural decortication. As the technology evolves, additional strides are being made, such as single-incision robotic thoracic surgery.[49,50] Ultimately, this progress will continue to lead to safer, less painful, and oncologically sound operations for our patients.

DISCLOSURE

Nothing to disclose (G. Schwartz); Intuitive Surgical (M. Sancheti); Intuitive Surgical (J. Blasberg).

REFERENCES

1. Melotti G, Piccoli M, Mullineris B, et al. Zenker diverticulectomy: first report of robot-assisted transaxillary approach. J Robot Surg 2015;9(1):75–8.

2. Compean SD, Gaur P, Kim MP. Robot assisted thoracoscopic resection of giant esophageal leiomyoma. Int J Surg Case Rep 2014;5(12):1132–4.

3. Elli E, Espat NJ, Berger R, et al. Robotic-assisted thoracoscopic resection of esophageal leiomyoma. Surg Endosc 2004;18(4):713–6.

4. Balci B, Kilinc G, Calik B, et al. Robotic-assisted transthoracic esophageal diverticulectomy. JSLS 2018;22(2) [pii:e2018.00002].

5. Pernazza G, Monsellato I, Pende V, et al. Fully robotic treatment of an epiphrenic diverticulum: report of a case. Minim Invasive Ther Allied Technol 2012;21(2): 96–100.

6. Crespin OM, Liu LWC, Parmar A, et al. Safety and efficacy of POEM for treatment of achalasia: a systematic review of the literature. Surg Endosc 2017;31(5): 2187–201.

7. Nakauchi M, Uyama I, Suda K, et al. Robot-assisted mediastinoscopic esophagectomy for esophageal cancer: the first clinical series. Esophagus 2019;16(1): 85–92.

8. Chang AC, Ji H, Birkmeyer NJ, et al. Outcomes after transhiatal and transthoracic esophagectomy for cancer. Ann Thorac Surg 2008;85(2):424–9.

9. Boone J, Borel Rinkes IH, van Hillegersberg R. Transhiatal robot-assisted esophagectomy. Surg Endosc 2008;22(4):1139–40.

10. Dunn DH, Johnson EM, Morphew JA, et al. Robot-assisted transhiatal esophagectomy: a 3-year single-center experience. Dis Esophagus 2013;26(2):159–66.

11. Horgan S, Berger RA, Elli EF, et al. Robotic-assisted minimally invasive transhiatal esophagectomy. Am Surg 2003;69(7):624–6.

12. Mori K, Yamagata Y, Aikou S, et al. Short-term outcomes of robotic radical esophagectomy for esophageal cancer by a nontransthoracic approach compared with conventional transthoracic surgery. Dis Esophagus 2016;29(5):429–34.

13. Levy G, Cordes MA, Farivar AS, et al. Transversus abdominis plane block improves perioperative outcome after esophagectomy versus epidural. Ann Thorac Surg 2018;105(2):406–12.

14. Kassis ES, Kosinski AS, Ross P Jr, et al. Predictors of anastomotic leak after esophagectomy: an analysis of the Society of Thoracic Surgeons general thoracic database. Ann Thorac Surg 2013;96(6):1919–26.

15. Kernstine KH, DeArmond DT, Shamoun DM, et al. The first series of completely robotic esophagectomies with three-field lymphadenectomy: initial experience. Surg Endosc 2007;21(12):2285–92.

16. Lehenbauer D, Kernstine KH. Robotic esophagectomy: modified McKeown approach. Thorac Surg Clin 2014;24(2):203–9, vii.

17. van der Horst S, de Maat MFG, van der Sluis PC, et al. Extended thoracic lymph node dissection in robotic-assisted minimal invasive esophagectomy (RAMIE) for patients with superior mediastinal lymph node metastasis. Ann Cardiothorac Surg 2019;8(2):218–25.

18. Cerfolio RJ, Bryant AS, Hawn MT. Technical aspects and early results of robotic esophagectomy with chest anastomosis. J Thorac Cardiovasc Surg 2013; 145(1):90–6.

19. Okusanya OT, Sarkaria IS, Hess NR, et al. Robotic assisted minimally invasive esophagectomy (RAMIE): the University of Pittsburgh Medical Center initial experience. Ann Cardiothorac Surg 2017;6(2):179–85.

20. Cerfolio RJ, Wei B, Hawn MT, et al. Robotic esophagectomy for cancer: early results and lessons learned. Semin Thorac Cardiovasc Surg 2016;28(1):160–9.

21. Wang Z, Zhang H, Wang F, et al. Robot-assisted esophagogastric reconstruction in minimally invasive Ivor Lewis esophagectomy. J Thorac Dis 2019;11(5):1860–6.

22. Greene CL, DeMeester SR, Augustin F, et al. Long-term quality of life and alimentary satisfaction after esophagectomy with colon interposition. Ann Thorac Surg 2014;98(5):1713–9 [discussion: 1719–20].

23. Kesler KA, Pillai ST, Birdas TJ, et al. "Supercharged" isoperistaltic colon interposition for long-segment esophageal reconstruction. Ann Thorac Surg 2013;95(4): 1162–8 [discussion: 1168–9].

24. Moore JM, Hooker CM, Molena D, et al. Complex esophageal reconstruction procedures have acceptable outcomes compared with routine esophagectomy. Ann Thorac Surg 2016;102(1):215–22.

25. Stephens EH, Gaur P, Hotze KO, et al. Super-charged pedicled jejunal interposition performance compares favorably with a gastric conduit after esophagectomy. Ann Thorac Surg 2015;100(2):407–13.
26. Petrov RV, Bakhos CT, Abbas AE. Robotic substernal esophageal bypass and reconstruction with gastric conduit-frequently overlooked minimally invasive option. J Vis Surg 2019;5 [pii:47].
27. Kingma BF, de Maat MFG, van der Horst S, et al. Robot-assisted minimally invasive esophagectomy (RAMIE) improves perioperative outcomes: a review. J Thorac Dis 2019;11(Suppl 5):S735–42.
28. Meredith K, Blinn P, Maramara T, et al. Comparative outcomes of minimally invasive and robotic-assisted esophagectomy. Surg Endosc 2020;34(2):814–82.
29. Sarkaria IS, Rizk NP, Goldman DA, et al. Early quality of life outcomes after robotic-assisted minimally invasive and open esophagectomy. Ann Thorac Surg 2019;108(3):920–8.
30. Straughan DM, Fontaine JP, Toloza EM. Robotic-assisted videothoracoscopic mediastinal surgery. Cancer Control 2015;22(3):326–30.
31. Ye B, Tantai JC, Li W, et al. Video-assisted thoracoscopic surgery versus robotic-assisted thoracoscopic surgery in the surgical treatment of Masaoka stage I thymoma. World J Surg Oncol 2013;11:157.
32. Yuan ZY, Cheng GY, Sun KL, et al. Comparative study of video-assisted thoracic surgery versus open thymectomy for thymoma in one single center. J Thorac Dis 2014;6(6):726–33.
33. Juanpere S, Cañete N, Ortuño P, et al. A diagnostic approach to the mediastinal masses. Insights Imaging 2013;4(1):29–52.
34. Asaf BB, Kumar A, Vijay CL. Robotic excision of paraesophageal bronchogenic cyst in a 9-year-old child. J Indian Assoc Pediatr Surg 2015;20(4):191–3.
35. Ribet ME, Copin MC, Gosselin B. Bronchogenic cysts of the mediastinum. J Thorac Cardiovasc Surg 1995;109(5):1003–10.
36. Cornwell LD, Echeverria AE, Samuelian J, et al. Video-assisted thoracoscopic lobectomy is associated with greater recurrence-free survival than stereotactic body radiotherapy for clinical stage I lung cancer. J Thorac Cardiovasc Surg 2018;155(1):395–402.
37. Chen L, Wu Y, Cai Y, et al. Comparison of programmed intermittent bolus infusion and continuous infusion for postoperative patient-controlled analgesia with thoracic paravertebral block catheter: a randomized, double-blind, controlled trial. Reg Anesth Pain Med 2019;44(2):240–5.
38. Rajaram R, Mohanty S, Bentrem DJ, et al. Nationwide assessment of robotic lobectomy for non-small cell lung cancer. Ann Thorac Surg 2017;103(4):1092–100.
39. Egberts JH, Moller T, Becker T. Robotic-assisted sleeve lobectomy using the four-arm technique in the DaVinci Si(R) and Xi(R) systems. Thorac Cardiovasc Surg 2019;67(7):603–5.
40. McDermott S, Fintelmann FJ, Bierhals AJ, et al. Image-guided preoperative localization of pulmonary nodules for video-assisted and robotically assisted surgery. Radiographics 2019;39(5):1264–79.
41. Ettinger DS, Wood DE, Aisner DL, et al. Non-small cell lung cancer, version 5.2017, NCCN clinical practice guidelines in oncology. J Natl Compr Canc Netw 2017;15(4):504–35.
42. Oh DS, Reddy RM, Gorrepati ML, et al. Robotic-assisted, video-assisted thoracoscopic and open lobectomy: propensity-matched analysis of recent premier data. Ann Thorac Surg 2017;104(5):1733–40.

43. Park BJ, Melfi F, Mussi A, et al. Robotic lobectomy for non-small cell lung cancer (NSCLC): long-term oncologic results. J Thorac Cardiovasc Surg 2012;143(2): 383–9.

44. Nelson DB, Mehran RJ, Mitchell KG, et al. Robotic-assisted lobectomy for non-small cell lung cancer: a comprehensive institutional experience. Ann Thorac Surg 2019;108(2):370–6.

45. Yang HX, Woo KM, Sima CS, et al. Long-term survival based on the surgical approach to lobectomy for clinical stage I nonsmall cell lung cancer: comparison of robotic, video-assisted thoracic surgery, and thoracotomy lobectomy. Ann Surg 2017;265(2):431–7.

46. Feczko AF, Wang H, Nishimura K, et al. Proficiency of robotic lobectomy based on prior surgical technique in the sts general thoracic database. Ann Thorac Surg 2019;108(4):1013–20.

47. Power AD, D'Souza DM, Moffatt-Bruce SD, et al. Defining the learning curve of robotic thoracic surgery: what does it take? Surg Endosc 2019;33(12):3880–8.

48. Tchouta LN, Park HS, Boffa DJ, et al. Hospital volume and outcomes of robot-assisted lobectomies. Chest 2017;151(2):329–39.

49. Gonzalez-Rivas D, Ismail M. Subxiphoid or subcostal uniportal robotic-assisted surgery: early experimental experience. J Thorac Dis 2019;11(1):231–9.

50. Park SY, Kim HK, Jang DS, et al. Initial experiences with robotic single-site thoracic surgery for mediastinal masses. Ann Thorac Surg 2019;107(1):242–7.

Robotic Foregut Surgery

Tanuja Damani, MD[a,b,*], Garth Ballantyne, MD[b]

KEYWORDS

- Robotic surgery • Heller myotomy • Antireflux surgery • Fundoplication • Achalasia
- Gastroesophageal reflux • Hiatal hernia

KEY POINTS

- Robotic-assisted surgery for benign esophageal disease is well described for the treatment of achalasia, gastroesophageal reflux, paraesophageal hernias, epiphrenic diverticula, and benign esophageal masses.
- Robotic Heller myotomy has been shown to have operative times, relief of dysphagia, and conversion rates comparable to laparoscopic approach, with a lower incidence of intraoperative esophageal perforation.
- The use of robotic platform for primary antireflux surgery is still under evaluation, due to prolonged operative time and increased operative costs, with no differences in postoperative outcomes or hospital stay.
- A small but growing number of studies have shown benefits of robotic surgery in complex reoperative foregut surgery with respect to decreased conversion rates, lower readmission rates, and improved functional outcomes.

INTRODUCTION

The approach to esophageal and foregut surgery continues to evolve with advances in technology. Prior to the 1990s, esophageal surgery was performed through large incisions in the abdomen, the chest, or both.[1] Traditional open surgery was subsequently replaced with laparoscopic surgery, with its benefits of smaller incisions, decreased pain, shorter hospital length of stay, fewer complications, and quicker recovery. Laparoscopic surgery, however, had several technical limitations, including a lack of 3-dimensional (3-D) visualization, limited range of motion due to fixed trocar sites and rigid instrumentation, amplification of physiologic tremor, and poor ergonomics.

In 2000, the Food and Drug Administration approved the da Vinci robot (Intuitive Surgical, Sunnyvale, California) for use in general surgical procedures in the United States, which overcame the technical barriers of laparoscopic surgery. In 2001, the first robot-assisted cholecystectomy was reported.[2] Since then, there has been wide adoption of robotic-assisted surgery in general surgical procedures.

[a] NYU Langone Health, 530 First Avenue, HCC Building, Suite 6C, New York, NY 10016, USA;
[b] NYU Grossman School of Medicine, New York, NY, USA
* Corresponding author.
E-mail address: Tanuja.damani@nyulangone.org

Surg Clin N Am 100 (2020) 249–264
https://doi.org/10.1016/j.suc.2019.11.002
0039-6109/20/© 2019 Elsevier Inc. All rights reserved.

surgical.theclinics.com

This article describes robotic approaches to benign esophageal pathologic conditions, including achalasia, gastroesophageal reflux disease (GERD), and hiatal hernia.

ROBOTIC HELLER MYOTOMY

Achalasia is an esophageal motility disorder that affects 0.4 to 1.1 per 100,000 persons annually.[3] The exact etiology is unknown, with suggestion of hereditary, degenerative, autoimmune, or infectious causes as possible etiologies for destruction of the ganglion cells of Auerbach myenteric plexus. It is a slowly progressive disease with primary symptom of dysphagia to solids and liquids. Other symptoms include regurgitation, chest pain, weight loss, aspiration, recurrent pneumonia, chronic cough, and heartburn. Diagnostic tools used in the work-up for achalasia include upper endoscopy and barium esophagram, with manometry being the goal standard diagnostic test. Endoscopy is important to rule out other causes of dysphagia, including malignancy, stricture, and infectious etiologies. Esophagram classically shows a bird's beak sign, with proximal esophageal dilation and distal narrowing. In patients with long-standing disease, it may show a massively dilated esophagus or sigmoid-shaped esophagus. The classic findings of manometry include a failure of relaxation of lower esophageal sphincter (LES) and aperistalsis of the distal esophagus.

Current treatment options include pneumatic dilation, botulinum toxin injection, surgical myotomy, and peroral endoscopic myotomy. Heller myotomy was first described by Ernest Heller in 1913 via a thoracotomy as an anterior and posterior esophageal myotomy.[4] This was modified in 1923 by Zaaijer[5] to an anterior myotomy. With the introduction of minimally invasive surgery and its benefits of decreased postoperative pain, shorter hospital stay, faster return to normal activities, and cosmetic outcome, laparoscopic Heller myotomy, first reported by Shimi and Pelligrini in 1993,[6,7] has become the gold standard treatment. Destruction of the nonrelaxing LES by myotomy and poor peristalsis of the esophagus, leading to diminished ability to clear the esophageal acid, can lead to postoperative reflux in a significant majority of patients. Thus, addition of a partial fundoplication is recommended based on current data for most patients, except those with megaesophagus or sigmoid-shaped esophagus, to decrease postoperative reflux.[8]

Robotic Heller myotomy was first reported by Melvin and colleagues[9] in 2001. Since then, multiple studies, albeit most being retrospective, single-center studies, have confirmed the safety and efficacy of a robotic Heller myotomy, with operative times comparable to a laparoscopic approach (**Table 1**). The relief of dysphagia also has been shown comparable between the 2 approaches.[10,14,16–18]

Surgical Technique

The camera port is placed at the umbilicus, or 2 cm above and 2 cm to the left of the umbilicus, in a straight line with the hiatus. Under direct visualization, the rest of the robotic ports and an assistant port are placed, as depicted (**Fig. 1**). A subxiphoid Nathanson liver retractor (Artisan Medical, Medford, NJ) is placed to elevate the left lateral segment of the liver.

The first step involves division of the gastrohepatic ligament using the robotic vessel sealer and identifying the right crus of the diaphragm. This dissection between the right crus and esophagus is then taken over anteriorly and the left crus is identified. Anterior dissection of the esophagus is performed in the mediastinum to mobilize it for 7 cm to 8 cm, and anterior vagus nerve is identified. The gastric fundus is mobilized by dividing the short gastric vessels using the vessel sealer, and the gastroesophageal

Table 1
Robot-assisted Heller myotomy for achalasia

Author, Year	No. of Patients	Mean Operating Time (min)	Conversions	Intraoperative Complications (%)	Postoperative Complications (%)	Mean Length of Stay (d)
Horgan et al,[10] 2005	59	141 ± 49	0	0	3.4	1.5
Melvin et al,[11] 2005	104	141	1	1.9	7.6	1.5
Galvani et al,[12] 2006	54	162	0	0	3.7	1.5
Iqbal et al,[13] 2006	19	NR	0	0	NR	NR
Huffmanm et al,[14] 2007	24	355 ± 23	0	0	0	2.8
Shaligram et al,[15] 2012	149	NR	NR	0	4	2.4
Sanchez et al,[16] 2012	13	79 ± 20	0	0	0	NR
Perry et al,[17] 2014	56	133 ± 29	NR	0	NR	1
Pallabazzer et al,[18] 2019	66	161 ± 40	0	0	0	NR
Kim et al,[19] 2019	37	158	0	2.7	NR	2.02

NR, not recorded.
Data from Refs.[10–19]

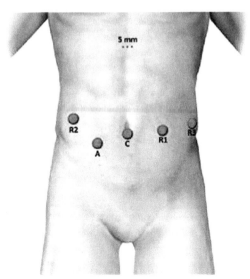

Fig. 1. Port placement for robotic Heller myotomy. C, A, assistant port; C, camera; R1, R2, R3, 3 working robot ports.

(GE) fat pad is removed to clearly expose the GE junction. If the plan is for a Toupet fundoplication, a retroesophageal window is completed.

The myotomy is begun 1 cm to 2 cm above the GE junction, between the 11 o'clock to 1 o'clock positions, with caudad and lateral traction on the esophagus. The longitudinal and circular muscle fibers are divided using the hook electrocautery and separated approximately 180°. The bulging submucosa is noted (**Fig. 2**). The myotomy is extended proximally to approximately 6 cm. The myotomy is then continued retrograde toward the GE junction and the cardia of the stomach. The oblique fibers of the stomach are clearly identified and divided for approximately 2 cm to 3 cm onto the cardia (**Fig. 3**). An upper endoscopy is performed to make sure that the LES is wide open and patulous on completion for the myotomy. An air leak test is performed as well to make sure there is no inadvertent full-thickness perforation.

A Dor fundoplication (180° anterior) or Toupet fundoplication (270° posterior) is then performed using 2-0 nonabsorbable braided sutures. The Toupet fundoplication has been shown a superior antireflux procedure[20] and allows keeping the myotomy edges separated, with the 3 o'clock position and 9 o'clock position sutures. The fundoplication is anchored to the left crus and the right crus as well.

Esophageal Perforation with Robotic-Assisted Myotomy

Although meta-analyses have shown no statistical difference between laparoscopic and robotic Heller myotomy with respect to operative times, estimated blood loss,

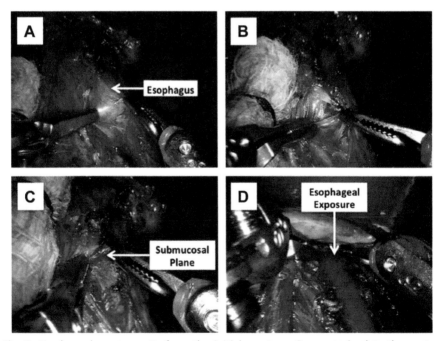

Fig. 2. Esophageal myotomy. Perform the initial myotomy 2 cm proximal to the gastroesophageal junction (*A*) using the hook or Maryland bipolar to divide the muscle fibers (*B*) and expose the submucosal plane (*C*). The esophageal dissection should proceed 6 cm proximally on the esophagus (*D*). (*From* Afaneh C, Finnerty B, Abelson JS, et al. Robotic-assisted Heller myotomy: A modern technique and review of outcomes. J Robotic Surg 2015; 9:101-108; with permission.)

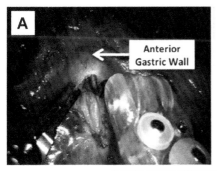
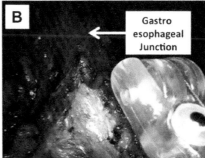
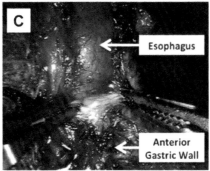

Fig. 3. Gastric myotomy. Gastric myotomy is made 3 cm distal to the gastroesophageal junction (A) and continued proximally (B) to join the esophageal myotomy (C). (*From* Afaneh C, Finnerty B, Abelson JS, et al. Robotic-assisted Heller myotomy: A modern technique and review of outcomes. J Robotic Surg 2015; 9:101-108; with permission.)

conversion to open surgery, length of hospital stay, relief of dysphagia, and long-term recurrence, the robotic approach has been found to be associated with a statistically significant lower rate of intraoperative esophageal perforations.[21] The reported rates of esophageal mucosal injury with laparoscopic myotomy in most studies varies between 5% and 15% (**Table 2**). Multiple studies, however, have shown a significantly lower incidence, mostly zero, of esophageal perforation with robotic approach (**Table 3**).

It is well known that most iatrogenic perforations occur at or distal to the GE junction, on the cardia of the stomach. Here, the oblique muscle fibers are very close to the mucosa without any well-defined plane. The magnified high-resolution 3-D vision, tremor filtration, and motion scaling provided by the da Vinci robotic platform allow meticulous visualization and division of each muscle fiber. The increase in the degrees of freedom of the robotic instruments allows the dissection to be performed from the esophagus to the stomach in a retrograde manner, without any excessive traction on the tissues. The lack of haptic feedback is compensated by the 3-D vision provided by the robot. These robotic platform factors help explain the decrease in esophageal perforation rates. It has also been suggested that the robotic platform may decrease early and late recurrences of achalasia by allowing a longer myotomy on both the esophageal and gastric sides.[19]

The decrease in iatrogenic perforations and potential for more durable results from a longer myotomy may help improve outcomes with a robotic approach. Larger prospective studies, preferably randomized controlled trails, are needed to better elucidate these findings.

Table 2
Rate of esophageal perforation during laparoscopic Heller myotomy

Author, Year	No. of Patients	Rate of Perforations (%)
Hunter et al,[22] 1997	40	15
Patti et al,[23] 1999	133	5
Bloomston et al,[24] 2004	111	7.2
Luketich et al,[25] 2001	62	9.7
Finley et al,[26] 2001	98	1.0
Zaninotto et al,[27] 2001	100	5
Sharp et al,[28] 2002	100	8.0
Chapman et al,[29] 2004	139	13.7
Douard et al,[30] 2004	52	5.8
Horgan et al,[10] 2005	62	16
Huffmanm et al,[14] 2007	37	8
Sanchez et al,[16] 2012	18	5.5
Perry et al,[17] 2014	19	15.8
Kim et al,[19] 2019	35	11.4

Data from Refs.[10,14,16,17,19,22–30]

Peroral endoscopic myotomy is showing promise in studies as a safe, efficacious, less invasive treatment of achalasia. Longer-term studies, as well as randomized studies between robotic and peroral approaches, are needed to assess outcomes and incidence of postoperative reflux.

ROBOTIC ANTIREFLUX SURGERY AND HIATAL HERNIA REPAIR

GERD, defined as reflux of gastric contents into the esophagus causing troublesome symptoms and/or complications,[31] has a prevalence of 10% to 20% and is the most common gastrointestinal diagnosis prompting an outpatient clinic visit.[32] The pathophysiology of GERD is secondary to the dysfunction of the antireflux barrier, made of the LES, the crural diaphragm, and the anatomic flap valve. The typical symptoms of GERD include heartburn, dysphagia, and regurgitation. The atypical symptoms of

Table 3
Rate of esophageal perforation during robotic Heller myotomy

Author, Year	No. Patients	Rate of Perforations (%)
Melvin et al,[11] 2005	104	0
Horgan et al,[10] 2005	59	0
Galvani et al,[12] 2006	54	0
Iqbal et al,[13] 2006	19	0
Huffmanm et al,[14] 2007	24	0
Sanchez et al,[16] 2012	13	0
Perry et al,[17] 2014	56	0
Pallabazzer et al,[18] 2019	66	0
Kim et al,[19] 2019	37	2.7

Data from Refs.[10–14,16–19]

GERD include cough, respiratory symptoms, chest pain, globus, throat clearing, and hoarseness.

Proton pump inhibitors (PPIs) have been the mainstay pharmacologic treatment of GERD. Breakthrough GERD symptoms on PPI therapy can be due to heterogeneous mechanisms, including increased transient LES relaxations, structural failure of the LES/defective antireflux barrier, reduced esophageal mucosal barrier function, impaired esophageal clearance, and inadequate acid suppression.[33] In addition to refractory GERD symptoms, recent concerns about adverse effects due to long-term PPI therapy, such as osteoporosis and nutritional deficiencies, and infectious complications, such as small bowel bacterial overgrowth and *Clostridium difficile* colitis,[34,35] have led to resurgence of interest in endoscopic and surgical antireflux procedures.

Diagnostic tests recommended by the Esophageal Diagnostic Advisory Panel for preoperative evaluation for antireflux surgery include upper endoscopy, barium esophagram, pH testing with or without impedance, esophageal manometry, and occasionally gastric emptying study.[36] Upper endoscopy is important to assess esophageal mucosal injury, such as esophagitis or Barrett esophagus, as well as to evaluate Hill grade GE flap valve and hiatal hernia. Barium esophagram provides anatomic and functional information, including presence and size of hiatal hernia, esophageal length, and esophageal stricture or diverticulum, as well as presence of GE reflux with provocative water siphon maneuver. Esophageal manometry is the most accurate and reliable method to assess function of the LES and esophageal peristalsis and, when coupled with impedance, measures effectiveness of bolus clearance with each swallow. Ambulatory pH testing is the gold standard diagnostic test for pathologic GERD. In addition to quantifying esophageal acid exposure, reflux in upright or supine position, and symptom association, when combined with multichannel intraluminal impedance, it can detect any type of reflux event (acid, weak acid, or nonacid).

Laparoscopic Nissen fundoplication, first performed by Dallemagne and colleagues[37] in 1991, is considered the gold standard surgical treatment of refractory GE reflux, with short-term and midterm results reported as excellent in 85% to 90% of patients, with less postoperative pain and shorter recovery than with conventional open fundoplication.[38,39] Several randomized control trials and meta-analyses have shown the same high level of reflux control with a posterior partial (Toupet) fundoplication as a total (Nissen) fundoplication, with similar or lower rates of postoperative dysphagia and a lower incidence of gas bloat syndrome[40–43]

With the widespread use of robotic surgery for several general surgery procedures, there has been increasing adoption of robotic-assisted antireflux surgery. The technical limitations of laparoscopic surgery include rigid nonarticulating instruments, poor ergonomics, and loss of depth perception. With the advantages of stable camera platform, 3-D imaging, increased maneuverability of the instruments, motion scaling, and tremor filtration, the rationale was that dissection and suturing in the narrow subdiaphragmatic and mediastinal spaces with a robot could be more expeditious and precise, potentially leading to improved patient outcomes.

Surgical Technique

The port placement for robotic fundoplication is similar to that for robotic Heller myotomy.

Dissection

Dissection is begun by opening the pars flaccida and identifying the right crus (**Fig. 4**) If a hiatal hernia is present, the avascular plane between the right crus and hernia sac is entered, while keeping traction on the stomach by grasping and pulling inferiorly.

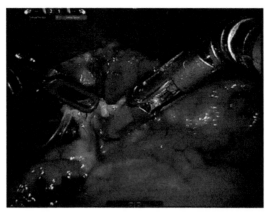

Fig. 4. Opening of the gastrohepatic ligament. (*From* Jensen JS, Antonsen HK, Durup J. Two years of experience with robotic-assisted anti—reflux surgery: A retrospective cohort study. Int J Surg 2017; 39:260-266; with permission.)

This dissection is completed around the arch of the crus to the left crus. With continued caudad traction on the hernia sac, dissection is carried out between the peritoneum and mediastinum in the extraperitoneal space. Care must be taken to not violate the pleura during this dissection. Once the entire hernia sac is dissected out of the mediastinum, it is removed to allow optimal visualization of the GE junction. A retroesophageal window is made, with placement of an umbilical tape or Penrose drain to provide traction on the lower esophagus. This allows intrathoracic dissection of the esophagus to as high as the inferior pulmonary vein. This extensive mediastinal mobilization of the esophagus is performed to obtain 2.5 cm to 3 cm of intra-abdominal esophagus without tension. The anterior and posterior vagus nerves are identified and preserved. In the case of a short esophagus, where the distance be-tween the angle of His to the crura is less than 3 cm without caudad traction on the esophagus, a wedge Collis gastroplasty is performed using a robotic stapler to lengthen the esophagus. A 46-50-French bougie is passed down the esophagus, hugging the lesser curvature of the stomach, during the wedge fundectomy (**Fig. 5**). The short gastric vessels then are divided to perform an adequately floppy wrap (**Fig. 6**).

Hiatal hernia repair

Hiatal closure is then performed with nonabsorbable sutures, making sure that an in-strument can be passed easily between the posterior esophagus and crural closure (**Fig. 7**). The newly created hiatus should allow sufficient expansion of the esophagus to prevent dysphagia when swallowing solid food. Depending on the hiatal defect and shape of the hiatus, sometimes anterior sutures can be added to avoid anterior angu-lation of the distal esophagus. It is helpful to decrease the pneumoperitoneum pres-sure to allow a tension-free closure of the hiatus. If this cannot be achieved or the crural pillars seem thin or attenuated, a synthetic biodegradable mesh reinforcement of the hiatus can be performed.

Fundoplication

The upper greater curvature of the fundus is passed behind the esophagus and a shoeshine maneuver performed to confirm sufficient gastric mobility for a tension-free wrap. A posterior 270° or 360° fundoplication is then performed on the distal

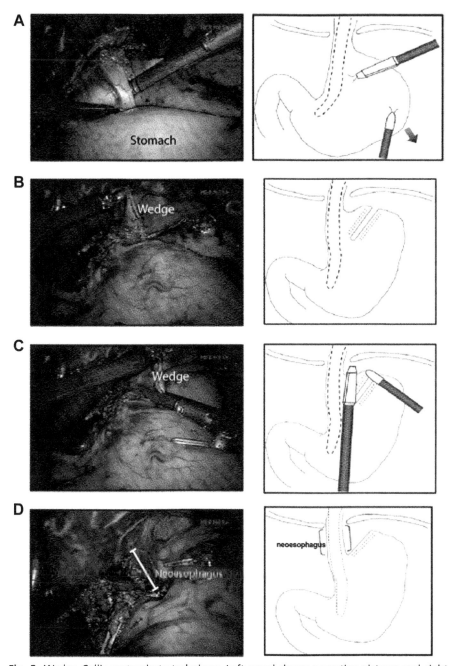

Fig. 5. Wedge Collis gastroplasty technique. Left panel shows operative pictures and right panel shows schematic diagrams. (*A*) The fundus is pulled inferolateral to expose the angle of His. A linear 45 mm robotic GIA stapler is positioned with the tip perpendicular to and on the bougie, then fired across the stomach. Arrow shows caudad and lateral traction on stomach during firing. (*B*) A small wedge of stomach, approximating a triangle, is created. (*C*) The wedge segment is held up and second linear Endo GIA stapler is placed parallel to the bougie and fired. (*D*) The completed wedge Collis gastroplasty with stapled gastric tube neoesophagus (*white line*). (*From* Hoang CD, Koh, PS, Maddaus MA. Short esophagus and esophageal stricture. Surg Clin N AM 2005; 85:433-451; with permission.)

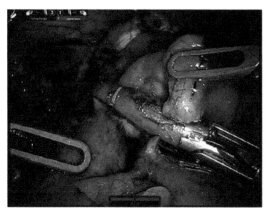

Fig. 6. Division of short gastric vessels. (*From* Jensen JS, Antonsen HK, Durup J. Two years of experience with robotic-assisted anti—reflux surgery: A retrospective cohort study. Int J Surg 2017; 39:260-266; with permission.)

esophagus with or without calibration using a 50-French to 60-French bougie. Usually 3 stitches are used for the fundoplication, keeping it short and floppy (**Fig. 8**). The fundoplication is then anchored to the left and right crura. A completion endoscopy is performed with a retroflexed view of the GE junction to assess adequacy of the wrap.

Comparison of Robotic vs. Laparoscopic-Assisted Fundoplication

Several studies, majority of them randomized controlled trials, have reported significantly longer total operative times for robotic-assisted fundoplication (RAF) compared with laparoscopic-assisted fundoplication (LAF) (**Table 4**), with the exception of 1 study,[44] with no significant difference in postoperative outcome, complication rate, hospital stay, and conversion or reoperation rates.

Multiple studies have also shown increased total costs of RAF compared with LAF,[44–48] but the results from systematic reviews and meta-analysis show no significant difference between the 2 groups.[52,53] There was noted to be significant heterogeneity of data on total cost, with no clear delineation, if the higher operating costs

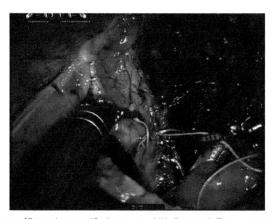

Fig. 7. Crural closure. (*From* Jensen JS, Antonsen HK, Durup J. Two years of experience with robotic-assisted anti—reflux surgery: A retrospective cohort study. Int J Surg 2017; 39:260-266; with permission.)

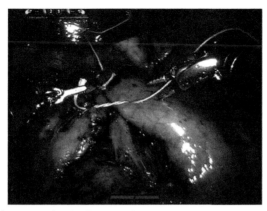

Fig. 8. Suturing the Nissen fundoplication. (*From* Jensen JS, Antonsen HK, Durup J. Two years of experience with robotic-assisted anti—reflux surgery: A retrospective cohort study. Int J Surg 2017; 39:260-266; with permission.)

were secondary to consumption of operating room resources, such as staff or expensive disposable instruments.

As familiarity with the robotic surgery platform increases and surgeons get past the learning curve, the operating time most likely will decrease. This has already been shown by Muller and colleagues,[44] who reported shorter total operating times compared with LAF (88 min vs 102 min), secondary to a single highly experienced surgeon performing all robotic procedures with a well-trained surgical team. Also, the effect of a learning curve has been demonstrated by Schraibman and colleagues,[54] where they used the robotic approach for complex/reoperative hiatal hernia repairs and reported a reduction in the mean operating time from 316 minutes to 195 minutes

Table 4
Operative times for robotic-assisted fundoplication versus laparoscopic-assisted fundoplication

Study, Year	No. Patients, Robotic-Assisted Fundoplication	No. Patients, Laparoscopic -Assisted Fundoplication	Operating Room Time (min), Robotic-Assisted Fundoplication	Operating Room Time (min), Laparoscopic-Assisted Fundoplication
Draaisma et al,[45] 2006	25	25	120	95
Cadiere et al,[46] 2001	10	11	76	52
Nakadi et al,[47] 2006	9	11	137	96 9
Morino et al,[48] 2006	25	25	131	91
Melvin et al,[49] 2002	20	20	141	97
Heemskerk et al,[50] 2007	11	11	176	135
Ceccarelli et al,[51] 2009	45	137	85	65

Data from Refs.[45–51]

after the first 5 procedures, with a setup time reduction from 20 minutes to 10 minutes. The total operation costs also are likely to decrease with more robotic platforms entering the market, leading to decreases in price of the system, maintenance costs, and semidisposable robotic instruments. Also, as surgeons/teams gain mastery in robotic-assisted surgery, the decreased operating time should translate into reduced operative costs.

When evaluating postoperative acid reflux parameters, similar postoperative pH results have been reported in both LAF and RAF groups.[45,48] Frazzoni and colleagues[55] have shown a modest improvement in median postoperative esophageal acid exposure in the robot-assisted group compared to the laparoscopic group. They have attributed this small therapeutic gain to a higher-powered analysis and to all surgical procedures performed by the same experienced surgeon in a standardized surgical technique. Also, no significant differences in quality of life and functional outcome have been reported up to 4 years out between the 2 groups.[56,57]

In summary, robotic-assisted antireflux surgery is safe and feasible. The proven additive value for the use of this expensive technology is controversial for primary antireflux surgery. Reoperative hiatal hernia/antireflux surgery, however, is technically more demanding, owing to extensive adhesiolysis and the need to dismantle the previous fundoplication. When approached laparoscopically, small studies have demonstrated higher conversion rates, higher rates of perforation and vagal nerve injury, higher postoperative complications, and inferior symptomatic relief.[58–60] With the improved ergonomics, visualization, and dexterity in small spaces, a growing literature has demonstrated its advantages in complex reoperative antireflux cases, with lower conversion rates, shorter hospital stay, lower readmission rates, higher preoperative symptom resolution, and functional outcomes.[61,62]

SUMMARY

Robotic-assisted esophageal surgery allows improved visualization, dexterity, and precision, which are especially beneficial in a narrow mediastinal or subdiaphragmatic space. There is controversy if these benefits, associated with a higher cost, translate into improved patient outcomes. In foregut surgery, the main advantage of robotics seem to be in procedures where better visualization and highly fine dissection is required, such as Heller myotomy, or in complex cases, such as reoperative hiatal hernia/antireflux surgery. Robotic surgery has its own well documented learning curve, however, and reserving it for complex cases may not allow surgeons to gain familiarity with and confidence in this technology. Further studies are needed to demonstrate learning curves, assess cost-effectiveness, and evaluate clinical benefit.

DISCLOSURE

The authors have nothing to disclose.

REFERENCES

1. Shah RD, D'amico TA. Modern impact of video-assisted thoracic surgery. J Thorac Dis 2014;6:S631–6.
2. Marescaux J, Leroy J, Gagner M, et al. Transatlantic robot-assisted telesurgery. Nature 2001;413:379–80.
3. Podas T, Eaden J, Mayberry M, et al. Achalasia: A critical review of epidemiologic studies. Am J Gastroenterol 1998;93:2345–7.

4. Brewer L. History of surgery of the esophagus. Am J Surg 1980;139:730–43.
5. Zaaijer J. Cardiospasm in the aged. Ann Surg 1923;77:615–7.
6. Shimi S, Nathanson L, Cuschieri A. Laparoscopic cardiomyotomy for achalasia. J R Coll Edinb 1991;36:152–4.
7. Pelligrini C, Wetter L, Patti M, et al. Initial experience with a new approach for the treatment of achalasia. Ann Surg 1992;216:291–6.
8. Richards WO, Torquati A, Holzman MD, et al. Heller myotomy versus Heller myotomy with Dor fundoplication for achalasia. Ann Surg 2004;240:405–12.
9. Melvin WS, Needleman BJ, Krause KR, et al. Computer-assisted robotic Heller myotomy: Initial case report. J Laparoendosc Adv Sur Tech A 2001;A11:251–3.
10. Horgan S, Galvani C, Gorodner MV, et al. Robotic-assisted Heller myotomy versus laparoscopic Heller myotomy for the treatment of esophageal achalasia: Multicenter study. J Gastrointest Surg 2005;9:1020–9.
11. Melvin WS, Dundon JM, Talamini M, et al. Computer-enhanced robotic telemetry surgery minimizes esophageal perforation during Heller myotomy. Surgery 2005; 138:553–8.
12. Galvani C, Gorodner MV, Moser F, et al. Laparoscopic Heller myotomy for achalasia facilitated by robotic assistance. Surg Endosc 2006;20:1105–12.
13. Iqbal A, Haider M, Desai K, et al. technique and follow-up of minimally invasive Heller myotomy for achalasia. Surg Endosc 2006;20:394–401.
14. Huffmanm LC, Pandalai PK, Boulton BJ, et al. Robotic Heller myotomy: A safe operation with higher postoperative quality-of-life indices. Surgery 2007;142: 613–20.
15. Shaligram A, Unnirevi J, Simorov A, et al. How does the robotic affect outcomes? A retrospective review of open, laparoscopic, and robotic Heller myotomy for achalasia. Surg Endosc 2012;26:1047–50.
16. Sanchez A, Rodriguez O, Nakhal E, et al. robotic-assisted Heller myotomy versus laparoscopic Heller myotomy for the treatment of esophageal achalasia: a case control study. J Robot Surg 2012;6:213–6.
17. Perry KA, Kanji A, Drosdeck JM, et al. Efficacy and durability of robotic Heller myotomy for achalasia: Patients symptoms and satisfaction at long-term follow-up. Surg Endosc 2014;28(1):3162–7.
18. Pallabazzer G, Peluso C, de Bertoli N, et al. Clinical and pathophysiological outcomes of the robotic-assisted Heller-Dor myotomy for achalasia: A single-center experience. J Robot Surg 2019. [Epub ahead of print].
19. Kim SS, Guillen-Rodriguez J, Little AG. Optimal surgical intervention for achalasia: Laparoscopic or robotic approach. J Robot Surg 2019;13930:397–400.
20. Khan M, Smylie A, Globe J, et al. randomized controlled trial of laparoscopic anterior versus posterior fundoplication for gastroesophageal reflux disease. ANZ J Surg 2010;80:500–5.
21. Milone M, Manigrasso M, Vertaldi S, et al. Robotic versus laparoscopic approach to treat symptomatic achalasia: Systematic review with meta-analysis. Dis esophagus 2019;0:1–8.
22. Hunter JG, Trus TL, Branum GD, et al. Laparoscopic Heller myotomy and fundoplication for achalasia. Ann Surg 1992;216:299.
23. Patti MG, Pelligrini CA, Horgan S, et al. Minimally invasive surgery for achalasia: an 8 year experience with 168 patients. Ann Surg 1999;230(4):587–93.
24. Bloomston M, Durkin A, Boyze HW, et al. Early results of Heller myotomy do not necessarily predict long-term outcome. Am J Surg 2004;187:403–7.
25. Luketich JD, Fernando HC, Christie NA, et al. outcomes after minimally invasive esophagomyotomy. Ann Thorac Surg 2001;72:1909–13.

26. Finley RJ, Clifton JC, Stewart KC, et al. Laparoscopic Heller myotomy improves esophageal emptying and the symptoms of achalasia. Arch Surg 2001;136: 892–6.

27. Zaninotto G, Costantini M, Molena D, et al. Minimally invasive surgery for esophageal achalasia. J Laparoendosc Adv Surg Tech A 2001;11(6):351–9.

28. Sharp K, Khaitan L, Scholz S, et al. 100 consecutive minimally invasive Heller myotomys: lessons learned. Ann Surg 2002;235:631–8.

29. Chapman JR, Joehl RJ, Murayama KM, et al. Achalasia treatment: improved outcome of laparoscopic myotomy with operative manometry. Arch Surg 2004; 139:508–13.

30. Douard R, gaudric M, Chaussade S, et al. Functional results after laparoscopic Heller myotomy for achalasia: A comparative study to open surgery. Surgery 2004;136:16–24.

31. Vakil N, van Zanten SV, Kahrilas P, et al. Montréal definition and classification of gastroesophageal reflux disease: A global evidence based consensus. Am J Gastroenterol 2006;101:1900–20.

32. Bredenoord AJ, Pandolfino JE, Smout AJPM. Gastro-oesophageal reflux disease. Lancet 2013;381:1933–42.

33. Gyawali CP, Roman S, Bredenoord AK, et al. Classification of esophageal motor findings in gastro-esophageal reflux disease: conclusions from an international consensus group. Neurogastroenterol Motil 2017;29.

34. Sheen E, Triadafilopoulos G. Adverse effects of long-term Proton Pump Inhibitor Therapy. Dig Dis Sci 2011;56:931–50.

35. Ali T, Roberts DN, Tierney W. Long-term safety concerns with proton pump inhibitors. Am J Med 2009;122:896–903.

36. Jobe BA, Richter JE, Hoppo T, et al. Preoperative diagnostic workup before antireflux surgery: and evidence an experience based consensus of esophageal diagnostic advisory panel. J Am Coll Surg 2013;217:586–97.

37. Dallemagne B, weerts JM, Jehaes C, et al. Laparoscopic Nissen fundoplication: preliminary report. Surg Laparosc Endosc 1991;1:138–43.

38. Ackroyd R, Watson DI, Majeed AW, et al. Randomized clinical trial of laparoscopic versus open fundoplication for gastro-esophageal reflux disease. Br J Surg 2004;91:975–82.

39. Chrysos E, Tsiaoussis J, Athanasakis E, et al. Laparoscopic versus open approach for Nissen fundoplication. A comparative study. Surg Endosc 2002; 16:1679–84.

40. Shaw JM, Bornman PC, Callanan MD, et al. Long-term outcome of laparoscopic Nissen and laparoscopic toupet fundoplication for gastroesophageal reflux disease: a prospective randomized trial. Surg Endosc 2010;24:924–32.

41. Hagedorn C, Lonroth H, Rydberg L, et al. Long-term efficacy of total (Nissen-Rossetti) and posterior partial (Toupet) fundoplication: Results of randomized clinical trial. J Gastrointest Surg 2002;6:540–5.

42. Hakanson BS, Lundell L, Bylund A, et al. Comparison of laparoscopic 270° posterior partial fundoplication versus total fundoplication for the treatment of gastroesophageal reflux disease: a randomized clinical trial. JAMA Surg 2019;154(6): 479–86.

43. Varin O, Velstra B, De Sutter S, et al. Total versus partial fundoplication in the treatment of gastroesophageal reflux disease: A meta-analysis. Arch Surg 2009;144:273–8.

44. Muller BP, Reiter MA, Wente MN, et al. Robot- assisted versus conventional laparoscopic fundoplication: Short-term outcome of a pilot randomized controlled trial. Surg Endosc 2007;21:1800–5.
45. Draaisma WA, Ruurda JP, Scheffer RC, et al. Randomised clinical trial of standard laparoscopic versus robotic-assisted laparoscopic Nissen fundoplication for gastro-esophageal reflux disease. Br J Surg 2006;93:1351–9.
46. Cadiere GB, Himpens J, Ertruyen M, et al. Evaluation of telesurgical (robotic) Nissen fundoplication. Surg Endosc 2001;15:918–23.
47. Nakadi IE, Melot C, Closset J, et al. Evaluation of da Vinci Nissen fundoplication: clinical results and cost minimization. World J Surg 2006;30:1050–4.
48. Morino M, Pellegrino L, Giaccone C, et al. Randomized clinical trial of robotic-assisted versus laparoscopic Nissen fundoplication. Br J Surg 2006;93:553–8.
49. Melvin WS, Needleman BJ, Krause KR, et al. Computer-enhanced versus standard laparoscopic antireflux surgery. J Gastrointest Surg 2002;6:11–6.
50. Hemmskerk J, van Gemert WG, Greve JWM, et al. Robotic-assisted versus conventional laparoscopic Nissen fundoplication: A comparative retrospective study on costs and time consumption. Surg Laparosc Endosc Percutan Tech 2007; 17:1–4.
51. Ceccarelli G, Patriti A, Biancafarina A, et al. Intraoperative and postoperative outcome of robotic-assisted and traditional laparoscopic Nissen fundoplication. Eur Surg Res 2009;43:198–203.
52. Zhang P, Tian J, Yang KH, et al. Robot-assisted laparoscope fundoplication for gastroesophageal reflux disease: a systematic review of randomized controlled trials. Digestion 2010;81:1–9.
53. Fan Y. Robotic Nissen fundoplication for gastroesophageal reflux disease: a meta-analysis of prospective randomized controlled trials. Surg Today 2014;44: 1415–23.
54. Schraibman V, Macedo ALV, Okazaki S, et al. Surgical treatment of hiatus hernia and gastroesophageal reflux disease and complex cases using robotic-assisted laparoscopic surgery: a prospective study/consistent experience in a single institution. J Robot Surg 2011;5:29–33.
55. Frazzoni M, Conigliaro R, Colli G, et al. Conventional versus robotic-assisted laparoscopic Nissen fundoplication: a comparison of postoperative acid reflux parameters. Surg Endosc 2012;26:1674–81.
56. Muller-Stich BP, Reiter MA, Mehrabi, et al. No relevant difference in quality of life and functional outcome at 12 months follow-up- a randomized control trial comparing robotic-assisted versus conventional laparoscopic Nissen fundoplication. Langenbecks Arch Surg 2009;394:441–6.
57. Hartmann J, Menenakos C, Ordemann J, et al. Long-term results of quality of life after standard laparoscopic versus robot-assisted laparoscopic fundoplications for gastro-esophageal reflux disease: a comparative clinical trial. Int J Med Robot 2009;5(1):32–7.
58. Van beck DB, Auyang ED, Soper NJ. Comprehensive review of laparoscopic redo fundoplication. Surg Endosc 2011;25:706–12.
59. Furnee EJB, Draaisma WA, Broeders IAMJ, et al. Surgical re-intervention after antireflux surgery for gastroesophageal reflux disease: a prospective cohort study in 130 patients. Arch Surg 2008;143:267–74.
60. Singhal S, Kirkpatric DR, Masuda T, et al. Primary and redo antireflux surgery: outcomes and lessons learned. J Gastrointest Surg 2018;22(2):177–86.

61. Elmously A, Gray KD, Ullmann TM, et al. Robotic reoperative antireflux surgery: Low perioperative morbidity and high symptom resolution. World J Surg 2018; 42:4014–21.
62. Tolboom RC, Draaisma WA, Broeders IAM. Evaluation of conventional laparo-scopic versus robot-assisted laparoscopic redo hiatal hernia and antireflux sur-gery: a cohort study. J Robotic Surg 2016;10:33–9.

Robotic Liver Resection

Kelly J. Lafaro, MD, MPH[a], Camille Stewart, MD[b], Abigail Fong, MD[b,c], Yuman Fong, MD[b,*]

KEYWORDS

- History of robotic liver surgery • Robotic liver surgery • Minimally invasive surgery
- Robotic hepatectomy • Robotic liver resection

KEY POINTS

- The robot-assisted surgical system has many advantages compared with laparoscopy, including better ergonomics for the surgeon; EndoWrist® articulated instruments; tremor filter; and a clear, three-dimensional, high-definition, magnified field of vision.
- Proposed limitations of robot-assisted liver surgery include concern for missed lesions caused by decreased haptic feedback, longer operative times, as well as increased technical difficulty of the procedure.
- Patients who benefit most from robot-assisted liver surgery include those with lesions in posterosuperior segments and for whom open surgery would require a large incision.

INTRODUCTION

History of Robotic Liver Surgery

Minimally invasive hepatobiliary surgery began in 1987 with the first laparoscopic cholecystectomy.[1,2] The first laparoscopic liver resection was reported by Reich and colleagues[3] in 1991 for excision of benign lesions. Over the next 2 decades, the use of laparoscopy in liver resection was reported on by multiple groups.[3–5] However, it was not until 2008, when the first consensus guidelines for laparoscopic liver surgery were published, that these new minimally invasive techniques were standardized.[6] Despite advances in instrumentation, including laparoscopic staplers and energy devices, laparoscopic liver resections were still limited by the rigid instruments with fixed maneuverability and two-dimensional vision resulting in high learning curves and significant open conversion rates.[7] These limitations are especially apparent in laparoscopic major hepatectomies, and for resections of lesions located in the posterior segments of the liver, which are difficult to reach.

Thus, the introduction of robotic technology was promising for these cases. While the laparoscopic techniques were maturing, the first robotic-assisted

[a] Department of Surgery, Johns Hopkins University School of Medicine, Blalock Building, 600 N. Wolfe St, Baltimore, MD 21205, USA; [b] Department of Surgery, City of Hope National Medical Center, 1500 East Duarte Road, Duarte, CA 91010, USA; [c] Department of Surgery, Cedars Sinai Medical Center, 8700 Beverly Blvd, Los Angeles, CA 90048, USA
* Corresponding author.
E-mail address: yfong@coh.org

Surg Clin N Am 100 (2020) 265–281
https://doi.org/10.1016/j.suc.2019.11.003
0039-6109/20/© 2019 Elsevier Inc. All rights reserved.

surgical.theclinics.com

cholecystectomies were performed by Himpens and colleagues[8] and Gagner and colleagues[9] in the early 1990s. This work was followed by the release of the da Vinci robotic surgical system in Europe in 1999 and its approval by the US Food and Drug Administration (FDA) in the United States in 2000.

The robot-assisted surgical system has many advantages compared with laparoscopy, including better ergonomics for the surgeon, EndoWrist® articulated instruments, tremor filter, and a clear three-dimensional (3D), high-definition, magnified field of vision. However, the system is criticized for the lack of tactile feedback as well as its high cost.

The first series of robotic-assisted laparoscopic liver resections was reported by Giulianotti and colleagues[10] in 2003. Since then, there have been multiple reports from several countries describing their own robotic liver experience[11–16]; however, these have all been single-center experiences. The field has continued to evolve and, in 2018, the first international consensus statement on robotic hepatectomy surgery was published.[17] Despite this, minimally invasive liver resections still make up a small fraction of all liver surgery.[18]

Indications for Robotic-Assisted Liver Surgery

Indications for robotic approach are the same as for laparoscopy and include:

- Primary tumors (hepatocellular carcinoma [HCC] and intrahepatic cholangiocarcinoma)
- Metastatic lesions from colorectal and breast cancers
- Benign tumors (enlarging hemangiomas, adenomas, focal nodular hyperplasia)
- Symptomatic lesions (cysts and abscesses)

However, the patients who most benefit from a robotic approach are those with posterosuperior segment lesions (a1, 4A, 7, 8), which would require a large incision when performed open, as well as tumors that are difficult to reach by conventional laparoscopic methods.[19,20]

In a recent retrospective study, Melstrom and colleagues[19] offered insight into the benefits of robotic surgery for so-called incision-dominant operations. This study evaluated 97 patients who underwent robotic liver resections, including 13 major resections and 84 minor resections, and including 51 inferior segmentectomies (segments 3, 4B, 5, and 6) as well as 33 posterosuperior segmentectomies (segments 1, 2, 4A, 7, and 8). Two-thirds of the patients were discharged within 3 days of the robotic procedure, including 3 patients subjected to hemihepatectomies, and 14 of the patients were discharged home the same day. Predictors of a hospital stay longer than 3 days included extent of resection ($P = .003$), occurrence of complications ($P = .009$), and operative time greater than 210 minutes ($P = .001$).[19] These data suggest that robotic approach allows outpatient liver surgery.

Nota and colleagues[20] performed a multinational, retrospective, propensity score–matched study that evaluated 51 robotic and 145 open posterosuperior liver resections performed between 2009 and 2016 by high-volume liver surgeons. The final 1:1 propensity-matched analysis of 31 robotic and 31 open resections of posterosuperior segments showed no differences in median operative time (222 minutes; interquartile ranges [IQRs], 164–505 vs 231 minutes and 190–301 minutes respectively; $P = .668$), estimated blood loss (200 mL; IQRs, 100–400 vs 300 mL and 125–750 mL respectively; $P = .212$), major complications rates (3% vs 10% respectively; $P = .612$), or readmission rates (10% vs 6% respectively; $P>.99$).[21]

Although these studies showed feasibility and safety of robotic-assisted liver surgery, the long-term oncologic outcomes have until recently been debated. Khan and colleagues[22] performed an international, multicenter, retrospective study of patients who underwent robotic-assisted surgery for HCC, cholangiocarcinoma, or gallbladder cancer between 2006 and 2016. This study included 61 major and minor resections (56% for HCC, 26% for cholangiocarcinoma, and 18% for gallbladder cancer) with a median follow-up time of 75 months.[22] R0 resection was achieved in 94%, 68%, and 81.8% respectively. Five-year overall survival (OS) was 56% and 3-year OS stratified by tumor type was 90% for HCC, 49% for cholangiocarcinoma, and 65% for gallbladder cancer, which was comparable with published long-term outcomes for both open and laparoscopic liver resection.[22]

ROBOTIC-ASSISTED VERSUS LAPAROSCOPIC LIVER SURGERY

To date, there are no randomized controlled trials to compare robotic with laparoscopic liver resection. However, there are several high-quality nonrandomized studies as well as meta-analyses comparing them. A recent meta-analysis performed by Guan and colleagues[23] examined 13 nonrandomized control studies, which included patients diagnosed with focal benign or malignant lesions, including HCC, cholangiocarcinoma, focal nodular hyperplasia, hemangioma, hepatic adenoma, and metastatic lesions, which reported at least 1 perioperative outcome of interest (operation time, intraoperative blood loss, blood transfusion rate, complications, conversion rate, R1 resection rate, and the hospital stays).[23] The meta-analysis included 938 patients (435 robotic hepatectomies vs 503 laparoscopic hepatectomies). The robotic hepatectomy group had decreased intraoperative blood loss by an average of 69.9 mL (95% confidence interval [CI], 27.1–112.7; $P<.001$); however, it also resulted in longer operative times of an average of 65.5 minutes (95% CI, 42.0–89.0 minutes; $P<.00001$) and a higher cost by a mean difference of $4,240 (95% CI, 3.08-5.39, $P<.00001$). There were no significant differences between the 2 groups in the other perioperative outcomes, including transfusion rate, complication rate, conversion rate, the R1 resection rate, or length of hospital stay.

A recent large, single-center, retrospective analysis of 173 major minimally invasive hepatectomies (57 robotic-assisted vs 116 laparoscopic) ultimately showed improved outcomes with less frequent postoperative intensive care unit admissions (43.9% vs 61.2% respectively; $P = .043$) as well as decreased 90-day readmission rates (7.0% vs 28.5% respectively; $P = .001$).[24] Fruscione and colleagues[24] found no significant difference in blood loss, operative times, or length of stay between the robotic-assisted and laparoscopic groups, suggesting a role for robotic-assisted techniques in major hepatic resections. Because robotic surgery is just an extension of the laparoscopic approach, expert laparoscopic surgery has similar outcomes to expert robotic surgery. As discussed later, the major advantages will be in ease of adoption and ergonomics. The robotic approach allows more surgeons to be minimally invasive surgeons, and allows more patients to benefit from minimally invasive surgery.

ADVANTAGES OF ROBOTICS IN LIVER SURGERY

There are several current advantages to robotic liver surgery, and also potential advantages in the future as technology develops (**Table 1**). These advantages are beyond the many arguments in favor of robotics in general that are related to surgeon comfort, including ergonomics with diminished surgeon fatigue,[25,26] issues related to hand dominance,[27] and superior visualization with a 3D view.[28] With the presence of wristed articulating instruments, robotic surgery may facilitate many incision-dominant liver surgeries to be performed in a minimally invasive fashion.[19] Specifically, incision-dominant liver surgeries are those in which a large incision is required to

Table 1
Advantages and limitations of robotic surgery

Advantages	Limitations
• Surgeon ergonomics	• Inability to palpate the liver
• Enables minimally invasive surgery for typically incision-dominant superior and posterior liver segment resections	• Increased incision size for larger specimen removal may negate benefits of smaller initial incisions
• Faster learning curve	• Additional operative time to dock and undock
• Facilitates use of indocyanine green imaging	• Potential for argon gas vascular embolization
• Potential for intraoperative liver navigation	• Increased cost

remove a small volume of liver parenchyma. Thus, it is the size of the incision that drives the extent and duration of recovery. Traditional laparoscopic instruments are limited in that they are rigid, and do not have wristed movement. This limitation has less impact on surgical interventions in the midabdomen, where there is more space and fewer boney constraints, but may be a significant hindrance for liver lesions that are more superior and posterior. In 2008, an expert panel came to the consensus that traditional laparoscopy was best suited for resection of tumors that were located in liver segments 2, 3, 4b, 5, and 6, and that were less than 5 cm and in the periphery of the liver.[6] The limited motion for traditional laparoscopic instruments was thought to make liver resections for the superior and posterior aspects of the liver, segments 1, 4a, 7, 8, significantly more difficult and thus not appropriate for minimally invasive surgery.[6] Lee and colleagues[29] and Teo and colleagues[30] both corroborated that superior and posterior resections were more challenging with traditional laparoscopy, reporting that operations took on average 1 to 2 hours longer, had greater estimated blood loss, and had higher rates of conversion to an open operation compared with the anterior and lateral laparoscopic liver resections.[29,30] Because of the additional instrument mobility that is possible, the robotic platform facilitates surgical resection of tumors in these superior and posterior segments that might otherwise not have been attempted with a traditional laparoscopic approach.[19,21] These properties extend the benefits of a minimally invasive approach to more patients, including lower estimated blood loss, less narcotic use, shorter length of hospitalization, and improved short-term quality of life.[11,14,31–33] Melstrom and colleagues[19] reported that two-thirds of patients that underwent robotic liver resections had hospitalizations of 3 days or less, with 33% having tumors in superior liver segments. Montalti and colleagues[34] questioned whether traditional laparoscopy could be used for superior and inferior liver tumors, by comparing laparoscopic with robotic liver resections for segments 1, 4a, 7, and 8 in a case-matched series. They reported no significant differences other than length of Pringle maneuver, which was longer in the robotic cohort.

A faster learning curve has also been suggested as an advantage for robotics in minimally invasive surgery.[35] With regard to liver surgery, evaluating the learning curve is challenging, because it is based on not only the surgical skill of the operator but also the complexity of the surgery, which has significant variation. Nevertheless, this has been reported subjectively,[34] and compared retrospectively in the literature.[36,37] Efanov and colleagues[36] compared laparoscopic and robotic liver resections from 2010 to 2016 and found that, as experience accrued with the robotic platform, the difficulty of the procedures increased. By comparison, the difficulty of laparoscopic liver resections was static over time.[37] Chong and colleagues[37] similarly evaluated procedures performed in 2003 to 2017 and also concluded that the robotic platform enabled more technically complex procedures. Validating this idea, Kluger and colleagues[38] reported that although the number of laparoscopic liver resections increased with experience from 1996 to 2008, the instances of resection with multiple tumors and resections with larger tumors were stable over the study period both in their institutional data and also in a multinational cohort.[38] These data imply that more challenging operations can be attempted with robotic surgery compared with laparoscopy, because learning is faster with the robotic platform. However, the results of the robotic studies were not adjusted for operative year and therefore may only be a reflection of increased comfort with minimally invasive liver surgery over time. Thus, it remains unclear how the learning curve affects the application of the robotic platform to liver surgery.

Another advantage offered by the robotic platform is enabling the use of near-infrared fluorescence (NIRF) imaging with indocyanine green (ICG). This method is a standard tool for the robotic surgical platform and can aid in the identification of vasculature, biliary anatomy, and liver tumors. ICG is an intravenously delivered agent that can be visualized when stimulated by polarized light. Console surgeons can easily switch between white light and near-infrared vision by using synchronized foot and hand movements (on the da Vinci Xi, pressing the camera pedal while pulling the hand clutch). After injection of 2.5 mg of ICG, the agent rapidly binds to albumin, and in this way highlights vasculature with a half-life of 2 to 5 minutes.[39] ICG is then selectively taken up by hepatocytes and then excreted unchanged into bile.[40] ICG injected into the portal vein to identify the vascular line of demarcation in robotic hepatectomies has been described.[41] ICG can also be used to visualize biliary structures 45 minutes after injection.[42] Further reports have shown that ICG is also taken up and retained preferentially by primary hepatic tumors compared with parenchyma.[43] For liver metastases, ICG fluorescence is also preferentially trapped within cytokeratin 7 (CK7)-positive hepatocytes compressed by the tumor, forming a rim around the tumor.[44] Thus, primary liver tumors appear bright, and metastases have a bright rim.[45] Studies comparing ICG imaging with preoperative CT, MRI, intraoperative palpation, and intraoperative ultrasonography show that ICG identifies more and smaller metastases than other modalities.[46,47] Although NIRF imaging is possible with other operative approaches, its presence as a switch on the robotic console simplifies its use (**Fig. 1**).

Many clinicians think that the greatest benefits of robotics in liver surgery are yet to come. The complexity of the intraparenchymal anatomy and absence of clear surface

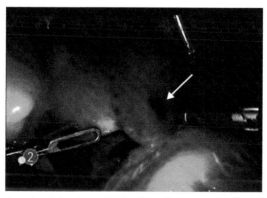

Fig. 1. Liver 2 minutes after injection of ICG, when the agent is still within the vasculature. The photopenic area (*white arrow*) is a hepatic cyst, and thus has no blood flow.

landmarks of the liver have prompted the extensive development of intraoperative navigation systems.[48,49] The ultimate goals of intraoperative navigational tools in hepatobiliary surgery are to provide feedback to surgeons regarding the position of the transection line versus the lesion of interest and major vasculature. This goal is intended to decrease the likelihood of a positive resection margin, decrease the risk of vascular injury, and increase the volume of preserved normal hepatic parenchyma. To achieve these goals, preoperatively obtained images must be processed and then intraoperatively registered with the patient and liver. Instruments must also be tracked during surgery to ensure their location relative to pertinent anatomy. Various optical and electromagnetic methods have been developed for instrument tracking during intraoperative navigation, which have variable accuracy and require significant additional equipment.[50–52] The use of the robotic platform eliminates this issue because the exact location of the robotic instruments is known at all times. Additional challenges exist with liver registration caused by the changes in liver shape that occur with laparoscopic conditions. Up to a 1.6 cm difference has been reported with 14-mm Hg insufflation pressure.[53] Efforts to develop computer algorithms that anticipate this change in shape are ongoing.[54] As the ability to register preoperative images with the intraoperative view improve, augmented reality with the robotic platform has the potential to take 3D hepatobiliary image reconstruction and intraoperative navigation to the next level. Soler and colleagues[55] described a method whereby 3D liver models were created using VR-Render software developed at IRCAD (Research Institute against Digestive Cancer; now called Virtual Patient, IRCAD, Strasbourg, France). Intrahepatic anatomic information was then overlaid when viewing the liver laparoscopically using a da Vinci robotic platform before surgery. This same group was then able to take this technology further, first by projecting the virtual liver model on the patient's abdominal skin to assist with port placement, and then with a computer scientist on hand, manually registering laparoscopic images with the preoperatively obtained 3D reconstructed image. The 3D reconstructed images were again superimposed on the laparoscopic view to facilitate identification of tumors and surrounding pertinent anatomy, and then manually adjusted as the liver was transected and deformed.[56] However, much of this technology is nascent and requires more prospective clinical evaluation before becoming the standard of care.

LIMITATIONS OF ROBOTICS IN LIVER SURGERY

There are several limitations to robotic liver surgery, and, as such, the robotic platform is not appropriate for all liver operations at this time. Some limitations pertain to minimally invasive surgery in general, including concern for missed lesions caused by the inability to feel the liver, and a theoretically increased risk of a positive margin caused by decreased haptic feedback, as well as the increased technical difficulty of the procedure.[6] However, data to support a difference in outcome based on the lack of hepatic feedback are limited and are skewed by a strong selection bias, as detailed earlier. Need for an additional attending surgeon has also been cited as a potential disadvantage for robotic liver surgery.[34] This important piece of information is often omitted from the existing literature, possibly because it is difficult to glean in a retrospective fashion. This limitation can be questioned depending on the availability of skilled registered nurse first assistants, surgical residents, and fellows; however, some investigators also describe using 2 assistants during robotic liver procedures.[57]

Note that some of the advantages related to expediency of recovery and postoperative pain related to a minimally invasive procedure may be lost if a large incision is required to remove the specimen. This point is particularly applicable to right hepatectomies and extended right hepatectomies. However, details regarding specimen size and incision size are also often omitted in literature discussing minimally invasive procedures. One report examining attitudes regarding incision size showed that 71% of patients thought their incisions were smaller with the robotic approach, as did 50% of hospital administrators, but this belief was held by only 5% of health care providers.[58] It was noted here that the smallest robotic ports, which are 8 mm, are larger than the smallest traditional laparoscopic ports, which are 5 mm. However, there are no current data regarding additional excisions for specimen extraction, likely because most data are retrospectively collected. This fact aside, there are series describing successful totally robotic right hepatectomies with low conversion rates, reasonable intraoperative blood loss, and limited postoperative morbidity.[57,59] A case-matched comparison that included 28 right hemihepatectomies for HCC did find that the robotic cohort continued to have decreased narcotic requirements, and a shorter length of hospitalization.[32] It has been noted that published reports of robotic formal hemihepatectomies are hampered by selection bias, and also may favor successes[6]; experts are aware of unpublished serious adverse events that have occurred because of these procedures, including mortalities. Therefore, significant caution should be exercised even in expert hands when embarking on robotic major hepatectomies.

Given the technical complexity of minimally invasive liver surgery, conversion to open is best viewed as prudent care, rather than a complication.[6] With traditional laparoscopy, a hand port can be useful for the control of bleeding without fully converting to an open operation. However, this option does not exist when using the robotic platform. As such, an additional limitation specific to robotic surgery is the extra time required to dock and to undock, which may be considered especially deleterious if an expedient conversion to an open procedure is required. Although it is known that some additional time is required for docking and undocking, the precise amount of time for this necessary step is often not quantified discreetly in comparisons of laparoscopic and robotic procedures. This observation is true even for well-executed randomized controlled trials comparing robotic with laparoscopic surgery. In the Robotic vs laparoscopic resection for rectal cancer (ROLARR) randomized trial for rectal cancer, the robotic operations were on average 38 minutes longer with the da Vinci Si robotic system, but there was no report of dock and undock time.[60] Other studies have reported initial dock times of 9 ± 3 minutes,[61] and combined dock and undock times of 25 minutes.[62] However, an inherent difficulty in assessing dock and undock time is that studies often do not report the particular da Vinci model used. Since da Vinci's initial model release, several iterations have been produced.[63] Although experience is expected to decrease time for docking and undocking, clinicians with experience spanning multiple models (S, Si, Si-e, Xi) understand that the ease of docking and undocking is different for each of the da Vinci robotic models released. As newer models improve ease of docking and undocking, this limitation will lessen.

Because of their unique coagulative properties, argon beam coagulators are often used in liver surgery. However, there is the potential for argon gas vascular embolization caused by the insolubility of argon gas in blood, which can then form gas bubbles in the blood stream.[64] It is thought that a theoretically increased risk of this adverse event exists with pneumoperitoneum, because of increased intra-abdominal gas accumulation.[6,65] Case reports have described patient deaths caused by use of argon beam coagulation on the liver[65,66]; however, most reports for this rare complication are in the setting of open surgery.[64] Nonetheless, recommendations have been for made for argon beam coagulator use with pneumoperitoneum. It is recommended that it be used for minor hemostasis only, always with a port open for venting, holding the tip at an oblique angle, limiting flow of argon to the lowest effective level, and moving the handpiece away after each activation.[6,65,67]

Beyond what was described earlier, the primary tangible limitation cited for robotic liver surgery is increased cost. Robotic surgery has been associated with an increased cost of 13% compared with laparoscopy,[68] in part caused by higher purchase and maintenance costs,[69] as well as more costly consumable surgical supplies.[70] However, decreased length of stay and fewer complications for robotic liver resections have resulted in overall cost being similar to or lower than open operations.[71,72] As such, recent meta-analysis concluded that robotic hepatectomies may have better perioperative outcomes and are not cost-prohibitive compared with open surgery; however, all included studies were retrospective.[73] The limitations of the existing data were highlighted in the International Consensus Statement on Robotic Hepatectomy Surgery in 2018,[17] in which the quality of the evidence evaluated was all considered low to very low. Thus, there is a strong need for more prospective data regarding robotic liver resections to fully understand the limitations of this approach.

TECHNICAL CONSIDERATIONS
Room, Operating Room Table, Patient, and Port Positioning

Before induction of anesthesia or positioning the patient, the operating room (OR) table should be positioned in an optimal location for robotic liver surgery. The robot will ultimately come toward the patient's left shoulder or left midabdomen with the da Vinci Xi, and toward the patient's head with the da Vinci Si, so the OR table should be moved toward the center of the room and positioned such that the anesthesia equipment is opposite to where the robot will approach (**Fig. 2**). Overhead lights should be positioned such that they will not interfere as the robot is navigated toward the patient for docking later.

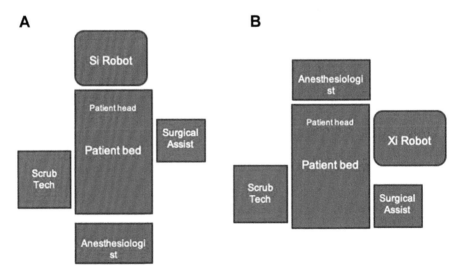

Fig. 2. Room setup for the Si and Xi da Vinci robots. (*A*) The robot is positioned at the patient's head when using the Si. The anesthesiologist must have a long connector for the ventilator. (*B*) The robot is positioned at the patient's left side when using the Xi, and anesthesiologist is at the head of the bed. Tech, technician.

After induction of anesthesia, patient positioning depends on the location of the lesion to be resected. For right posterior segments (6 and 7), the patient should be positioned left lateral decubitus with the right arm resting on an airplane, and the hand at the level of the patient's forehead. This position facilitates traction on the right triangular ligament, and improves visualization of the inferior vena cava if needed. For tumors in segments 1 to 5 and 8, the authors prefer the patient to be positioned supine with arms tucked, and a footboard; however, some clinicians place the patient supine with legs apart (so-called French position) to create a space for the bedside assistant. The OR table should then be positioned in reverse Trendelenburg to facilitate traction on the suspensory ligament. Additional padding should be placed over the patient's thighs, because the robotic arms can be almost parallel to the legs and can push into them. The patient should be widely prepped from the nipple line to the pubic bone in case there needs to be an emergent conversion to open surgery. During the preprocedural timeout, a plan for emergent conversion should always be discussed. This plan includes removing all of the instruments before undocking the robot to prevent system errors, and having laparoscopic instruments open and available to put pressure on the areas of bleeding as the robot is being undocked.

Once the patient is positioned, prepped, and draped, the abdomen is insufflated, and ports are placed (**Fig. 3**). For the Si, ports are placed in a curvilinear fashion around the target anatomy with spacing at least 8 cm apart, whereas, for the Xi, ports are placed in a straight line across the abdomen with spacing at least 5 cm apart. For procedures with a small volume of liver parenchyma being resected, the authors sometimes opt to only use 3 robotic arms, pushing the first arm up and away. Of note, with the da Vinci Xi, the camera and instruments can easily be switched from port to port. Ports should be 18 to 20 cm from the target anatomy. Unlike many other robotic procedures, the accessory port can be placed between the robotic camera and the target anatomy but should be at least 5 cm from other ports. It can be used for suction or retraction. Given the amount of surgical smoke created while dividing the liver, some surgeons prefer to use a smoke evacuation system as well. For the Xi robot, docking is performed such that the target anatomy, camera port, and robotic tower

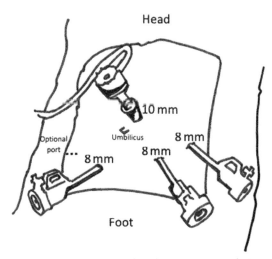

Fig. 3. Port placement. For the Si, ports are placed in a curvilinear fashion around the target anatomy with spacing at least 8 cm apart, whereas, for the Xi, ports are placed in a straight line across the abdomen with spacing at least 5 cm apart.

form a straight line (see **Fig. 2**). For the Si robot, docking is performed such that the target anatomy is between the camera port and the robotic tower (see **Fig. 2**). The upper abdomen anatomic location should be selected on the Xi tower, which causes the robotic arms to swing toward the patient's head, facing toward the feet.

After docking, the instruments are inserted. If drop-in ultrasonography is going to be used at the start of the operation, the authors start by inserting ProGrasp forceps, because these have a high grip strength and are less likely to drop the handle of the drop-in ultrasonography. The TilePro display can be used so that the console surgeon visualizes both the laparoscopic field and the ultrasonography image while at the console (**Fig. 4**). Once the lesion of interest has been characterized on ultrasonography, hot shears are used to demarcate the intended lines of transection. Ultrasonography is then used to again visualize the lesion of interest in correlation with the cautery marks on the liver, which can also be seen on the ultrasonography images. At this point, the initial instruments are removed and replaced with a Cadiere, which has low grip strength and is better suited for gently manipulating or grasping the liver, and also the vessel sealer, which can be used to divide the liver parenchyma and seals vessels up to 7 mm in diameter. Surgeons may wish to place a vessel loop around the liver hilum, which is clipped to secure it in place and then retracted as needed to limit hilar flow. The authors prefer to divide the liver with a crush clamp technique using the unactivated vessel sealer, which is then reapplied and activated to divide the vessels.

SAFETY IN ROBOTIC LIVER SURGERY

As robotically assisted operations become more common, safety concerns and concerns over how to best protect patients have arisen along with them. The realities of a

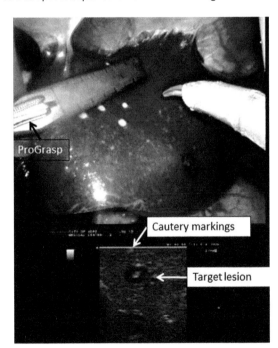

Fig. 4. Use of drop-in ultrasonography manipulated by forceps, and visualized at the robotic console with the Tile Pro feature. The cautery marks can be seen at the surface over the liver lesion.

large robot occupying the space over the patient, lack of a large incision, and an unscrubbed surgeon not at the bedside create new safety challenges because the limited access to the patient can delay the start of effective treatment of a life-threatening emergency, with possibly harmful outcome.[74] An approach to preparing for emergent situations in robotic surgery is discussed here.

Emergent, Urgent, and Elective Conversion to Open Operation

Converting from robotic to open operation can be done on an emergent, urgent, or elective basis. Emergent conversions are necessary if the patient experiences life-threatening distress such as cardiac arrest, carbon dioxide pulmonary embolus, or tension pneumothorax. Urgent conversions can result from situations such as hemorrhage unable to be controlled robotically, or other issues that need to be addressed quickly. Elective conversions result from situations such as difficult dissection caused by scar tissue, need for tools or access not available on the robot, and questions regarding anatomy of suboptimal visualization or tissue margins.

Preoperative Planning

Planning rescue strategies is an essential part of any major operation and is especially important in robotic surgery. In general, it takes longer to convert to open surgery from robotic than from laparoscopic surgery because extra time is needed for the robot to be undocked, the room to be reconfigured for open surgery, and the surgeon to scrub in.

It is essential that all team members participate in planning and preparing rescue strategies in order to maximize team readiness to act when needed to optimize patient outcomes. Open, clear communication among all operative team members allows the greatest likelihood of safe, effective, efficient delivery of patient care; helps set expectations for the operation; and helps the team prepare for any situation they may face in the OR.

Operative planning and team preparation begin long before the procedure. Preoperative orders should communicate patient positioning, equipment, and anticipated blood products needed. Optimizing room setup on the day of surgery is important because the robot, the robotic tower, and the console are bulky and can limit access to the patient, so positioning equipment, cords, and personnel to maximize the ability to move around the room and access the patient is necessary. OR work flow should be organized to establish good intravenous access and monitoring of the patient before docking the robot and limiting access to the patient. Spending time planning organization before the procedure can help prevent struggles with equipment and delays in navigating around the robot.

Team Emergency Planning Briefing

Team briefings have become standard practice in ORs to improve safety.[75]

Team briefings in robotic surgery should also include emergency planning timeouts that include:

- The level of concern for hemorrhage (especially in liver surgery patients, who often have higher bleeding risk)
- Patient cardiopulmonary risk level
- Likelihood of conversion
- Planning for conversion (team member expectations and roles)

Plans should be made for the most likely situations that would result in conversion, as well as the most catastrophic, in order to be ready to respond quickly to an emergency. A basic conversion plan before starting the procedure can minimize delay in patient care if conversion is needed (**Box 1**).

Other urgent scenarios that should be planned for preoperatively include hemorrhage and cardiac arrest. Preoperative plans for responding to hemorrhage or cardiac arrest should be made to include, in addition to the basic conversion plan:

- Who will provide manual tamponade, if possible
- Who will begin chest compressions/resuscitation
- In procedures with high likelihood of hemorrhage, consideration should be made for placement of GelPort preoperatively to allow for manual tamponade if needed

Simulation

Simulation of and training for response to emergency situations can help prepare OR teams to respond quickly and minimize patient harm. Simulation is now a standard part of critical care, trauma, and emergency room response to treatment of critically unstable patients.[76–78] Similarly, simulation in emergency robotic situations has been studied and shown to improve time to beginning chest compressions in cardiac arrest to seconds (5–10 seconds).[75,79–83] Including such simulations as part of robotic training should be considered.

Conversion

When undocking the robot and/or converting to open surgery, it is important to minimize the risks of inadvertently harming the patient with the robot. Especially in urgent/emergent procedures, in which there can be significant stress and movement in the OR during conversion, it is important to remove all instruments from the patient before attempting to undock as well as to avoid entanglement or disconnection of power cords until after undocking. Failure to do these things can slow the conversion process and potentially cause harm to the patient. It is also important to remove needles, sponges, and other foreign objects from the belly as quickly as is safe. Leaving them in the abdomen may save time in the moment but increases the risk of lost foreign objects that might require much time later to locate and remove.

Optimizing safety in robotic surgery can be achieved using the same principles as are common more broadly in both laparoscopic and open surgery: planning, communication, and preparation. Although there are fundamental differences between robotic and laparoscopic conversions, with additional obstacles in robotics, they can be managed safely with proper planning. Ensuring that the operative team understands the steps that need to be taken in order to respond to an adverse event and that the equipment needed to respond is present in the room can help avoid negative patient outcomes.

Box 1
Elements of basic conversion plan

- Desired open surgical instruments, retractors, sutures staples
- Desired electricity devices (Bovie, LigaSure, bipolar, and so forth)
- Planned incision
- Patient positioning
- Who will undock the robot
- How the room will be reconfigured, if needed

SUMMARY

Robotic-assisted liver surgery has emerged as an alternative approach to laparoscopic and open techniques, offering small incisions, better visualization, and articulated instruments, which overcome the shortcomings of laparoscopic and open liver surgery. Careful patient selection as well as stringent safety protocols are imperative for successful robotic-assisted liver surgery. The technology is continuously evolving and the development of new robotic systems and instruments will allow the development of new procedures and expertise within liver surgery.

DISCLOSURE

The authors have nothing to disclose.

REFERENCES

1. Litynski GS. Profiles in laparoscopy: Mouret, Dubois, and Perissat: the laparoscopic breakthrough in Europe (1987-1988). JSLS 1999;3:163–7.
2. Muhe E. Long-term follow-up after laparoscopic cholecystectomy. Endoscopy 1992;24:754–8.
3. Reich H, McGlynn F, DeCaprio J, et al. Laparoscopic excision of benign liver lesions. Obstet Gynecol 1991;78:956–8.
4. Katkhouda N, Fabiani P, Benizri E, et al. Laser resection of a liver hydatid cyst under videolaparoscopy. Br J Surg 1992;79:560–1.
5. Cherqui D, Husson E, Hammoud R, et al. Laparoscopic liver resections: a feasibility study in 30 patients. Ann Surg 2000;232:753–62.
6. Buell JF, Cherqui D, Geller DA, et al, World Consensus Conference on Laparoscopic Surgery. The international position on laparoscopic liver surgery: the Louisville Statement, 2008. Ann Surg 2009;250:825–30.
7. Lee SY, Goh BKP, Sepideh G, et al. Laparoscopic liver resection difficulty score-a validation study. J Gastrointest Surg 2019;23:545–55.
8. Himpens J, Leman G, Cadiere GB. Telesurgical laparoscopic cholecystectomy. Surg Endosc 1998;12:1091.
9. Gagner M, Begin E, Hurteau R, et al. Robotic interactive laparoscopic cholecystectomy. Lancet 1994;343:596–7.
10. Giulianotti PC, Coratti A, Angelini M, et al. Robotics in general surgery: personal experience in a large community hospital. Arch Surg 2003;138:777–84.
11. Kingham TP, Leung U, Kuk D, et al. Robotic liver resection: a case-matched comparison. World J Surg 2016;40:1422–8.
12. Ji WB, Wang HG, Zhao ZM, et al. Robotic-assisted laparoscopic anatomic hepatectomy in China: initial experience. Ann Surg 2011;253:342–8.
13. Lai EC, Yang GP, Tang CN. Robot-assisted laparoscopic liver resection for hepatocellular carcinoma: short-term outcome. Am J Surg 2013;205:697–702.
14. Tsung A, Geller DA, Sukato DC, et al. Robotic versus laparoscopic hepatectomy: a matched comparison. Ann Surg 2014;259:549–55.
15. Goh BKP, Lee LS, Lee SY, et al. Initial experience with robotic hepatectomy in Singapore: analysis of 48 resections in 43 consecutive patients. ANZ J Surg 2019;89:201–5.
16. Choi GH, Chong JU, Han DH, et al. Robotic hepatectomy: the Korean experience and perspective. Hepatobiliary Surg Nutr 2017;6:230–8.
17. Liu R, Wakabayashi G, Kim HJ, et al. International consensus statement on robotic hepatectomy surgery in 2018. World J Gastroenterol 2019;25:1432–44.

18. Stiles ZE, Behrman SW, Glazer ES, et al. Predictors and implications of un-planned conversion during minimally invasive hepatectomy: an analysis of the ACS-NSQIP database. HPB (Oxford) 2017;19:957–65.
19. Melstrom LG, Warner SG, Woo Y, et al. Selecting incision-dominant cases for ro-botic liver resection: towards outpatient hepatectomy with rapid recovery. Hepa-tobiliary Surg Nutr 2018;7:77–84.
20. Nota CL, Woo Y, Raoof M, et al. Robotic versus open minor liver resections of the posterosuperior segments: a multinational, propensity score-matched study. Ann Surg Oncol 2019;26:583–90.
21. Nota C, Molenaar IQ, van Hillegersberg R, et al. Robotic liver resection including the posterosuperior segments: initial experience. J Surg Res 2016;206:133–8.
22. Khan S, Beard RE, Kingham PT, et al. Long-term oncologic outcomes following robotic liver resections for primary hepatobiliary malignancies: a multicenter study. Ann Surg Oncol 2018;25:2652–60.
23. Guan R, Chen Y, Yang K, et al. Clinical efficacy of robot-assisted versus laparo-scopic liver resection: a meta analysis. Asian J Surg 2019;42:19–31.
24. Fruscione M, Pickens R, Baker EH, et al. Robotic-assisted versus laparoscopic major liver resection: analysis of outcomes from a single center. HPB (Oxford) 2019;21:906–11.
25. Tarr ME, Brancato SJ, Cunkelman JA, et al. Comparison of postural ergonomics between laparoscopic and robotic sacrocolpopexy: a pilot study. J Minim Inva-sive Gynecol 2015;22:234–8.
26. Szeto GP, Poon JT, Law WL. A comparison of surgeon's postural muscle activity during robotic-assisted and laparoscopic rectal surgery. J Robot Surg 2013;7:305–8.
27. Mucksavage P, Kerbl DC, Lee JY. The da Vinci((R)) surgical system overcomes innate hand dominance. J Endourol 2011;25:1385–8.
28. Wilhelm D, Reiser S, Kohn N, et al. Comparative evaluation of HD 2D/3D lapa-roscopic monitors and benchmarking to a theoretically ideal 3D pseudodisplay: even well-experienced laparoscopists perform better with 3D. Surg Endosc 2014;28:2387–97.
29. Lee W, Han HS, Yoon YS, et al. Comparison of laparoscopic liver resection for he-patocellular carcinoma located in the posterosuperior segments or anterolateral segments: a case-matched analysis. Surgery 2016;160:1219–26.
30. Teo JY, Kam JH, Chan CY, et al. Laparoscopic liver resection for posterosuperior and anterolateral lesions-a comparison experience in an Asian centre. Hepatobili-ary Surg Nutr 2015;4:379–90.
31. Croner RS, Perrakis A, Hohenberger W, et al. Robotic liver surgery for minor he-patic resections: a comparison with laparoscopic and open standard proced-ures. Langenbecks Arch Surg 2016;401:707–14.
32. Chen PD, Wu CY, Hu RH, et al. Robotic versus open hepatectomy for hepatocel-lular carcinoma: a matched comparison. Ann Surg Oncol 2017;24:1021–8.
33. Fretland AA, Dagenborg VJ, Waaler Bjornelv GM, et al. Quality of life from a ran-domized trial of laparoscopic or open liver resection for colorectal liver metasta-ses. Br J Surg 2019;106(10):1372–80.
34. Montalti R, Scuderi V, Patriti A, et al. Robotic versus laparoscopic resections of posterosuperior segments of the liver: a propensity score-matched comparison. Surg Endosc 2016;30:1004–13.
35. Moore LJ, Wilson MR, Waine E, et al. Robotic technology results in faster and more robust surgical skill acquisition than traditional laparoscopy. J Robot Surg 2015;9:67–73.

36. Efanov M, Alikhanov R, Tsvirkun V, et al. Comparative analysis of learning curve in complex robot-assisted and laparoscopic liver resection. HPB (Oxford) 2017;19:818–24.
37. Chong CCN, Lok HT, Fung AKY, et al. Robotic versus laparoscopic hepatectomy: application of the difficulty scoring system. Surg Endosc 2019. [Epub ahead of print].
38. Kluger MD, Vigano L, Barroso R, et al. The learning curve in laparoscopic major liver resection. J Hepatobiliary Pancreat Sci 2013;20:131–6.
39. Cherrick GR, Stein SW, Leevy CM, et al. Indocyanine green: observations on its physical properties, plasma decay, and hepatic extraction. J Clin Invest 1960;39:592–600.
40. Faybik P, Hetz H. Plasma disappearance rate of indocyanine green in liver dysfunction. Transplant Proc 2006;38:801–2.
41. Marino MV, Builes Ramirez S, Gomez Ruiz M. The application of indocyanine green (ICG) staining technique during robotic-assisted right hepatectomy: with video. J Gastrointest Surg 2019;23(11):2312–3.
42. Daskalaki D, Fernandes E, Wang X, et al. Indocyanine green (ICG) fluorescent cholangiography during robotic cholecystectomy: results of 184 consecutive cases in a single institution. Surg Innov 2014;21:615–21.
43. Zhang YM, Shi R, Hou JC, et al. Liver tumor boundaries identified intraoperatively using real-time indocyanine green fluorescence imaging. J Cancer Res Clin Oncol 2017;143:51–8.
44. van der Vorst JR, Schaafsma BE, Verbeek FP, et al. Near-infrared fluorescence sentinel lymph node mapping of the oral cavity in head and neck cancer patients. Oral Oncol 2013;49:15–9.
45. Ishizawa Y, Aizawa S, Okudera D, et al. A case of advanced gastric cancer with liver metastases successively treated with S-1/CDDP combination therapy followed by curative resection. Gan To Kagaku Ryoho 2012;39:289–92 [in Japanese].
46. Handgraaf HJM, Boogerd LSF, Hoppener DJ, et al. Long-term follow-up after near-infrared fluorescence-guided resection of colorectal liver metastases: a retrospective multicenter analysis. Eur J Surg Oncol 2017;43:1463–71.
47. Boogerd LS, Handgraaf HJ, Lam HD, et al. Laparoscopic detection and resection of occult liver tumors of multiple cancer types using real-time near-infrared fluorescence guidance. Surg Endosc 2017;31:952–61.
48. Kingham TP, Pak LM, Simpson AL, et al. 3D image guidance assisted identification of colorectal cancer liver metastases not seen on intraoperative ultrasound: results from a prospective trial. HPB (Oxford) 2018;20:260 7,
49. Banz VM, Muller PC, Tinguely P, et al. Intraoperative image-guided navigation system: development and applicability in 65 patients undergoing liver surgery. Langenbecks Arch Surg 2016;401:495–502.
50. Yaniv Z, Wilson E, Lindisch D, et al. Electromagnetic tracking in the clinical environment. Med Phys 2009;36:876–92.
51. Maier-Hein L, Tekbas A, Seitel A, et al. In vivo accuracy assessment of a needle-based navigation system for CT-guided radiofrequency ablation of the liver. Med Phys 2008;35:5385–96.
52. Hinds S, Jaeger HA, Burke R, et al. An open electromagnetic tracking framework applied to targeted liver tumour ablation. Int J Comput Assist Radiol Surg 2019;14(9):1475–84.
53. Clements LW, Collins JA, Weis JA, et al. Deformation correction for image guided liver surgery: an intraoperative fidelity assessment. Surgery 2017;162:537–47.

54. Heiselman JS, Clements LW, Collins JA, et al. Characterization and correction of intraoperative soft tissue deformation in image-guided laparoscopic liver surgery. J Med Imaging (Bellingham) 2018;5:021203.

55. Soler L, Nicolau S, Pessaux P, et al. Real-time 3D image reconstruction guidance in liver resection surgery. Hepatobiliary Surg Nutr 2014;3:73–81.

56. Pessaux P, Diana M, Soler L, et al. Towards cybernetic surgery: robotic and augmented reality-assisted liver segmentectomy. Langenbecks Arch Surg 2015;400:381–5.

57. Giulianotti PC, Sbrana F, Coratti A, et al. Totally robotic right hepatectomy: surgical technique and outcomes. Arch Surg 2011;146:844–50.

58. Ahmad A, Ahmad ZF, Carleton JD, et al. Robotic surgery: current perceptions and the clinical evidence. Surg Endosc 2017;31:255–63.

59. Chen PD, Wu CY, Hu RH, et al. Robotic major hepatectomy: is there a learning curve? Surgery 2017;161:642–9.

60. Jayne D, Pigazzi A, Marshall H, et al. Effect of robotic-assisted vs conventional laparoscopic surgery on risk of conversion to open laparotomy among patients undergoing resection for rectal cancer: the ROLARR randomized clinical trial. JAMA 2017;318:1569–80.

61. Sarlos D, Kots L, Stevanovic N, et al. Robotic compared with conventional laparoscopic hysterectomy: a randomized controlled trial. Obstet Gynecol 2012;120: 604–11.

62. Waters JA, Canal DF, Wiebke EA, et al. Robotic distal pancreatectomy: cost effective? Surgery 2010;148:814–23.

63. Tsuda S, Oleynikov D, Gould J, et al. SAGES TAVAC safety and effectiveness analysis: da Vinci (R) surgical system (Intuitive Surgical, Sunnyvale, CA). Surg Endosc 2015;29:2873–84.

64. Sankaranarayanan G, Resapu RR, Jones DB, et al. Common uses and cited complications of energy in surgery. Surg Endosc 2013;27:3056–72.

65. Stojeba N, Mahoudeau G, Segura P, et al. Possible venous argon gas embolism complicating argon gas enhanced coagulation during liver surgery. Acta Anaesthesiol Scand 1999;43:866–7.

66. Ousmane ML, Fleyfel M, Vallet B. Venous gas embolism during liver surgery with argon-enhanced coagulation. Eur J Anaesthesiol 2002;19:225.

67. Palmer M, Miller CW, van Way CW 3rd, et al. Venous gas embolism associated with argon-enhanced coagulation of the liver. J Invest Surg 1993;6:391–9.

68. Barbash GI, Glied SA. New technology and health care costs–the case of robot-assisted surgery. N Engl J Med 2010;363:701–4.

69. Turchetti G, Palla I, Pierotti F, et al. Economic evaluation of da Vinci-assisted robotic surgery: a systematic review. Surg Endosc 2012;26:598–606.

70. Higgins RM, Frelich MJ, Bosler ME, et al. Cost analysis of robotic versus laparoscopic general surgery procedures. Surg Endosc 2017;31:185–92.

71. Daskalaki D, Gonzalez-Heredia R, Brown M, et al. Financial impact of the robotic approach in liver surgery: a comparative study of clinical outcomes and costs between the robotic and open technique in a single institution. J Laparoendosc Adv Surg Tech A 2017;27:375–82.

72. Sham JG, Richards MK, Seo YD, et al. Efficacy and cost of robotic hepatectomy: is the robot cost-prohibitive? J Robot Surg 2016;10:307–13.

73. Wong DJ, Wong MJ, Choi GH, et al. Systematic review and meta-analysis of robotic versus open hepatectomy. ANZ J Surg 2019;89:165–70.

74. Thompson J. Myocardial infarction and subsequent death in a patient undergoing robotic prostatectomy. AANA J 2009;77:365–71.

75. Ziewacz JE, Arriaga AF, Bader AM, et al. Crisis checklists for the operating room: development and pilot testing. J Am Coll Surg 2011;213:212–7.e10.
76. Arriaga AF, Bader AM, Wong JM, et al. Simulation-based trial of surgical-crisis checklists. N Engl J Med 2013;368:246–53.
77. Brazil V, Purdy E, Alexander C, et al. Improving the relational aspects of trauma care through translational simulation. Adv Simul (Lond) 2019;4:10.
78. Steinemann S, Berg B, Skinner A, et al. In situ, multidisciplinary, simulation-based teamwork training improves early trauma care. J Surg Educ 2011;68:472–7.
79. Huser AS, Muller D, Brunkhorst V, et al. Simulated life-threatening emergency during robot-assisted surgery. J Endourol 2014;28:717–21.
80. Holzman RS, Cooper JB, Gaba DM, et al. Anesthesia crisis resource management: real-life simulation training in operating room crises. J Clin Anesth 1995; 7:675–87.
81. Yee B, Naik VN, Joo HS, et al. Nontechnical skills in anesthesia crisis management with repeated exposure to simulation-based education. Anesthesiology 2005;103:241–8.
82. Birkmeyer JD. Strategies for improving surgical quality–checklists and beyond. N Engl J Med 2010;363:1963–5.
83. Haynes AB, Weiser TG, Berry WR, et al, Safe Surgery Saves Lives Study Group. A surgical safety checklist to reduce morbidity and mortality in a global population. N Engl J Med 2009;360:491–9.

Robotic Biliary Surgery

Karen Chang, MD, Fahri Gokcal, MD, Omar Yusef Kudsi, MD, MBA, FACS*

KEYWORDS

- Robotic cholecystectomy • Robotic common bile duct exploration • Gallbladder
- Infrared-ICG cholangiography • Robotic hepaticojejunostomy

KEY POINTS

- Robotic cholecystectomy has potential advantages of ease of dissection and visualization over laparoscopic cholecystectomy in benign and malignant gallbladder disease.
- Choledocholithiasis can be addressed, in a safe and reproducible manner in one setting during a robotic cholecystectomy.
- Difficult cholecystectomies can be performed using a robotic approach with potential benefits of less conversion to open techniques while maintaining a critical view of safety.
- Use of infrared indocyanine green cholangiography during robotic cholecystectomy aids in biliary anatomy visualization, which can contribute to a decreased open conversion rate.
- Robotic cholecystectomy can be performed using either a multiport or a single port approach, depending on patient characteristics and pathology.

INTRODUCTION

Surgery for symptomatic gallbladder disease is one of the most common procedures performed by a general surgeon. Today, laparoscopic cholecystectomy is the gold standard for benign gallbladder disease, replacing open cholecystectomy. With the advancement of robotic surgery techniques, robotic cholecystectomy is a fast-growing alternative to laparoscopic cholecystectomy. The robotic approach combines a 3-dimensional view with wristed instruments, allowing for fine dissection in a minimally invasive fashion, which may lead to decreased rates of conversion and complications.[1] In addition, robotic cholecystectomy can be combined with common bile duct exploration to address complicated gallbladders in a single setting. This article first provides a literature review of reported outcomes after robotic biliary surgery. Then, a technical overview of single-port and multiport approaches to robotic cholecystectomy including the approach for benign bile duct disease using the da Vinci Surgical System (Intuitive Surgical, Inc, Sunnyvale, CA).

Good Samaritan Medical Center, Tufts University School of Medicine, 1 Pearl Street, Suite 2000, Brockton, MA 02301, USA
* Corresponding author.
E-mail address: omar.kudsi@tufts.edu

Surg Clin N Am 100 (2020) 283–302
https://doi.org/10.1016/j.suc.2019.12.002
0039-6109/20/Published by Elsevier Inc.

surgical.theclinics.com

BENIGN GALLBLADDER DISEASES

The most common indications for robotic cholecystectomy are symptomatic gall-bladder disease, including gallstones and polyps. Multiple published reports conclude that robotic cholecystectomy can be successfully performed via either multiport of single port access, which are summarized in **Table 1**.[1–26] The vast majority of these studies are about single site robotic cholecystectomy (SSRC). SSRC allows for a safe dissection, with good exposure of Calot's triangle comparable to a multiport laparoscopic cholecystectomy. Advantages of improved cosmesis are a benefit of SSRC.[18,20] One potential drawback is the increased risk of incisional hernia secondary to a larger incision. According to our literature review (see **Table 1**), we found that only 4 incisional hernias were reported after SSRC. However, this occurrence rate may be due to the lack of long-term results in most of the studies.

The adoption of robotic cholecystectomy over laparoscopic cholecystectomy is also limited owing to the increased cost. Robotic cholecystectomy has similar outcomes to laparoscopic cholecystectomy, but has been shown to have a higher cost.[2,24] However, a study from 2016 comparing 117 robotic cholecystectomies with 281 laparoscopic cholecystectomies showed that, in a hospital with an infrastructure already in place for robotic surgery, the procedural cost of robotic approach is less due to decreased supplies and less operating room time with increased experience.[27]

Complex gallbladders, where the anatomy requires extensive dissection, is where the enhanced visualization of the robotic approach is advantageous. Magge and colleagues[28] reviewed the advantages of a robotic approach to Mirizzi syndrome with cholecystocholedochal fistulas. In these cases, the dissection is difficult with a laparoscopic approach given the severe inflammation that limits the critical view of safety; often, a subtotal cholecystectomy is performed as the safest procedure. Their institution uses a multiport robotic approach after endoscopic stenting; the robotic platform allows for enhanced visualization with the ability to obtain exposure of the gallbladder from the common bile duct that is similar to that of open surgery.

GALLBLADDER CANCER

Incidental gallbladder cancer is rare, accounting for 0.19% to 2.10% of all patients undergoing laparoscopic cholecystectomy for benign gallbladder disease.[29–31] Patients with incidental gallbladder cancer have a better prognosis than nonincidentally discovered disease with appropriate staging and R0 resection.[32,33] If gallbladder cancer is suspected preoperatively, laparoscopic cholecystectomy had not been recommended routinely.[32] However, a meta-analysis involving a total of 1217 cases concluded that laparoscopic cholecystectomy did not worsen the prognosis of patients with early gallbladder cancer.[34] In a 10-year prospective cohort study, extended laparoscopic cholecystectomy, including lymphadenectomy or simple cholecystectomy, was found in a total 45 patients to be safe with favorable oncological outcomes in patients with early gallbladder cancer who do not have invasion of the liver or extrahepatic bile duct.[35] Furthermore, robotic approaches for gallbladder cancer with diagnosed different stages, both in the incidental and nonincidental settings, have also been reported from various institutions[36–41] (**Table 2**). A comparison of outcomes for minimally invasive approaches versus open approaches is needed.

BENIGN BILIARY OBSTRUCTIONS (CHOLEDOCHOLITHIASIS/STRICTURE)

Choledocholithiasis, benign strictures and biliary injury, contribute to the majority of biliary tract disorders that are indications for exploration of the biliary system.[42]

Table 1
Available studies involving robotic procedures for GBC

Authors, Year	No. of Case(s) with GBC in the Study	Tumor Stage (No. of Cases)	Robotic Procedure (No. of Cases)	Study Finding/Conclusion
Liu et al,[36] 2012	11 GBC in a total of 60 studied cases	T1 (0) T2 (0) T3 (4) T4 (7)	Excision of gallbladder tumor and RNYHJ (2) Cholecystectomy (3) Cholecystectomy, internal biliary drainage (1) Cholecystectomy, T-tube biliary drainage (5)	Two of 60 (3.3%) port site metastasis was observed (none of them were a GBC)/ Biliary malignancy can be selected as an indication of robotic surgery
Chandarana et al,[37] 2017	14 proven or suspected GBC in a total of 25 studied cases	N/A	Simple cholecystectomy (with perihilar lymphadenectomy) (4) Radical cholecystectomy (with a 2.5- to 3.0-cm wedge of liver in the gallbladder fossa and perihilar lymphadenectomy) (8) Revision cholecystectomy (1) Simple cholecystectomy with left adnexectomy (1)	In the entire cohort, 5 patients required the conversion to open, the median lymph nodes was 7/Robotic surgery even for hepatobiliary oncology is feasible and can be performed safely
Araujo et al,[38] 2019	3 incidental GBCs	T1b (1) N/A for other 2 cases	Bisegmentectomy (IVb/V) with perihilar lymphadenectomy (3)	None of harvested lymph nodes was involved metastasis, absence of residual disease/Bisegmentectomy with perihilar lymphadenectomy could be safely done by using a robot, without jeopardizing oncologic outcomes
Goja et al,[39] 2017	1 incidental GBC in a total of 10 studied cases	Stage 2b (1)	Radical cholecystectomy with anatomic segment IVb and V resection and perihilar lymphadenectomy (1)	A bile leak was occurred from the cystic duct stump in this patient/Versatility of the robotic system allows ease of use for both liver resections and biliary reconstruction

(continued on next page)

Table 1
(continued)

Authors, Year	No. of Case(s) with GBC in the Study	Tumor Stage (No. of Cases)	Robotic Procedure (No. of Cases)	Study Finding/Conclusion
Shen et al,[40] 2012	2 incidental GBCs in a total of 5 studied cases; other 3 cases preoperatively diagnosed as a stage of ≤T3	Stage 2 (2) Stage 3 (3)	Radical resection (cholecystectomy as well as all hepatic tissue behind 2 cm of the gallbladder) bed with perihilar lymphadenectomy (5)	In only 1 patient, reginal lymph nodes were a 3/3 positive/Five patients with GBC were successfully treated by radical resection using a robotic surgical system
Sucandy et al,[41] 2019	4 GBC in a total of 80 studied cases	N/A	N/A	5% cases underwent robotic hepatectomy owing to GBC/Robotic hepatectomy is safe and feasible, with favorable short-term outcomes for both benign and malignant tumors and with a low open conversion rate

Abbreviations: GBC, gallbladder cancer; N/A, not available; RNYHJ, Roux-N-Y hepaticojejunostomy.
Data from Refs.[36–41]

Table 2
Available studies on robotic cholecystectomy

Authors, Reference Year	Design		n	Access Type	Total Operating Time in (min) Mean ± SD, or Mean/Median (Range)	No of Intraoperative Events	Postoperative Complication
Breitenstein et al,[2] 2008	Case control	Robotic	50	Multiport	54.6 ± 31.6	No conversions 12 GB perforation	1 bile leakage
		Laparoscopic	50	Multiport	50.2 ± 29.2	No conversion 9 GB perforation	1 jejunal perforation
Kroh et al,[3] 2011	Case series		13	Single port	107 ± 53.8	In 1 patient additional port No complications No conversions	No complications
Wren and Curet,[4] 2011	Case control	Robotic	10	Single port	105.3 (82–139)	1 open conversions No complications No conversions	2 urinary retention
		Laparoscopic	10	Multiport	106.1 (70–142)	No conversions No complications	2 urinary retention
Morel et al,[5] 2011	Case series		28	Single port	80 (45–195)	No conversions No complications	No complications
Konstantinidis et al,[6] 2012	Case series		45	Single port	84.5 ± 25.5	In 3 patients additional port No complications No conversions	1 hemorrhage (liver bed oozing)
Spinoglio et al,[7] 2012	Case control	Robotic	25	Single port	62.7 ± 16.6	No conversions No complications	No complications
		Laparoscopic	25	Single port	83.2 ± 21.1	No conversions No complications	No complications

(continued on next page)

Table 2
(continued)

Authors, Reference Year	Design	n	Access Type	Total Operating Time in (min) Mean ± SD, or Mean/Median (Range)	No of Intraoperative Events	Postoperative Complication
Pietrabissa et al,[8] 2012	Multicenter prospective observational	100	Single port	71 ± 19	2 open conversions 7 minor gas-leak 7 GB perforations 5 hemorrhage (liver bed oozing)	N/A
Buzad et al,[9] 2013	Case control	Robotic 20	Single port	84.6 ± 20.5	No conversions No complications	1 pain, constipation
		Laparoscopic 10	Single port	85.5 ± 11.8	No conversions No complications	1 wound infection
Ayloo and Choudhury,[10] 2014	Case series	31	Single port	81.4 ± 21	2 additional port No conversions No complications	1 wound infection
Vidovszky et al,[11] 2014	Case series	95	Single port	88.63 ± 32	1 cystic duct avulsion 24 GB perforation 3 minor bleeding No conversions	3 CBD sludge/stone 2 pain/constipation 1 infected biloma
Uras et al,[12] 2014	Case series	36	Single port	61.8 (45–130)	1 additional port 3 technical problems No conversions No complications	1 incisional hernia

Study	Study type	Approach		n	Port	Operative time	Conversions	Complications
Ayloo et al,[13] 2014	Case control	Robotic		147	Multiport	95.7 ± 38.3	2 open conversions No complications	1 CBD stone 1 CBD injury 1 subhepatic abscess 1 pain 1 pancreatitis 1 pseudocyst infection 1 bile leakage 1 urinary retention
		Laparoscopic	179		Multiport	89.6 ± 33.7	3 open conversions No complications	
Svoboda et al,[14] 2015	Case series (patients with BMI ≥30 kg/m²)			112	Single port	69.8 ± 26	No conversions No complications	1 incisional hernia
Chung et al,[15] 2015	Case control	Robotic		70	Single port	111.5 ± 31.1	1 Open conversion Complication N/A	Hematoma CBD stone
		Laparoscopic	70		Multiport	106 ± 41	11 Open conversions Complication N/A	2 Pancreatitis 1 Pain
Bibi et al,[16] 2015	Case series			102	Single port	109 (36–375)	3 Laparoscopic conversions 1 Open conversion No complications	2 Anemia 1 Ileus 1 Pneumonia
Gonzalez et al,[17] 2016	Case series, multicenter			465	Single port	52 (43–65)	6 Additional ports 4 Laparoscopic conversions	2 Bile leakage 9 Infections 2 Wound disruptions
Kudsi et al,[18] 2016	Multicenter prospective randomized trial	Robotic		83	Single port	61 ± 27.5	No conversions No complications	2 Wound infections 1 IBD attack 1 DVT, PE
		Laparoscopic	53		Multiport	44 ± 19	No conversions No complications	1 bile leakage 1 wound infection

(continued on next page)

Table 2
(continued)

Authors, Reference Year	Design		n	Access Type	Total Operating Time in (min) Mean ± SD, or Mean/Median (Range)	No of Intraoperative Events	Postoperative Complication
Li et al,[1] 2017	Case control	Robotic	78	Single port	75.7 ± 31.3	No conversions No complications	1 Incisional hernia 2 Medical (local ileus, diarrhea)
		Laparoscopic	367	Multiport	64.47 ± 30.61	7 Open conversions No complications	2 Incisional hernias 10 Wound infections 9 GB removal-related (CBD stone, stricture, leakage, subhepatic fluid) 54 Medical (atelectasis, tachycardia, UTI, local ileus, diarrhea)
Lee et al,[19] 2017	Case series		30	Single port (glove port)	53.8 ± 15.2 (console time)	No conversions No complications	No complications
Pietrabissa et al,[20] 2016	Prospective randomized double-blind trial	Robotic	30	Single port	98 ± 43	No conversions 4 Bile spillages 3 Minor bleeding (liver bed oozing)	2 Wound infections, one of them incisional hernia
		Laparoscopic	30	Multiport	87 ± 30	No conversions 5 Bile spillages 2 Minor bleeding (liver bed oozing)	No wound infections

Study	Case type	Approach	n	Port	Operative time	Conversions/ports	Complications
Lim et al,[21] 2017	Case control[a]	Robotic	37	Single port	132 ± 36	5 GB perforations / No conversions	5 Wound infections
		Laparoscopic	60	Multiport (suprapubic)	53 ± 20	6 Additional ports / 7 GB perforations / No Conversion	1 Intra-abdominal abscess / 1 Abdominal collection
Su et al,[22] 2017	Case control	Robotic	51	Single port	71.3 ± 48.88	No conversions / 5 GB perforations	N/A
		Laparoscopic	63	Single port	74.7 ± 30.16	2 Additional ports / 12 GB perforations	2 Bile leakage
Balachandran et al,[23] 2017	Case control	Robotic	415	Single port	89.4 ± 27.8	12 Laparoscopic conversions / 13 Open conversions	1 Bile leakage / 29 Wound related / 43 Medical (pain, ileus, UTI)
		Laparoscopic	263	Multiport	92.6 ± 31.9	2 Additional ports / 13 Open conversions	2 Bile leakage / 9 Wound related / 14 Medical (pain, ileus, UTI)
Strosberg et al,[24] 2017	Case control	Robotic	140	Multiport	74.5 (47–293)	1 Open conversion / Complication N/A	3 Bile leakage / 1 wound infection
		Laparoscopic	97	Multiport	556 (35–244)	7 Open conversions / Complication N/A	1 Bile leakage / 1 Wound infection
Jang et al,[25] 2019	Case control (patients with BMI ≥25 kg/m²)	Robotic	39	Single port	107.92 ± 24.95	2 Conversions / 6 GB perforations / No complications	No complications
		Laparoscopic	78	Single port	60.99 ± 17.81	2 conversions / 10 Additional ports / 9 GB perforations	5 Complication (mostly wound infection)

Abbreviations: BMI, body mass index; CBD, common bile duct; DVT, deep venous thrombosis; GB, gallbladder; IBD, inflammatory bowel disease; N/A, not available; PE, pulmonary emboli; UTI, urinary tract infection.

[a] Le Roy et al.[26]'s study was used as control group.

Data from Refs.[1-26]

Endoscopic approaches are commonly used as alternatives to operative intervention. A single-stage approach to clear the bile duct is recommended when common duct stones are identified during an operation to treat cholelithiasis over a 2-stage approach using endoscopic retrograde cholangiography with sphincterotomy for common bile duct clearance owing to lower cost, shorter hospital stay, and less associated morbidity.[42] Robotic surgery for common bile duct exploration is safe and effective; currently, it is recommended owing to better visualization and easier closure of the choledochotomy. Furthermore, robotic exploration of the common bile duct is one of the available alternatives for biliary intervention in case of a complex choledocholithiasis or in case of technical difficulty in transoral biliary access secondary to altered foregut anatomy.[42–46] Results after robotic compared with open common bile duct exploration comparing 37 patients showed longer hospital stays for the open group, and longer operating times for the robotic group, with a small percentage of patients in both groups requiring postoperative endoscopic intervention to remove retained stones and/or sludge.[46] In another study, Almamar and colleagues[44] found that robotic common bile duct exploration for ERCP refractory choledocholithiasis compared with open surgery had longer operating times and increased operating costs but fewer complications, a shorter length of stay, and a lower overall cost. Similarly, Gilbert and colleagues[47] shared their experience of 12 consecutive patients who underwent fully robotic choledochoduodenostomy with side-to-side or end-to-side anastomosis for benign common bile duct obstruction after endoscopic failure; 1 patient developed cholangitis, and no other long-term complications were reported. The robotic platform also allows for a safe and easier periduodenal dissection over laparoscopy that assists in the management of common bile duct strictures that are not amenable to nonoperative management.[43] Further studies are warranted for long-term results.

EXTRAHEPATIC BILE DUCT INJURIES

Bile duct injury is a rare, dreaded complication of cholecystectomy that can lead to significant morbidity. During the era of laparoscopic cholecystectomy, the incidence increased to 0.4% to 0.7% compared with 0.1% to 0.2% for open cholecystectomy.[48] The primary cause of bile duct injury is often attributed to the misinterpretation of biliary anatomy, accounting for upwards of 80% of all injuries.[49] Multiple strategies and techniques have been described to decrease injury rates including achieving the critical view of safety, intraoperative cholangiography, dissection techniques (infundibular, anterograde, etc), landmark techniques (Rouvière's sulcus,[50] Calot's node[51]) and the use of near-infrared fluorescent cholangiography.[52–55] Iatrogenic bile duct injury continues to be a major concern in cholecystectomy, even with the technical advantages of robotic technology. Long-term and multicenter studies are needed to determine if robotic technology can afford a decrease in the bile duct injury.

The repair of major bile duct injuries not amenable to primary repair requires a tension-free bilioenteric anastomosis. Multiple techniques of robotic hepaticojejunostomy have been described, entailing the use of interrupted or continuous sutures for the anastomosis, and constructing an end-to-end or side-to-side anastomosis. Cuendis-Velázquez and colleagues[56] described a Roux-en-Y robotic hepaticojejunostomy in a total of 30 patients with bile duct injury with a hand sewn anastomosis constructed using two 4-0 monofilament absorbable barbed sutures in a running fashion, one anteriorly and the other posteriorly. This technique differs from the laparoscopic approach, where interrupted sutures are placed. In the same center, patients undergoing and robotic hepaticojejunostomy (n = 35) versus laparoscopic hepaticojejnostomy (n = 40) owing to bile duct injury were found to be similar in terms of safety; more important, the efficacy of primary patency within 90 days were similar, and leak rates were the same.[57] Giulianotti and colleagues[58] reported outcomes of 14 patients who underwent robotic hepaticojejunostomy where the anastomosis was constructed using a posterior running suture of 5-0 polydioxanone suture and anterior interrupted stitches with the same 5-0 or 6-0 polydioxanone suture. Results showed no conversions to open surgery, with 1 patient with a hepaticojejunostomy leak within 30 days postoperatively with subsequent recurrent episodes of cholangitis and another patient with cholangitis beyond 30 days. Although many surgeons prefer running sutures in the minimally invasive approaches, it is believed that separated sutures warrant a better anastomosis owing to the heterogenous nature of the bile duct.[59] Marino and colleagues[60] have recently reported the outcomes of a total of 12 patients who underwent robotic bile duct injury repair with hepaticojejunostomy anastomosis. In one patient, a stenosis of the anastomosis with ensuing cholangitis was developed, and the patient was reoperated, performing a revision of the anastomosis by the robotic approach. According to authors, the repair of common bile duct injury is one of the best indications for robotic surgery. Although technically feasible, studies are needed to show similar outcome of minimally invasive repair of bile duct injuries when compared with open approaches.

INDOCYANINE GREEN IN ROBOTIC BILIARY SURGERY

Safety is paramount during robotic cholecystectomy. In addition to adhering to the principles to obtain a critical view of safety, fluorescent imaging is available on the robotic platform to augment biliary anatomy. Indocyanine green (ICG) is a vital dye that can be administered intravenously that binds to plasma proteins.[61] When ICG is stimulated by near infrared (NIR) light integrated on the robotic system, biliary and vascular anatomy is visualized in real time during surgery without transecting any biliary structures.[48,62] NIR-ICG cholangiography is useful for identifying extrahepatic biliary anatomy to obtain the critical view, identification of aberrant biliary anatomy, evaluation of nonbiliary anatomy, and identification of variants of cystic duct and common bile duct anatomy.[48,63] In our practice, NIR-ICG has been helpful in performing portal lymphadenectomy for incidental gallbladder cancer. Additionally, NIR-ICG has been suggested to be advantageous in lowering the conversion to open cholecystectomy.[63–65] In our series, we observed 1% conversion to open during robotic cholecystectomy before the routine use of NIR-ICG.

TECHNICAL OVERVIEW OF ROBOTIC CHOLECYSTECTOMY
Preoperative Planning and Patient Selection

- Both single and multiport approaches can be used for symptomatic cholelithiasis, acute and chronic cholecystitis, gallbladder polyps, and biliary dyskinesia.
- Patients with suspected Mirizzi syndrome, suspected bile duct stones, and known aberrant anatomy would benefit from a multiport approach.
- The single port technique should be used with patients with a normal body mass index, concern for cosmesis, and with less complicated pathology.
- The robotic single-site platform allows a perfect triangulation to open the Calot's triangle as in a multiport robotic cholecystectomy to achieve the critical view of safety.
- ICG needs to be injected intravenously a minimum of 30 minutes before fluorescent imaging can be optimally used. The dosage is 2.5 mg (1 mL).

Multiport Technique

1. Four ports are used; 3 ports for instruments and 1 for the camera.
2. The exact room configuration may vary depending on size of the room and location of permanent fixtures. The operating table can be turned 90° from standard position to avoid crowding between the patient-side cart of the robot and anesthesia equipment.
3. The patient is placed in the supine position with the arms extended. After inserting the trocar in proper positions, the robot is docked depending on the model of the robot.
4. Trocars are placed in a straight line at least 10 cm away from the target anatomy, providing a 6 to 8 cm distance between to each other to avoid robotic arm interference (**Fig. 1**). Port positions can be altered to a certain extent based on the patient's body habitus and the preference of the surgeon.
   - The choice for the EndoWrist instruments as well as the choice of camera (30° or 0°) may change per surgeon's preference. We generally perform the procedure using a 0° camera, a bipolar Maryland grasper, a prograsp, and a monopolar curved scissors, alternating with use of a Hem-o-Lok clip applier (see **Fig. 1**).
5. The dissection begins by grasping Hartmann's pouch and retracting the infundibulum of the gallbladder laterally.
6. Rouvière's sulcus (present 82% of the livers), a naturally occurring cleft in the right lobe, can be used as an anatomic landmark for beginning the dissection of Calot's triangle. The risk of common bile duct injury during initial dissection is very low in any attempt at anterior and above of this landmark (**Fig. 2**). NIR-ICG cholangiography can be used to delineate the biliary anatomy.
7. Three main criteria are required to identify the cystic duct while performing the initial dissection to achieve the 'critical view of safety' (**Fig. 3**):
   - Calot's triangle is cleared of fatty tissue.
   - The lower third of the gallbladder is separated from its bed to expose the cystic plate.
   - Two and only 2 structures should be seen entering the gallbladder.

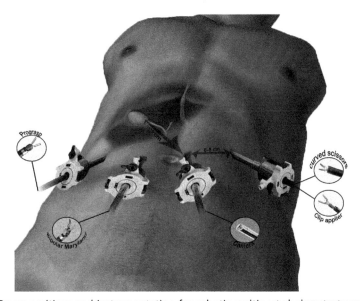

Fig. 1. Trocar positions and instrumentation for robotic multiport cholecystectomy.

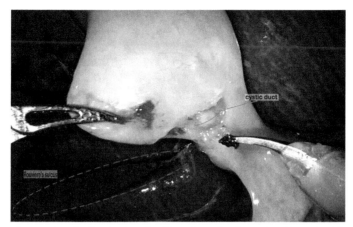

Fig. 2. Rouviere's sulcus for beginning the dissection of Calot's triangle and to identify cystic duct.

8. A bipolar fenestrated Maryland grasper is extremely useful during the dissection to obtain this critical view.
9. Once the critical view of safety is achieved, the Hem-o-lock clips are used to clip the cystic duct and artery. In most cases, 2 clips are applied on both the proximal and distal sides of the cystic duct. The cystic artery requires only one clip on the proximal side; the distal side can be controlled with bipolar cautery (**Fig. 4**).
10. At this point, if there was preoperative concern for common bile duct stones, transcystic common bile duct exploration (TCCBDE) is attempted if the intraoperative cholangiography is amenable to transcystic common bile duct exploration.
11. To perform an intraoperative cholangiogram, a cholangiogram catheter (CC) is placed through an angiocatheter in the right upper quadrant. The cystic duct is partially transected, clipping the proximal duct and then introducing the CC into the distal duct, in the direction of the common bile duct. The CC is secured with a clip across the CC and distal cystic duct. The number 1 arm is then undocked to use the C-arm, taking care to not interfere with the other robotic

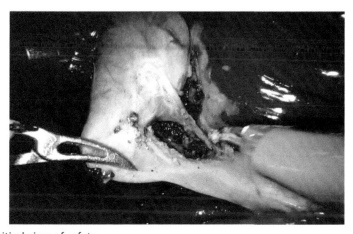

Fig. 3. Critical view of safety.

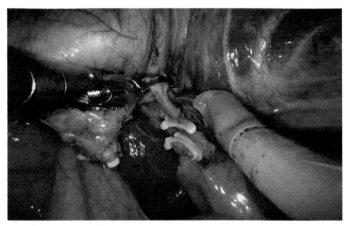

Fig. 4. Clip application to cystic duct and artery.

arms. The CC is injected to obtain images of the biliary tree. If no bile duct stones are visualized, the catheter is removed and another clip is placed on the distal cystic duct. The remaining distal cystic duct is then divided.

12. The gallbladder is then dissected from its bed using a monopolar cautery. During this step, the surgeon should be aware of whether there is aberrant duct of Luschka, because uncontrolled traction of the gallbladder can result its perforation.

13. After the cholecystectomy is completed, the liver bed is checked once more if there is oozing from dissection area. If needed, bleeding control is achieved by using bipolar or monopolar cautery.

14. After gallbladder removal, if required, the fascial defect is closed by using an absorbable suture to avoid an incisional hernia.

Single Port Technique

1. To insert the single port, a 3-cm vertical incision in the umbilicus followed by a transverse incision in the fascia is made. To exclude the presence of intra-abdominal adhesions, a digital exploration is performed after entering the peritoneal cavity. The single-site port can be placed through the umbilical incision (**Fig. 5**) with unfolded or folded clamp technique.

2. The instruments used in SSRC are flexible to allow introduction into curved cannulas which will be placed in channels in a single port. We prefer the 300-mm curved cannula whenever possible with a 0° camera. What is very important is the distance between the tip of cannula and surgical target. We have found that a 6- to 8-cm distance provides the ideal control of those instruments (**Fig. 6**).

3. Effective retraction of the fundus by bedside assistant is crucial for safely completion of SSRC. For this purpose, a long laparoscopic grasper can be used to allow the assistant's hands to be farther away from the robotic arms.

4. Similar steps to those described above are performed to remove the gallbladder using single site instruments. For the purpose of dissection in this procedure, we prefer the use of a hook cautery.

5. After removal of the gallbladder, the fascial defect should be closed. We prefer the use of running absorbable barbed suture (0-Stratafix, Ethicon, Sommerville, NJ) to close the defect. In the setting of preexisting umbilical hernia, we do not use mesh. Finally, in the setting of limited retraction and exposure, an additional port is advised.

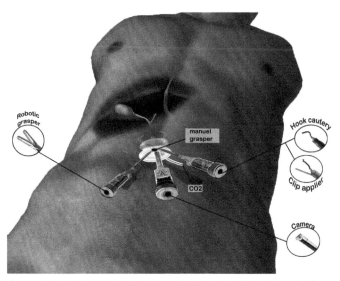

Fig. 5. Single-port and instrumentation for robotic single-site cholecystectomy.

Robotic Common Bile Duct Exploration

If common bile duct stones are visualized, transcystic common bile duct exploration can be attempted using multiple techniques involving a choledochoscope and balloon catheter.[42] Robotic common bile duct exploration is used if common bile duct stones are unable to be cleared via transcystic common bile duct exploration.

1. An additional 8-mm trocar is placed in the left lateral abdomen for the third robotic arm.
2. Remove the CC, leaving the transected distal duct in place.
3. Dissect the cystic duct to the common bile duct, using IR-ICG, then meticulously dissect the common bile duct to the level of the duodenum.
4. Choledochotomy is then performed; we prefer a 1-cm vertical incision above the duodenum. A transverse incision may also be used.

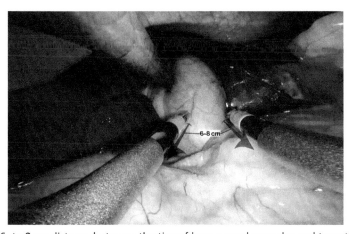

Fig. 6. A 6- to 8-cm distance between the tips of long-curved cannulas and target anatomy.

5. The fourth arm is used to retract the liver with a sponge. Using Cadiere forceps common bile duct stones are swept up or down toward the choledochotomy for extraction.
6. A 4F Fogarty balloon catheter is used to sweep additional stones.
7. Choledochoscopy is performed to visualize the entire length of the common bile duct.
8. Arm 1 is then undocked and completion cholangiogram is performed. If remaining stones are found, repeat step 6 and use TCCBDE techniques to remove residual stones.
9. If the completion cholangiogram shows no remaining common bile duct stones and contrast flows freely into the duodenum, the choledochotomy incision is closed using an absorbable 4-0 monofilament barbed suture. The completion cholangiogram is performed again.
10. The gallbladder is then removed according to steps 13 and 14 in the Multiport Technique section. A closed suction drain is placed in the subhepatic space for drainage.

Robotic Hepaticojejunostomy

1. Trocars are placed in a straight line in the same configuration as a multiport chole-cystectomy. A 5-mm assistant trocar is placed in the left upper quadrant for the laparoscopic liver retractor to avoid robotic arm interference.
2. If performing at the same time during a cholecystectomy, the gallbladder is left in place, with the cystic duct and artery clipped.
3. If performing for bile duct injury, IR-ICG is used to delineate anatomy, along with intraoperative cholangiography as needed.
4. The hilum is evaluated to assess anatomy, using the same instrumentation as RCBDE; the hepatic ducts are dissected and prepared for reconstruction.
5. Once the bile duct is ready for reconstruction, a proximal loop of jejunum is used to create a 70-cm Roux limb, dividing the jejunum and mesentery. A side-to-side enteroenterostomy of the jejunal loops is created using a 60-cm stapler. The enterotomies are closed in a continuous fashion using monofilament 3-0 barbed suture. The mesenteric defect is also closed using monofilament 3-0 barbed suture.
6. An end-to-side hepaticojejunostomy is fashioned using 2 sutures in a running fashion. The posterior aspect of the anastomosis is created by running 4-0 mono-filament barbed suture then completed by running another 4-0 monofilament barbed suture on the anterior aspect. If there is any concern for bile duct quality, interrupted sutures may be placed.
7. The gallbladder is then removed according to steps 13 and 14 in the Multiport Technique section. A closed suction drain is placed in the subhepatic space for drainage.

SUMMARY

Robotic cholecystectomy is a safe and feasible minimally invasive option for benign gallbladder disease. Literature is limited about the robotic approach for malignant gall-bladder disease; further studies comparing outcomes with open surgery are needed. The robotic platform offers advantages of improved visualization and range of motion owing to wristed instruments, enabling experienced surgeons to tackle complex cases in a minimally invasive fashion. Robotic cholecystectomy can be combined with common bile duct exploration to address complicated gallbladders in a single setting. Selection of a multiport versus SSRC technique depends on patient characteristics and pathology. NIR-ICG cholangiography aids in improved visualization of biliary anatomy and identification of aberrant anatomy and accessory ducts. The combination of NIR-ICG with the robotic approach allows for a minimally invasive option for challenging gallbladder pathology and bile duct disease. Biliary reconstruction is also technically feasible in cases of bile duct injury; further studies comparing this approach to open procedures are needed.

DISCLOSURE

Drs F. Gokcal and K. Chang have no conflicts of interest or financial ties to disclose. Dr O.Y. Kudsi has received a teaching course and/or consultancy fees from Intuitive Surgical, Bard-Davol, and W. L. Gore & Associates outside the submitted work.

REFERENCES

1. Li YP, Wang SN, Lee KT. robotic versus conventional laparoscopic cholecystectomy: a comparative study of medical resource utilization and clinical outcomes. Kaohsiung J Med Sci 2017;33(4):201–6.
2. Breitenstein S, Nocito A, Puhan M, et al. Robotic-assisted versus laparoscopic cholecystectomy: outcome and cost analyses of a case-matched control study. Ann Surg 2008;247(6):987–93.
3. Kroh M, El-Hayek K, Rosenblatt S, et al. First human surgery with a novel single-port robotic system: cholecystectomy using the da Vinci single-site platform. Surg Endosc 2011;25(11):3566–73.
4. Wren SM, Curet MJ. Single-port robotic cholecystectomy: results from a first human use clinical study of the new da Vinci single-site surgical platform. Arch Surg 2011;146(10):1122–7.
5. Morel P, Hagen ME, Bucher P, et al. Robotic single-port cholecystectomy using a new platform: initial clinical experience. J Gastrointest Surg 2011;15(12):2182–6.
6. Konstantinidis KM, Hirides P, Hirides S, et al. Cholecystectomy using a novel Single-Site((R)) robotic platform: early experience from 45 consecutive cases. Surg Endosc 2012;26(9):2687–94.
7. Spinoglio G, Lenti LM, Maglione V, et al. Single-site robotic cholecystectomy (SSRC) versus single-incision laparoscopic cholecystectomy (SILC): comparison of learning curves. First European experience. Surg Endosc 2012;26(6):1648–55.
8. Pietrabissa A, Sbrana F, Morelli L, et al. Overcoming the challenges of single-incision cholecystectomy with robotic single-site technology. Arch Surg 2012;147(8):709–14.
9. Buzad FA, Corne LM, Brown TC, et al. Single-site robotic cholecystectomy: efficiency and cost analysis. Int J Med Robot 2013;9(3):365–70.
10. Ayloo S, Choudhury N. Single-site robotic cholecystectomy. JSLS 2014;18(3). https://doi.org/10.4293/JSLS.2014.00266.
11. Vidovszky TJ, Carr AD, Farinholt GN, et al. Single-site robotic cholecystectomy in a broadly inclusive patient population: a prospective study. Ann Surg 2014; 260(1):134–41.
12. Uras C, Boler DE, Erguner I, et al. Robotic single port cholecystectomy (R-LESS-C): experience in 36 patients. Asian J Surg 2014;37(3):115–9.
13. Ayloo S, Roh Y, Choudhury N. Laparoscopic versus robot-assisted cholecystectomy: a retrospective cohort study. Int J Surg 2014;12(10):1077–81.
14. Svoboda S, Qaqish TR, Wilson A, et al. Robotic single-site cholecystectomy in the obese: outcomes from a single institution. Surg Obes Relat Dis 2015;11(4):882–5.

15. Chung PJ, Huang R, Policastro L, et al. Single-site robotic cholecystectomy at an inner-city academic center. JSLS 2015;19(3) [pii:e2015.00033].

16. Bibi S, Rahnemai-Azar AA, Coralic J, et al. single-site robotic cholecystectomy: the timeline of progress. World J Surg 2015;39(10):2386–91.

17. Gonzalez A, Murcia CH, Romero R, et al. A multicenter study of initial experience with single-incision robotic cholecystectomies (SIRC) demonstrating a high success rate in 465 cases. Surg Endosc 2016;30(7):2951–60.

18. Kudsi OY, Castellanos A, Kaza S, et al. Cosmesis, patient satisfaction, and quality of life after da Vinci Single-Site cholecystectomy and multiport laparoscopic cholecystectomy: short-term results from a prospective, multicenter, randomized, controlled trial. Surg Endosc 2017;31(8):3242–50.

19. Lee H, Lee DH, Kim H, et al. Single-incision robotic cholecystectomy: a special emphasis on utilization of transparent glove ports to overcome limitations of single-site port. Int J Med Robot 2017;13(3). https://doi.org/10.1002/rcs.

20. Pietrabissa A, Pugliese L, Vinci A, et al. Short-term outcomes of single-site robotic cholecystectomy versus four-port laparoscopic cholecystectomy: a prospective, randomized, double-blind trial. Surg Endosc 2016;30(7):3089–97.

21. Lim C, Bou Nassif G, Lahat E, et al. Single-incision robotic cholecystectomy is associated with a high rate of trocar-site infection. Int J Med Robot 2017;13(4). https://doi.org/10.1002/rcs.1856.

22. Su WL, Huang JW, Wang SN, et al. Comparison study of clinical outcomes between single-site robotic cholecystectomy and single incision laparoscopic cholecystectomy. Asian J Surg 2017;40(6):424–8.

23. Balachandran B, Hufford TA, Mustafa T, et al. A comparative study of outcomes between single-site robotic and multi-port laparoscopic cholecystectomy: an experience from a tertiary care center. World J Surg 2017;41(5):1246–53.

24. Strosberg DS, Nguyen MC, Muscarella P 2nd, et al. A retrospective comparison of robotic cholecystectomy versus laparoscopic cholecystectomy: operative outcomes and cost analysis. Surg Endosc 2017;31(3):1436–41.

25. Jang EJ, Roh YH, Kang CM, et al. single-port laparoscopic and robotic cholecystectomy in obesity (>25 kg/m(2)). JSLS 2019;23(2) [pii:e2019.00005].

26. Le Roy B, Fetche N, Buc E, et al. Feasibility prospective study of laparoscopic cholecystectomy with suprapubic approach. J Visc Surg 2016;153(5):327–31.

27. Bedeir K, Mann A, Youssef Y. Robotic single-site versus laparoscopic cholecystectomy: which is cheaper? a cost report and analysis. Surg Endosc 2016;30(1):267–72.

28. Magge D, Steve J, Novak S, et al. performing the difficult cholecystectomy using combined endoscopic and robotic techniques: how I do it. J Gastrointest Surg 2017;21(3):583–9.

29. Pitt SC, Jin LX, Hall BL, et al. Incidental gallbladder cancer at cholecystectomy: when should the surgeon be suspicious? Ann Surg 2014;260(1):128–33.

30. Konstantinidis IT, Deshpande V, Genevay M, et al. Trends in presentation and survival for gallbladder cancer during a period of more than 4 decades: a single-institution experience. Arch Surg 2009;144(5):441–7 [discussion: 447].

31. Kwon AH, Imamura A, Kitade H, et al. Unsuspected gallbladder cancer diagnosed during or after laparoscopic cholecystectomy. J Surg Oncol 2008;97(3):241–5.

32. Qadan M, Kingham TP. Technical Aspects of Gallbladder Cancer Surgery. Surg Clin North Am 2016;96(2):229–45.

33. Smith GC, Parks RW, Madhavan KK, et al. A 10-year experience in the management of gallbladder cancer. HPB (Oxford) 2003;5(3):159–66.

34. Zhao X, Li XY, Ji W. laparoscopic versus open treatment of gallbladder cancer: a systematic review and meta-analysis. J Minim Access Surg 2018;14(3):185–91.
35. Yoon YS, Han HS, Cho JY, et al. Is laparoscopy contraindicated for gallbladder cancer? a 10-year prospective cohort study. J Am Coll Surg 2015;221(4):847–53.
36. Liu QD, Chen JZ, Xu XY, et al. Incidence of port-site metastasis after undergoing robotic surgery for biliary malignancies. World J Gastroenterol 2012;18(40): 5695–701.
37. Chandarana M, Patkar S, Tamhankar A, et al. Robotic resections in hepatobiliary oncology - initial experience with Xi da Vinci system in India. Indian J Cancer 2017;54(1):52–5.
38. Araujo RLC, de Sanctis MA, Coelho TRV, et al. Robotic surgery as an alternative approach for reoperation of incidental gallbladder cancer. J Gastrointest Cancer 2019. https://doi.org/10.1007/s12029-019-00264-3.
39. Goja S, Singh MK, Soin AS. Robotics in hepatobiliary surgery-initial experience, first reported case series from India. Int J Surg Case Rep 2017;33:16–20.
40. Shen BY, Zhan Q, Deng XX, et al. Radical resection of gallbladder cancer: could it be robotic? Surg Endosc 2012;26(11):3245–50.
41. Sucandy I, Schlosser S, Bourdeau T, et al. Robotic hepatectomy for benign and malignant liver tumors. J Robot Surg 2019. [Epub ahead of print]. https://doi.org/ 10.1007/s11701-019-00935-0.
42. Helton WS, Ayloo S. Technical aspects of bile duct evaluation and exploration: an update. Surg Clin North Am 2019;99(2):259–82.
43. Benzie AL, Sucandy I, Spence J, et al. Robotic choledochoduodenostomy for benign distal common bile duct stricture: how we do it. J Robot Surg 2019; 13(6):713–6.
44. Almamar A, Alkhamesi NA, Davies WT, et al. Cost analysis of robot-assisted chol- edochotomy and common bile duct exploration as an option for complex chole- docholithiasis. Surg Endosc 2018;32(3):1223–7.
45. Roeyen G, Chapelle T, Ysebaert D. Robot-assisted choledochotomy: feasibility. Surg Endosc 2004;18(1):165–6.
46. Alkhamesi NA, Davies WT, Pinto RF, et al. Robot-assisted common bile duct exploration as an option for complex choledocholithiasis. Surg Endosc 2013; 27(1):263–6.
47. Gilbert A, Doussot A, Ortega-Deballon P, et al. Robot-assisted choledochoduo- denostomy: a safe and reproducible procedure for benign common bile duct obstruction. Dig Surg 2017;34(3):177–9.
48. Cpinoglio G. ICG fluorescence In: Kim KC, editor. In: Robotics in general surgery. New York: Springer; 2014. p. 461–76.
49. Connor S, Garden OJ. Bile duct injury in the era of laparoscopic cholecystectomy. Br J Surg 2006;93(2):158–68.
50. Hugh TB, Kelly MD, Mekisic A. Rouviere's sulcus: a useful landmark in laparo- scopic cholecystectomy. Br J Surg 1997;84(9):1253–4.
51. Ferzli G, Timoney M, Nazir S, et al. Importance of the node of Calot in gallbladder neck dissection: an important landmark in the standardized approach to the lapa- roscopic cholecystectomy. J Laparoendosc Adv Surg Tech A 2015;25(1):28–32.
52. Renz BW, Bosch F, Angele MK. Bile duct injury after cholecystectomy: surgical therapy. Visc Med 2017;33(3):184–90.
53. Pesce A, Latteri S, Barchitta M, et al. Near-infrared fluorescent cholangiography - real-time visualization of the biliary tree during elective laparoscopic cholecystec- tomy. HPB (Oxford) 2018;20(6):538–45.

54. Strasberg SM, Hertl M, Soper NJ. An analysis of the problem of biliary injury during laparoscopic cholecystectomy. J Am Coll Surg 1995;180(1):101–25.
55. Fletcher DR, Hobbs MS, Tan P, et al. Complications of cholecystectomy: risks of the laparoscopic approach and protective effects of operative cholangiography: a population-based study. Ann Surg 1999;229(4):449–57.
56. Cuendis-Velázquez A, Bada-Yllan O, Trejo-Avila M, et al. Robotic-assisted Roux-en-Y hepaticojejunostomy after bile duct injury. Langenbecks Arch Surg 2018; 403(1):53–9.
57. Cuendis-Velazquez A, Trejo-Avila M, Bada-Yllan O, et al. A new era of bile duct repair: robotic-assisted versus laparoscopic hepaticojejunostomy. J Gastrointest Surg 2019;23(3):451–9.
58. Giulianotti PC, Quadri P, Durgam S, et al. Reconstruction/repair of iatrogenic biliary injuries: is the robot offering a new option? short clinical report. Ann Surg 2018;267(1):e7–9.
59. Mercado MA. Comment on "reconstruction/repair of iatrogenic biliary injuries: is the robot offering a new option? short clinical report. Ann Surg 2019;269(4):e47.
60. Marino MV, Mirabella A, Guarrasi D, et al. Robotic-assisted repair of iatrogenic common bile duct injury after laparoscopic cholecystectomy: surgical technique and outcomes. Int J Med Robot 2019;15(3):e1992.
61. Yoneya S, Saito T, Komatsu Y, et al. Binding properties of indocyanine green in human blood. Invest Ophthalmol Vis Sci 1998;39(7):1286–90.
62. Spinoglio G, Bertani E, Borin S, et al. Green indocyanine fluorescence in robotic abdominal surgery. Updates Surg 2018;70(3):375–9.
63. Maker AV, Kunda N. A technique to define extrahepatic biliary anatomy using robotic near-infrared fluorescent cholangiography. J Gastrointest Surg 2017;21(11): 1961–2.
64. Gangemi A, Danilkowicz R, Elli FE, et al. Could ICG-aided robotic cholecystectomy reduce the rate of open conversion reported with laparoscopic approach? A head to head comparison of the largest single institution studies. J Robot Surg 2017;11(1):77–82.
65. Sharma S, Huang R, Hui S, et al. The utilization of fluorescent cholangiography during robotic cholecystectomy at an inner-city academic medical center. J Robot Surg 2018;12(3):481–5.

Robotic Pancreatic Surgery for Solid, Cystic, and Mixed Lesions

Alexander S. Rosemurgy, MD*, Sharona Ross, MD,
Kenneth Luberice, MD, Harrison Browning, MD,
Iswanto Sucandy, MD

KEYWORDS

- Robotic • Robotic surgery • Pancreatectomy • Pancreatic cancer

KEY POINTS

- The application of the robotic platform to complex abdominal surgery and the treatment of pancreatic cancer is safe and feasible.
- Proper operating room setup and port placement helps facilitate the robotic pancreatectomy.
- The robotic platform has secured a role in pancreaticoduodenectomy and distal pancreatectomy and splenectomy.
- Understanding the molecular profiling of pancreatic cancer tumorigenesis is essential for targeting strategies.
- Use of the robot for the surgical management of benign, premalignant, and malignant solid lesions, cystic lesions, and mixed lesions, and yields the same benefits as minimally invasive surgery.

INTRODUCTION

It was not until the early 2000s that a robotic approach was applied to pancreatic surgery. The robotic da Vinci Xi system (Intuitive Surgical, Sunnyvale, CA) has proved to be both safe and feasible.[1] As individual surgeon experience with robotic surgery increases and technology further improves, it is thought that a robotic approach to pancreatic surgery will significantly improve patient outcomes and, possibly, long-term survival.[2–4]

Digestive Health Institute, AdventHealth Tampa, 3000 Medical Park Drive, Suite 500, Tampa, FL 33613, USA
* Corresponding author.
E-mail address: arosemurgy@hotmail.com

Surg Clin N Am 100 (2020) 303–336
https://doi.org/10.1016/j.suc.2019.12.006
0039-6109/20/© 2020 Elsevier Inc. All rights reserved.

surgical.theclinics.com

Pancreatic Cancer Epidemiology

Pancreatic cancer is estimated to be the third leading cause of cancer death in the United States.[5–7] Most pancreatic cancers are diagnosed in patients older than 65 years of age; it is a near certainty that its incidence will increase with the aging demographics in the United States. At the time of diagnosis, a distinct minority of pancreatic cancers are deemed to be resectable.[2,6–8] The only potential cure to pancreatic cancer is complete surgical resection with adjunctive chemotherapy.[9] Thus, the 5-year survival rate for pancreatic cancer is approximately 6% worldwide.[5–8,10–13]

Although this article explains our practice's experience with robotic operations of the pancreas, we think that a thorough understanding of pancreatic cancer and its precursor lesions, as well as its molecular markers, is vital to understanding holistic care.

Tumor Markers

Many tumor-associated antigens have been studied in connection with pancreatic adenocarcinoma. It is important to have a preoperative measure to serve as a baseline value, because this will serve as context in following the response to neoadjuvant therapy, surgery, and adjuvant therapy. Common tumor markers associated with pancreatic cancer that should be measured include carcinoembryonic antigen (CEA), carbohydrate antigen 125 (CA 125), and carbohydrate antigen 19-9 (CA 19-9). The increase of serum levels of CA 19-9 can be nonspecific (eg, biliary obstruction) but can be of prognostic value, assist in determining the need for neoadjuvant therapy, and can be a marker of recurrence. It is now thought that a preoperative CA 19-9 level greater than 500 U/mL, in the absence of another explanation, is a prognostic marker of poor outcome.[14] In 1 prospective study, patients that had decreasing serial CA 19-9 serum levels and a postresection serum level of less than 180 U/mL had significantly longer median survival compared with patients with persistently increased CA 19-9 serum levels (hazard ratio, 3.53; $P<.0001$).[15,16] Continued postoperative measurements should be obtained before adjuvant chemotherapy and periodically during and after as part of a surveillance protocol. One caveat is that patients that are Lewis non-A and non-B do not produce CA 19-9.

Traditionally, CA 125 has been the biomarker most useful in surveillance of ovarian cancer and colorectal adenocarcinoma. However, in a recent meta-analysis, CA 125 with CA 19-9 serum levels was found to significantly increase the sensitivity and specificity of identifying pancreatic cancer recurrence relative to either biomarker alone. It has also been determined that CA 125 level becomes abnormally high in patients developing postoperative distant metastasis. Although neither of these biomarkers, alone or together, is yet able to diagnose pancreatic cancer, they are becoming increasingly valuable in postoperative surveillance[14] (Fig. 1A, B).

Pancreatic Exocrine Neoplasms, Solid Tumors

When people talk about pancreatic cancer, they are talking about ductal or exocrine adenocarcinoma of the pancreas, because 85% of pancreatic cancers are of the ductal adenocarcinoma type.[2,6,8,16] Two-thirds of these neoplasms occur in the head or uncinate process of the pancreas. The remaining neoplasms are in the body (15%), tail (10%), or diffusely dispersed throughout the pancreatic gland (multifocal).[2,11,17] It is important to acknowledge other types of pancreatic tumors because

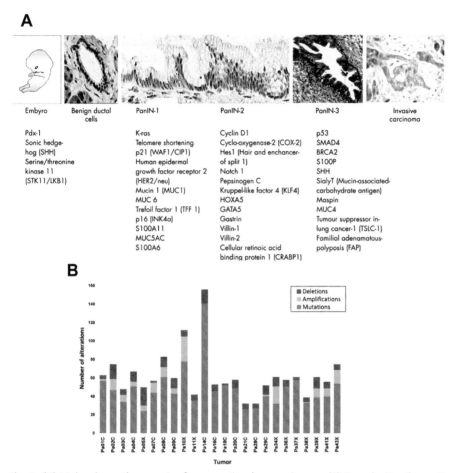

Fig. 1. (A) Molecular pathogenesis of pancreatic adenocarcinoma. (B) Complexity of genetic mutations in pancreatic tumors. There are 20,661 genes and an average of 63 alterations per patient, mostly point mutations. (From [A] Ghaneh P, Costello E, Neoptolemos JP. Biology and management of pancreatic cancer. Gut. 2007; 58(8):1134-1152; and [B] Jones S, Zhang X, Parsons DW, et al. Core signaling pathways in human pancreatic cancers revealed by global genomic analyses. Science. 2008;321(5897): 1801-1806; with permission.)

their unique characteristics and genetics can alter their presentation and management.

Pancreatic intraepithelial neoplasia (PanIN) is a term that is used to describe premalignant lesions with varying degrees of cellular atypia. These lesions have been classified as 1A, 1B, 2, and 3 based on the extent of atypia, as well as identified genetic mutations. The predominant mutation detected in 75% to 90% of all pancreatic carcinoma specimens is K-Ras (some clinicians think it cannot be a pancreatic cancer without a K-Ras mutation). K-Ras mutations cause constitutive activation and subsequent downstream signaling for cell proliferation. Early PanIN-1 specimens show this mutation before any architectural atypia, suggesting that it occurs early in the development of carcinoma. In metastatic colorectal cancer and non–small cell lung cancer, K-Ras mutations are associated with resistance to epidermal growth factor receptor–based monoclonal antibodies (eg, panitumumab and cetuximab). Other mutations seen in later stages are Tp53, p16/CDKN2A, and Mucin 1, and others (see **Fig. 1**).

Other carcinoma types, such as adenosquamous carcinoma and acinar cell carcinoma, are extremely rare, constituting about 1% of pancreatic malignancies. Although it is beneficial to understand they exist, their management is much the same as ductal adenocarcinoma, as is their prognosis.

Ampullary neoplasms may be premalignant (adenoma) or malignant (carcinoma). These neoplasms arise from within the ampulla of Vater and, as such, may be of intestinal and/or pancreaticobiliary cell origin. These neoplasms carry a better prognosis than pancreatic ductal adenocarcinoma, with a 10-year survival rate of 35%, and they are mentioned only because they are often confused for pancreatic adenocarcinomas. These cancers have a different tumor biology and tend to present earlier because of obstructive symptoms. Neoplastic tumors arising in the ampulla are more likely to obstruct the pancreatic and biliary outflow, resulting in clinically apparent symptoms leading to their earlier diagnosis. Tumors of the ampulla of Vater with biopsies negative for malignancy but positive for p53 are likely to be carcinomas. These lesions should be removed operatively, although lesions less than 2 cm with no duodenal invasion may be removed via endoscopic excision, following American Gastroenterological Association guidelines.[8]

When computed tomography (CT) findings are inconclusive or a mass is not definitively seen, endoscopic ultrasonography (EUS) with a fine-needle aspiration/biopsy (FNA) may be appropriate. EUS-FNA is 80% to 90% sensitive and nearly 100% specific for the diagnosis of pancreatic malignancy.[18] An engaged cytopathologist is of great aid. In large solid pancreatic tumors, or tumors deemed unresectable, EUS-FNA is undertaken to provide certainty of diagnosis before administering chemotherapy. In small (<15 mm diameter) solid pancreatic tumors, or tumors deemed resectable, the benefit of EUS-FNA preoperatively versus resection without biopsy-confirmed diagnosis is less straightforward; not all patients require a preoperative EUS with or without FNA. Although relatively safe with a complication rate of less than 2%, EUS can be complicated by bleeding, pancreatitis, and a plethora of other, albeit infrequent, complications.[18] There is minimal to no evidence of pancreatic tumor seeding occurring during EUS-FNA, unlike percutaneous biopsy, which is indicated only in patients deemed to be unresectable. Considering the safety of EUS-FNA, some clinicians think that all small (<15 mm diameter) solid pancreatic tumors should be biopsied using EUS-FNA before surgical resection because the reported incidence of disorders other than adenocarcinoma, such as neuroendocrine tumors, is as high as 5% to 13%.[18] In a recent multicenter retrospective study, 60% of small solid pancreatic lesions were diagnosed as lesions other than adenocarcinoma on final pathology, such as autoimmune pancreatitis and pancreatic neuroendocrine tumors.[19]

Pancreatic Exocrine Neoplasms, Cystic/Mixed Tumors

Incidental discovery of fluid-filled pancreatic lesions is becoming far more common with the increased usage of CT and MRI modalities. Incidental findings during imaging of the chest, abdomen, and/or pelvis of a cystic pancreatic lesion occur in 2.2% of CT examinations and 19.6% of MRI examinations[20,21]; 70% of these lesions are asymptomatic and most are benign or of very low malignant potential. However, all of these lesions warrant sufficient identification because approximately half have no malignant potential, whereas the malignant potential of some types of lesions is as high as 68%.[20,22] A symptomatic lesion dictates surgical intervention and resection.

MRI/magnetic resonance cholangiopancreatography has benefit compared with CT for cystic pancreatic lesions by providing superior characterization of cyst morphology, including septa and nodular components. However, CT offers benefits of low cost, high availability, and clinician familiarity. EUS can be used for characterization of cystic pancreatic lesions with the benefit of sampling of cystic fluid and biopsy/FNA, when needed.

Pancreatic pseudocysts are the most commonly found cystic lesions in the pancreas. These pseudocysts lack an epithelial lining and are, therefore, not true cysts and are nonneoplastic. They most commonly occur as a complication of acute pancreatitis, chronic pancreatitis (especially caused by alcohol), or a disrupted pancreatic duct. EUS can be used to characterize these lesions through imaging characteristics and, most particularly, characterization of contained fluid, which should be high in amylase and low in CEA (generally <196U/mL). The management of these lesions, when symptomatic, involves drainage of the fluid into the gastrointestinal lumen via endoscopic procedure, if possible, or operative intervention, given persistence and notable size.

Serous cystic neoplasms (SCNs) account for approximately one-third of all pancreatic cystic lesions and are neoplastic lesions of low-grade malignant potential, with less than 1% undergoing malignant change.[16,23] They most commonly occur after the sixth to seventh decades of life, with 80% occurring in women. They are most commonly located in the head of the pancreas (40%), followed by the body (34%) and tail (26%). Most are asymptomatic, although large (>4 cm) serous cysts may cause mass effect resulting in abdominal pain, a bloating sensation, early satiety, and possibly jaundice.[8,20,21] Imaging of pancreatic serous cystic neoplasms classically has a well-circumscribed, lobulated, and honeycombed appearance. A central stellate, fibrous, and calcified scar is highly specific for serous cysts but is only present in about 30% of patients.[20,21] Serous cysts, also called microcystic neoplasms, can appear similar to pseudocysts that are loculated. EUS-FNA fluid analysis showing fluid amylase level less than 250 U/L (with a low CEA level) can help differentiate serous cysts from pseudocysts.[21] Asymptomatic cysts can typically be left alone with regular follow-up, although cysts larger than 7 cm should be removed because of the increased risk of malignancy. Other risk factors for malignancy and indications for extirpation include rapid growth in diameter (>5 mm/y on average) and the symptoms caused by the SCN. Of note, SCNs are associated with inactivation of the von Hippel-Lindau (VHL) gene, VHL disease, and other sporadic tumors, including pancreatic neuroendocrine tumors.[20,23]

Mucinous cystic neoplasms (MCNs) represent a spectrum of lesions, including low-grade neoplastic mucinous cystadenomas (72% of MCNs), mucinous cystic tumors of intermediate malignant potential (11% of MCNs), mucinous cystic tumors with carcinoma in situ (6% of MCNs), and mucinous cystadenocarcinomas (12% of MCNs).[20] As a group, these represent 45% of all pancreatic cystic neoplasms. MCNs occur more often in women, and more commonly during the fourth to fifth decades of life. They are most commonly located in the pancreatic tail (72%), followed by the body (13%), and least commonly the head (6%).[20] Diagnosis of an MCN is most commonly made with abdominal CT followed by EUS-FNA. They are most commonly macrocystic, unilocular lesions (80%). On presentation, MCNs are typically large, with an average diameter of 6to 11 cm. Imaging studies vary from innocuous-appearing lesions with smooth borders to more ominous-appearing lesions with insidious margins, mural nodules, and pancreatic duct dilatation. Peripheral calcifications are another sign of malignant transformation. Chance of malignancy is best determined by morphologic changes such as cyst size or rapid increases in cyst size, pancreatic duct dilation, and intramural nodules. Focal wall thickening greater than 3 mm, cyst size greater than 3 cm, and pancreatic duct dilatation (particularly focal and larger than 8 mm) are all associated with higher likelihood of the presence of adenocarcinoma and therefore warrant resection.[24] The presence of ovarian-type stroma on biopsy and fluid analysis showing low amylase level and increased CEA level (>196 U/mL) help confirm the diagnosis.[25] However, biopsy and fluid analysis cannot exclude the presence of malignancy within the lesion, or any cystic lesions of the pancreas.[8,20] Because of the risk of malignancy of these lesions, it is recommended that they be resected once identified, unless they are very small and have been stable on repeated imaging. It is important that, during resection, the cystic capsule is not violated to prevent seeding of the surrounding tissue.[8,20,24] Patients with benign-appearing cystic and small (<2–3 cm) masses or those who are not operative candidates (eg, extreme cardiopulmonary issues) may opt for surveillance rather than resection. Appropriate surveillance programs should rely on repeated imaging, with only infrequent EUS undertaken if anticipating a change in management.

Solid pseudopapillary neoplasms (SPNs) of the pancreas are unique pancreatic neoplasms devoid histologically of all pancreatic exocrine and endocrine cells.[20] SPNs account for about 9% of all pancreatic cystic neoplasms and most commonly occur in women less than the age of 40 years. This age and gender predilection is thought to be caused by the progesterone receptor presence and estrogen receptor presence in these neoplasms. Interestingly, there is a loose association with hepatitis B and C Virus, although the viral role in tumorigenesis is not known.[26] Most SPNs are slow-growing, but relentless, neoplastic lesions of very-low-grade malignant potential. Imaging of these lesions denotes a heterogeneous appearance, with solid, papillary, and cystic areas. The cystic areas denote internal hemorrhage and central necrosis. Calcifications can be seen diffusely in 30%. Although CT appearance is usually enough to make the diagnosis, MRI appearance accentuates the cystic nature of the tumor and gives a pathognomonic appearance. Management of these lesions is by resection, even though malignancy rates are low, occurring in just 10% to 15%. Without resection, the tumor masses just grow and grow. It is important to resect with clear margins and no capsule violation to ensure cure, which should be expected.[26]

Intraductal papillary mucinous neoplasms (IPMNs) are neoplastic tumors containing intraductal epithelial cells that produce mucin. Primarily located within the head or uncinate process of the pancreas, IPMNs are divided by anatomic location, size, involvement with the pancreatic ductal system, and tumor characteristics. Lesions commonly involve the main pancreatic duct (MD-IPMN), branch pancreatic duct (BD-IPMN), or a combination of the two (MT-IPMN), although the latter type of IPMN is considered less frequently to be a distinct entity, and tumors of this type are increasingly considered to be BD-IPMN. MD-IPMNs are more likely to be malignant (62% malignant), given a notable size (>2 cm), than BD-IPMN (6%–46% malignant),[8] but all BD-IPMN lesions are stratified based on presentation of worrisome features and high-risk stigmata.[27] The revised Fukuoka guidelines recommend the Sendai guidelines, which advocated resection of BD-IPMNs with at least 1 of 5 criteria for suspected malignancy (the Sendai criteria), and resection of all MD-IPMNs, just as did the Sendai guidelines.[27]

For BD-IPMNs there are considerations for operative intervention (noted later): the presence of positive pancreatic juice cytology (high CEA and low amylase levels), the presence of mural nodules, cyst size greater than 3 cm, dilatation of the main pancreatic duct (to >5 mm), and notable abdominal pain. The importance of the size criterion is controversial, because 13% to 22% of resected BD-IPMNs greater than 3 cm without mural nodules are malignant; to us, this incidence of cancer seems high. To avoid unnecessary operative intervention, the Fukuoka guidelines moved the size criterion from high-risk stigmata to a category of worrisome features.

For Branch Pancreatic Duct Intraductal Papillary Mucinous Neoplasm

High-risk stigmata

- Obstructive jaundice in a patient with a cystic lesion of the head of the pancreas.
- Enhancing mural nodule larger than 5 mm.
- Main pancreatic duct dilatation greater than 10 mm (best predictor of high-grade dysplasia or invasion[28]).

Worrisome features

- Pancreatitis.
- Cyst size larger than 3 cm.
- Thickened, enhancing cyst walls.
- Nonenhancing mural nodule less than 5 mm.
- Main pancreatic duct diameter 5 to 9 mm.
- Abrupt change in main pancreatic duct caliber with distal pancreatic parenchymal atrophy.
- Lymphadenopathy.
- Increased serum level of CA 19-9.
- Cyst growth rate greater than 5 mm in 2 years.

The histologic subclassification of IPMNs into gastric, intestinal, pancreaticobiliary, and oncocytic types has been introduced in the Fukuoka guidelines. Most BD-IPMNs were of gastric type, whereas most MD-IPMNs were of intestinal type. The prognosis of BD-IPMNs is better than with MD-IPMNs, and, thereby, the histologic subtypes are correlated with the prognosis.

It is currently recommended that all MD-IPMNs be resected because of the high risk of malignancy. BD-IPMN resections are less straightforward, although current recommendations state that a BD-IPMN greater than 3 cm and BD-IPMN less than 3 cm with any of the high-risk stigmata noted earlier should undergo resection. Those without high-risk stigmata and few to no worrisome features need to have the risk-benefit weighed before pancreatic resection of the IPMN, whereas those with 2 or more of the worrisome features should be strongly encouraged to undergo operative resection,[29] despite considerations of increased risk of perioperative morbidity and mortality in patients undergoing operations for IPMN compared with those for ductal adenocarcinoma.[27,29] As stated, overall, patients with invasive IPMNs have a favorable prognosis compared with those with ductal adenocarcinoma because of the less aggressive biological nature of the disease.[30]

Following resection of an IPMN, patients should undergo long-term surveillance for recurrent disease as well as additional new lesions forming within the pancreatic remnant, because of a phenomenon known as the field (multicentric) cancerization and clonality defect; there is a field defect associated with IPMN. Pancreatic cancers are generally accepted as being the stepwise progression from precursor lesions, with IPMN being a type of precursor lesion. However, unique to IPMN is the discovery that a single IPMN lesion is the result of the coalescence of multiple primary neoplastic lesions caused by different mutations.[31] Therefore, IPMNs can be regarded as poly-clonal and/or oligoclonal because a single tumor is composed of multiple, independently derived, monoclonal cell populations. The gene most commonly associated with neoplastic mutation is K-Ras, resulting in ductal hyperplasia. This mutation had its highest prevalence in patients with a history of pancreatic ductal adenocarcinoma or chronic pancreatitis. This mutation is evident even in a normal-appearing pancreas, suggesting it is a very early mutation in the spectrum of pancreatic cancer. K-Ras mutations are also associated with inactivation of the p16 tumor-suppressor gene.[31] These series of mutations and polyclonality help to explain the high rate of recurrence after resection (20%),[17] which significantly increases with higher levels of cell dysplasia. The presence of an IPMN and its field defect also increases the risk of the entire pancreas being prone to accumulation of distinct genetic mutations that will eventually evolve into cancer.[17] For patients with BD-IPMN, pancreatic ductal adenocarcinoma is found distal to and distinct from the primary lesion in 3% to 9% of patients.[32]

OPERATIVE CONSIDERATIONS
Pancreatic Cancer Diagnosis

There are no recommendations for screening for pancreatic neoplasms in the general population, and the impact of screening on patients considered high risk remains unclear.[2,6–8,16] As such, most pancreatic neoplasms (up to 95%[18]) are diagnosed either incidentally on imaging obtained for another reason or in response to the onset of suspicious clinical signs and symptoms. Signs and symptoms that increase suspicion for underlying malignancy include, but are not limited to, dull epigastric abdominal pain, weight loss, jaundice, steatorrhea, silver-colored stool (Thomas sign), dyspepsia, early satiety, nausea, migratory thrombophlebitis (Trousseau sign of malignancy), and painless and palpable gallbladder (Courvoisier sign). Other concerning findings include the sudden onset of type 2 diabetes mellitus (DMT2) and/or pancreatitis in people older than 55 years and the sudden inability to control previously controlled DMT2.[2,6,16] These largely nonspecific symptoms and signs denote the insidious nature of pancreatic cancer, thus explaining why most diagnosed cancers are advanced and unresectable at the time of diagnosis.

Initial evaluation should begin with triphasic helical CT with cross-sectional imaging with 1-mm thin slices, also known as pancreatic protocol CT.[16] CT scan is the preferred initial imaging modality because of its ability to reliably differentiate between normal contrast-enhanced parenchyma and the hypodense lesion of adenocarcinoma, as well as to stage the cancer and assess for resectability with 70% to 85% specificity.[16] CT scanning undertaken with the pancreatic protocol clearly shows the important vasculature, adjacent organs, regional lymph node basins, and common places for distant metastases (eg, the liver).

Staging at Diagnosis

Initial staging is determined preoperatively by imaging studies, including EUS.[8]

- Ten percent are diagnosed with a localized stage before any extension beyond primary site and without invasion or encasement of regional blood vessels (eg, portal vein).
- Twenty-nine percent are diagnosed with localized disease after spread to regional lymph nodes or beyond the primary site and, thus, are inoperable at this time.
- Fifty-two percent are diagnosed with distant metastasis.

Final postoperative staging is determined once final pathology is able to examine the specimen.

Criteria for Operative Resectability/Unresectability

Unresectable disease

- Liver metastasis (any size)/distant metastasis[8,11,16]
- Involvement of greater than 180° of the celiac axis, hepatic artery, or superior mesenteric artery (SMA)
- Celiac lymph node involvement[a]
- Hepatic hilar lymph node involvement[a]
- Peritoneal implants
- Ascites with positive peritoneal cytology[b]
- Distant metastasis
- Arterial vascular encasement

Borderline Resectable Disease

- Abutment of less than 180° of the circumference of the SMA, celiac axis, or hepatic artery[13]
- Only a short segment of venous occlusion that can be reconstructed by vascular repair or grafting (eg, left renal vein)

Conversion from a Robotic Operation to an Open Approach

Conversion from robotic to open approach should not be viewed as a failure, but good judgment. In high-volume centers, experienced surgeons generally have few conversions, although the optimal frequency of conversions has not been established.[34] Appropriate and thorough preoperative work-up and planning help to prevent most intraoperative surprises. Patient factors that promote poor candidacy for a robotic approach include obesity, previous intra-abdominal operations (often with mesh), advanced cancers, major vascular involvement, and poor overall health; these are also factors that deter open operations.

Our intraoperative indications for conversion from robotic to open approach include[34]:

- Failure to progress for greater than 15 minutes for any reason (most common).
- Significant intraoperative bleeding or uncontrolled bleeding, real or potential.
- Intolerance to carbon dioxide pneumoperitoneum.
- Unanticipated need for major vascular resection and reconstruction.
- Excessive difficulties to complete safe biliary, pancreatic, or enteral reconstructions.

---

[a] Locally advanced disease and lymph node involvement is not always a contraindication for resection and is subject to surgeon judgment. Invasion of the duodenum and/or distal stomach can be resected with a pancreaticoduodenectomy with concomitant distal gastrectomy or distal pancreatectomy with concomitant gastric resection, as needed. Peripancreatic lymph nodes and lymph nodes along the porta hepatis can be swept down and resected with the pancreatic specimen. However, metastatic disease to lymph nodes (ie, N1) portends a very poor prognosis.

[b] Positive peritoneal cytology is a contraindication to resection based on guidelines published by the National Comprehensive Cancer Network (NCCN) as an equivalent finding of stage IV distant metastasis regardless of other findings. Patients with positive peritoneal cytology had significantly greater tumor burden and a dismal prognosis with median survival of only 6 weeks. Therefore, peritoneal washings showing positive cytology equates to M1 disease, and induction of chemotherapy should not be delayed.[33]

It is appropriate to acknowledge that there is always a reason why a robotic operation is converted to open; what might be converted in one center might not in another. This acknowledgment conveys some sense that the reason for conversion will affect outcomes after the conversion and in the postoperative period and beyond. Our institution found that operative mortality was much higher following conversion, reflecting the foreboding impact of factors leading to conversion (eg, large tumor/advanced T-status tumor). Operations completed robotically yield a mortality less than 3%. Operations converted to open led to a mortality that was nearly 1 in 4.[34]

Perioperative Planning

Management of pancreatic cancer relies heavily on the presence of symptoms, location of the neoplasm, its imaging characteristics, histology (if biopsy is obtained), estimated cancer stage, genomic profile (with tissue), and the operative candidacy of the patient. The authors follow an enhanced recovery after surgery (ERAS) protocol for all robotic pancreatectomies. Patients are given preoperative education on the protocol by a team member in our clinic after a decision to operate is made. The multidisciplinary team of surgeons, physician extenders, perioperative nursing staff, residents, fellows, and anesthesiologists (and their certified registered nurse anesthetists) are all familiar with the ERAS protocol. Preoperatively, the patient agrees to smoking/alcohol cessation, weight loss as needed, diet, and exercise regimen (increasing exercise by 10% per day), diabetes education classes, targeted use of incentive spirometry, and nutritional optimization with Impact Advanced Recovery (Nestle HealthCare Nutrition, Florham Park, NJ), (a nutritional drink taken 3 times a day for 5 days and ending the night before the operation to boost their immune system and nutritional status).

In addition, patients meet with members of the anesthesiology team to discuss their perioperative analgesia management plan (ie, intrathecal injection of 10 mL of Duramorph before induction, oral Celebrex/gabapentin, and intravenous [IV] Tylenol preoperatively and postoperatively). Twelve milligrams of alvimopan is administered 30 minutes to 5 hours preoperatively and followed by 12 mg twice daily beginning postoperative day (POD) 1 for 7 days, as needed (maximum total treatment: 15 doses [180 mg total]), for perioperative nausea and vomiting control. It is our opinion that preoperative education (by all members of the multidisciplinary team) of the patient on what to expect has led to early recovery and increased patient satisfaction. With this ERAS plan, we have been able to reduce our length of stay after robotic pancreatectomy to 5 days but are nearing a median of 4 days.

Operating Room Setup

The patient is placed supine on the operating table. Compression stockings and sequential compression devices are used in all patients to prevent deep vein thrombosis. After endotracheal intubation, general anesthesia is established, and then a nasogastric tube and a Foley catheter are placed. Both arms are extended with all pressure points padded for patient safety and comfort. The patient's abdomen is widely prepped with alcohol before a Betadine-impregnated plastic drape is applied. The operating room table is then positioned in 9° to 12° reverse Trendelenburg position with a slight left lateral tilt (4°). The da Vinci Xi robotic system is docked with the boom coming over the patient's right shoulder. The bedside surgeon stands on the patient's right and the scrub tech stands to the patient's left. This arrangement enables easy access to the robotic arms for instrument exchanges. Two surgeon consoles (dual consoles) are placed in such a way that the surgeon at the console has direct visualization of the patient. We use dual consoles for the education and training of fellows and residents. Preoperative imaging studies are displayed on a monitor and placed next to the surgeon's console for easy reference by all team members during the operation.

OPERATIVE STEPS: DISTAL PANCREATECTOMY WITH SPLENECTOMY
Step 1. Operating Room Setup and Port Placement

Before making any incisions, approximately 5 to 8 mL of 0.25% Marcaine (AstraZeneca, Wilmington, DE) with epinephrine (1:1000) is injected into the umbilicus and all robotic port sites for pain relief/prevention. We believe this helps decrease postoperative pain. The abdomen is entered via an 8-mm incision in the umbilicus, and pneumoperitoneum is established (up to 15 mm Hg). After diagnostic laparoscopy, without notable findings, three 8-mm robotic trocars, an Advanced Access Gelpoint (Applied Medical, Rancho Santo Margarita, CA), and one 5-mm AirSeal Access Port (ConMed Inc, Utica, NY) are placed under laparoscopic visualization (**Fig. 2**). The placement site for each trocar is very important. The liver retractor is placed through the right upper quadrant AirSeal port and is secured to the surgical drape using Kocher clamps. The da Vinci Xi robotic system is brought over the patient's right shoulder and is docked with the bed in the reverse Trendelenburg position, as mentioned, with a slight left lateral tilt.

Trocar placement

- At the umbilicus: 8-mm trocar for the robotic camera (**Fig. 3**). Do not make this too big or trocar/camera migration and/or loss of pneumoperitoneum will occur.

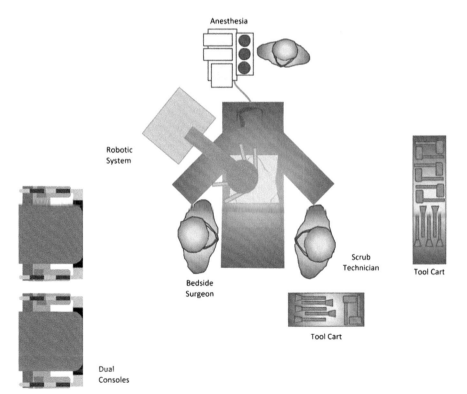

Fig. 2. Operating room setup.

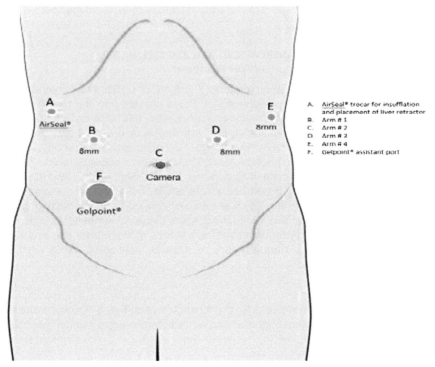

Fig. 3. Distal pancreatectomy with splenectomy port placement. (*Courtesy of* S. Ross, MD, Tampa, FL.)

- Just to the right of the right midclavicular line at the level of the umbilicus: 8-mm robotic trocar (for arm 1).
- Midway between these 2 trocars and caudal to the umbilicus: advanced Access Gelpoint (for bedside surgeon and specimen extraction).
- At the left midclavicular line at the level of the umbilicus: 12-mm robotic trocar (for arm 3; 12 mm to accommodate the robotic stapler).
- At the left anterior axillary line, cephalad to the umbilicus: 8-mm robotic trocar (for arm 4).
- At the right anterior axillary line at the costal margin: 5-mm AirSeal port (for insufflation and a liver retractor).

Step 2. Exposure of the Pancreas Body and Tail

Robotic arm 1: fenestrated bipolar device.
  Robotic arm 2: camera.
  Robotic arm 3: vessel sealer.
  Robotic arm 4: atraumatic bowel grasper.
  The splenic flexure is first mobilized widely (**Fig. 4**) from the mid–transverse colon to the proximal descending colon. Next, the gastrocolic omentum is divided in stellate fashion along the greater curvature of the stomach (**Fig. 5**). Short gastric vessels and their associated mesentery are divided, generally with an extended vessel sealer or cautery (**Fig. 6**). With the stomach fully mobilized, we reposition the liver retractor to retract both the left lobe of the liver and the stomach together, lifting the stomach to

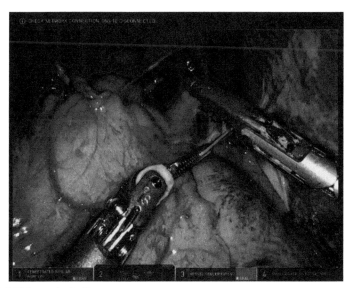

Fig. 4. Mobilizing splenic flexure.

expose the celiac trunk and the body and tail of the pancreas (**Figs. 7** and **8**). The dissection is undertaken to localize the celiac trunk and its branches, as needed.

Step 3. Mobilization of the Pancreas

Robotic arm 1: fenestrated bipolar device.
   Robotic arm 2: camera.
   Robotic arm 3: vessel sealer (alternating with hook cautery).
   Robotic arm 4: atraumatic bowel grasper.

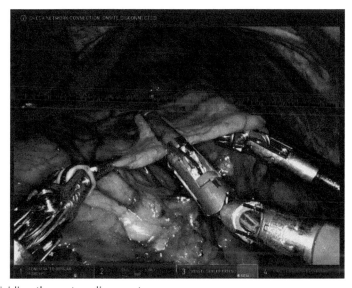

Fig. 5. Dividing the gastrocolic omentum.

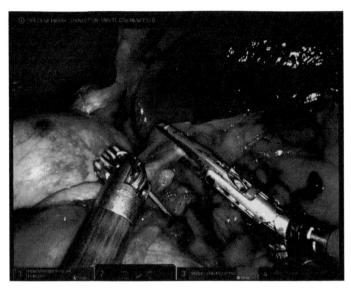

Fig. 6. Ligating the short gastric arteries.

With the gastrocolic omentum opened and the stomach reflected in the cephalad direction by the liver retractor, the pancreas is brought into view. The inferior border of the pancreas is identified and dissected using hook cautery or vessel sealer. The dissection is carried to the caudal tip of the spleen. We begin to lift the pancreas up (ventral) off the more dorsal tissues. This dissection is usually avascular but is more difficult with larger tumors. If the operation is being undertaken for neoplasm, we use intraoperative ultrasonography frequently to locate the lesion, ensuring that no areas of transection include tumor (**Fig. 9**).

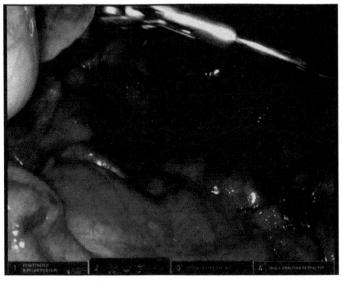

Fig. 7. Retracting stomach and liver.

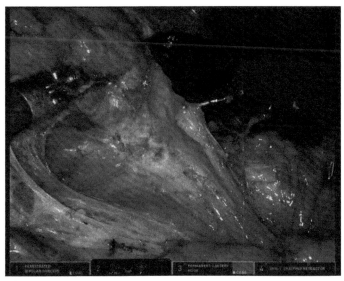

Fig. 8. Mobilizing the pancreas.

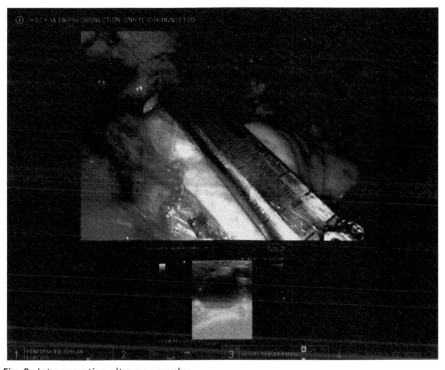

Fig. 9. Intraoperative ultrasonography.

Step 4. Pancreatectomy: Dividing the Pancreas

Robotic arm 1: fenestrated bipolar device (alternating with a vessel sealer).
  Robotic arm 2: camera.
  Robotic arm 3: vessel sealer (alternating with hook cautery)/robotic stapler.
  Robotic arm 4: atraumatic bowel grasper.
  The dissection is carried along the caudal edge of the pancreas, lifting it ventrally. This dissection is carried to patient's right, as needed, which allows the identification of the superior mesenteric vein posteriorly if the dissection is carried far enough to the patient's right. For body tumors, transection may need to be ventral to the portal vein. That being the case, the common hepatic artery is then identified to avoid injury. The pancreas is divided with a robotic stapler (**Fig. 10**). The dissection is carried along the common hepatic artery heading toward the celiac trunk. We then reflect (lift and displace the pancreas caudally) the body and tail of the pancreas away to reveal the splenic artery and vein, each of which are divided. The splenic vein is divided with a stapler and the splenic artery may be controlled with clips or a stapler. In some situations, both the splenic artery and/or vein can be ligated simultaneously with a vascular stapler. This dissection is carried out to the tail of the pancreas. The spleen is fully mobilized, in part by dividing the lienorenal ligament using electrocautery, providing full mobilization of the spleen. The spleen is never handled until late in the operation, after splenic artery division, to avoid bleeding while the operation is completed.

Step 5. Oversewing Pancreatic Transection Staple Line

The remnant edge of the pancreas is oversewn with needle holders in arms 1 and 3. The authors used 150-mm (6-inch) 3-0 V-Loc suture to oversew the staple line, in a cephalad toward caudal direction (**Fig. 11**). It is important not to fracture the pancreas parenchyma by applying excess force on the needle holders. The pancreatic staple line is then buried onto the retroperitoneal adipose tissue to provide further buttress.

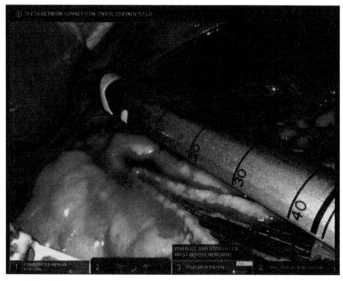

Fig. 10. Transecting the pancreas.

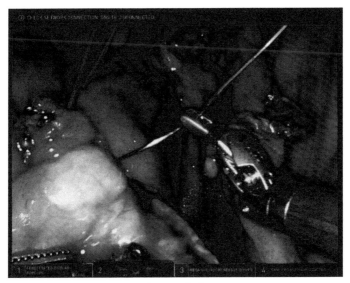

Fig. 11. Oversewing pancreatic transection staple line.

Step 6. Specimen Removal

The specimen, including body and tail of the pancreas as well as the spleen, is removed via an Endo Catch bag through the gel port (**Fig. 12**). An omental pedicle flap and/or a mobilized falciform ligament flap are wrapped around any remaining pancreatic tissue in the area of the celiac trunk to protect the tissues and minimize risk of pancreatic leak.

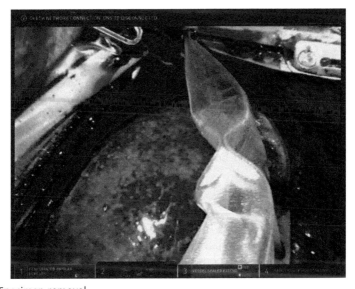

Fig. 12. Specimen removal.

Step 7. Placement of Closed Suction Drain and Closure

At this point, the robot can be undocked. The diaphragm is irrigated liberally with a solution of 7.5 mL of 0.25% Marcaine in 250 mL of normal saline to minimize postoperative pain. We place a closed-suction 10-French Jackson-Pratt (JP) drain along the transection line of remaining pancreas, when indicated by a thick gland or a soft gland. The drain is brought out through the anterior axillary line incision. All port site incisions are injected with 20 mL of Exparel (Pacira Pharmaceuticals, Parsippany, NJ) in 30 mL of normal saline before closure to further minimize postoperative pain. All incisions are closed along anatomic layers. The fascia is closed with absorbable monofilament sutures, whereas the skin is reapproximated with interrupted 3-0 absorbable sutures. All incision sites are covered by Steri-Strips and sterile silver dressings and covered by a watertight Tegaderm dressing. This process allows patients to shower at home after discharge for the 5 to 7 days postoperatively before follow-up in clinic.

DISTAL PANCREATECTOMY WITH SPLENIC PRESERVATION

Distal pancreatectomy with concomitant splenectomy is mandatory in the presence of malignancy. However, when benign or, more likely, low-grade neoplastic lesions are being resected, it may be possible to preserve the spleen. In our practice, we seldom preserve the spleen because almost all distal pancreatectomies are undertaken for cancer and there is no compelling evidence that supports preservation of the spleen. Our opinion is that the possibility of increased risk, cost, and mean blood loss in the operating room do not justify the presumed benefit of spleen preservation.[35] However, some pancreatic neuroendocrine tumors can be resected with splenic preservation.

Kimura Technique

The most common approach to spleen preservation in the setting of a distal pancreatectomy is the Kimura technique.[36] This technique completely preserves the spleen, splenic vessels, and splenic lymph nodes. Although technically challenging, the preservation of native vasculature minimizes the risk of immediate postoperative complications involving the spleen, although splenic vein thrombosis, splenic infarct, and splenic abscess remain concerns.

Warshaw Technique

The Warshaw technique involves segmental resection of both the splenic artery and vein while preserving the spleen. This technique requires preservation of the short gastric vessels. Although blood flow in the spleen is segmental, preservation of the short gastric vessels and the gastroepiploic arcade and left gastroepiploic vessels, if possible, should result in splenic viability and function. There is a higher risk of splenic infarct in this technique compared with the Kimura technique, especially in patients with splenomegaly, making this a relative contraindication. There is also a risk of developing gastric varices (ie, left-sided portal hypertension) and their associated risk of bleeding.[37]

Distal Pancreatectomy with Celiac Axis Resection (Modified Appleby Technique)

The Appleby technique was originally described for gastric carcinoma that involved celiac axis resection and complete gastric resection. However, the modified version used for pancreatic cancer is the combination of distal pancreatectomy, splenectomy, and resection of the celiac axis and common hepatic artery while preserving the proper hepatic artery and gastroduodenal artery, through which collateral flow from the SMA perfuses the liver.[38] Some surgeons elect to embolize the common hepatic artery before this operation to cause an enhancement of flow through the gastroduodenal artery and the proper hepatic artery.[39] Associated postoperative complications for this procedure include gastric ischemia, hepatic ischemia, pancreatitis, pancreatic insufficiency, and mesenteric ischemia (thrombotic or embolic).

OPERATIVE STEPS: PYLORUS-PRESERVING PANCREATICODUODENECTOMY
Step 1. Operating Room Setup and Port Placement

Before making the incision, approximately 5 to8 mL of 0.25% Marcaine (AstraZeneca, Wilmington, DE) with epinephrine (1:1000) is injected into the umbilicus and all port sites for local anesthesia. We believe this helps decrease postoperative pain. The abdomen is entered via 8-mm incision in the umbilicus, and pneumoperitoneum is established (up to 15 mm Hg). After diagnostic laparoscopy, without notable findings, three 8-mm robotic trocars, an Advanced Access Gelpoint (Applied Medical, Rancho Santo Margarita, CA), and one 5-mm AirSeal Access Port (ConMed Inc, Utica, NY) are then placed under laparoscopic visualization. The placement site for each trocar is very important. The liver retractor is placed via the right upper quadrant AirSeal port and secured to the surgical drape using Kocher clamps. The da Vinci Xi robotic system is brought over the patient's right shoulder and is docked with the bed in the reverse Trendelenburg position (8°–12°) with a slight left lateral tilt (4°).

Trocar placement

- Just to the right of the right midclavicular line at the level of the umbilicus: 8-mm robotic trocar (robotic arm 1) (**Fig. 13**).

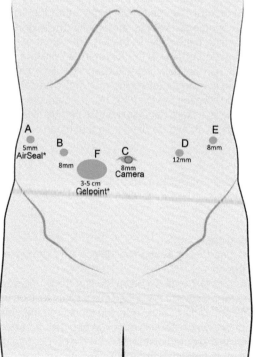

A. AirSeal* trocar for insufflation and placement of liver retractor
B. Arm # 1
C. Arm # 2
D. Arm # 3
E. Arm # 4
F. Gelpoint* assistant port

Fig. 13. Pylorus-preserving pancreaticoduodenectomy port placement. (*Courtesy of* S. Ross, MD, Tampa, FL.)

- At the umbilicus: 8-mm trocar for the robotic camera (robotic arm 2).
- At the left midclavicular line, at the level of the umbilicus: 12-mm robotic trocar (to accommodate a robotic staple) (robotic arm 3).
- At the left anterior axillary line, cephalad to the umbilicus: 8-mm robotic trocar (robotic arm 4).
- At the right anterior axillary line, at the costal margin: AirSeal Access Port (not interfering with robotic arm 1) (for insufflation and placement of the liver retractor).
- Midway between the umbilical and midclavicular line trocars and caudal to the umbilicus: Advanced Access Gelpoint (for bedside surgeon and specimen extraction).

Step 2. Kocher Maneuver

Robotic arm 1: fenestrated bipolar device.
Robotic arm 2: camera.
Robotic arm 3: hook cautery.
Robotic arm 4: atraumatic bowel grasper.
The Advanced Access Gelpoint is used as a suctioning device and atraumatic graspers are used by the bedside surgeon.

Because the nature of any written report does not allow for simultaneous activities, it is important to note that a Kocher maneuver should be undertaken first in the operation. With adequate anterosuperior retraction of the liver by the liver retractor, the hepatic flexure of the colon is mobilized caudally, as needed. In general, the colon is best left alone. The C loop of the duodenum is exposed and widely mobilized, working proximal to distal along the ventral surface of the inferior vena cava and the lateral edge of the duodenum. The duodenum is grasped with an atraumatic bowel grasper in robotic arm 4 and retracted ventrally and, especially, to the left, with great care to avoid injury to the duodenum. The dissection begins in the foramen of Winslow. The dissection continues until the left renal vein is easily identified and the ligamentum of Treitz is divided. The proximal jejunum is brought under the root of the mesentery. The jejunum is then divided with a robotic stapling device (**Fig. 14**); we mark the proximal end of the jejunum for later reference to ensure our dissection is carried along the appropriate portion of jejunum. The jejunum should be placed so that it can easily be retrieved later.

Step 3. Porta Hepatis Dissection

Robotic arm 1: fenestrated bipolar device.
Robotic arm 2: camera.
Robotic arm 3: hook cautery.
Robotic arm 4: atraumatic bowel grasper.
The Advanced Access Gelpoint is used as a suctioning device and atraumatic graspers are used by the bedside surgeon.

The robotic camera remains in robotic arm 2 until we begin closing trocar incisions (ie, the whole operation). The gastrohepatic ligament is opened in a stellate fashion using robotic hook cautery (**Fig. 15**). The common hepatic artery is identified, the characteristic overlying common hepatic artery lymph node is removed and sent for frozen section analysis (**Fig. 16**), and the artery is dissected distally toward the proper hepatic artery. The gastroduodenal artery (GDA) is identified and circumferentially dissected (**Fig. 17**) before placement of 2 Hem-o-lok clips both proximally and distally. A thorough review of a triphasic CT scan and/or three-dimensional (3D) imaging

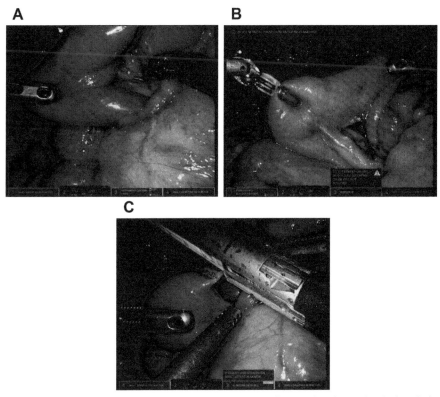

Fig. 14. Division of the jejunum. (*A*) The ligamentum of Treitz has been divided and the jejunum has been delivered to the right of the root of the mesentery. (*B*) A defect in the jejunal mesentery has been made with cautery in anticipation of applying the blue-load stapler. (*C*) The staple has been applied and the jejunum has been divided.

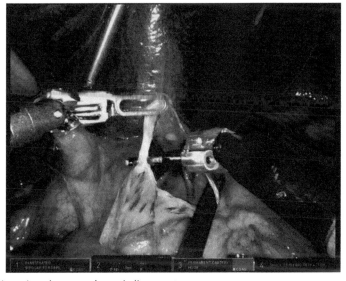

Fig. 15. Dissecting the gastrohepatic ligament.

A   **B**

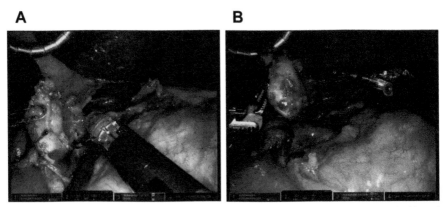

Fig. 16. Removal of lymph node overlying the common hepatic artery. (*A*) Removal of lymph node overlying the common hepatic artery; it is readily apparent after mobilization (*B*).

preoperatively is mandatory to rule out the presence of an accessory or replaced right hepatic artery, which is anticipated in this location.

Before division, the GDA is routinely test clamped (**Fig. 18**), and the pulsation in the hepatic artery is visually assessed to confirm that the artery being divided is not a replaced hepatic artery and to exclude a significant celiac artery stenosis. Once the GDA has been divided using robotic scissors (**Fig. 19**), the portal vein, which is located medially and dorsally, comes into view with a bit of dissection dorsal to and medial to the GDA.

Step 4. Division of the Duodenum/Pancreatic Exposure/Pancreas Division

Robotic arm 1: fenestrated bipolar device.
  Robotic arm 2: camera.

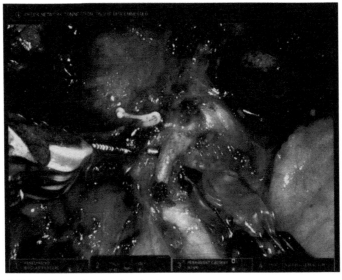

Fig. 17. Mobilizing the gastroduodenal artery.

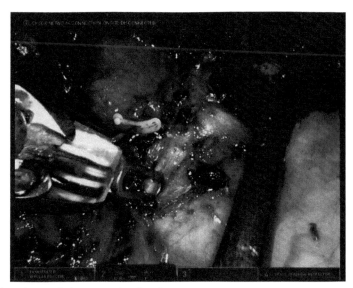

Fig. 18. Test clamp of the gastroduodenal artery.

Robotic arm 3: vessel sealer (alternating with hook cautery), scissors, hook cautery, robotic stapler.

Robotic arm 4: atraumatic bowel grasper.

We begin to divide the gastrocolic omentum while the stomach is reflected in the cephalad direction (**Fig. 20**). The gastrocolic omentum is opened near the midpoint along the greater curve of the stomach, most often across from the incisura angularis. This exposure places the right gastroepiploic vein at a near right angle to the superior

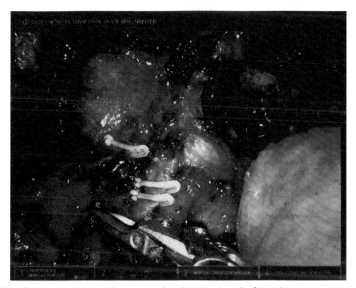

Fig. 19. Clips being applied to the gastroduodenal artery before division.

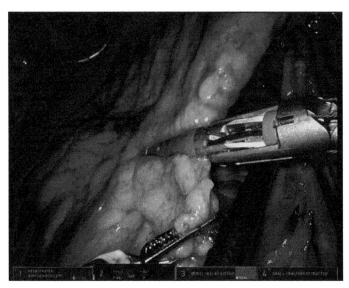

Fig. 20. Dividing the gastrocolic omentum.

mesenteric vein, to facilitate later clipping and division. As the omentum is opened, the pancreas comes into view. The right gastroepiploic vein is double clipped and divided as it is encountered in the subpyloric area.

The dissection is carried to the duodenum and it is divided with a stapler about 3 to 4 cm distal to the pylorus; the more length the better (**Fig. 21**). The dissection is then carried along the inferior border of the pancreas to expose the superior mesenteric vein (SMV). Branches feeding into the SMV can direct this dissection. Once the SMV is identified, the dissection is carried along its ventral surface going cephalad

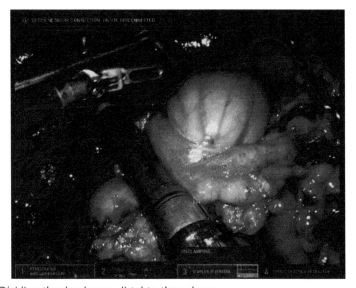

Fig. 21. Dividing the duodenum distal to the pylorus.

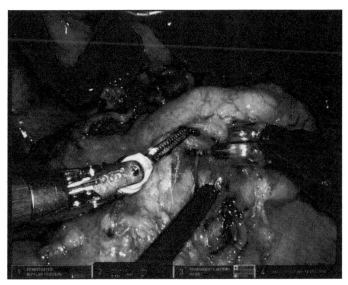

Fig. 22. Making a tunnel underneath the pancreas.

and lifting the pancreas up (ventrally) as the dissection continues. A tunnel behind the neck of the pancreas is carefully developed using robotic hook cautery while gently elevating the pancreas ventrally using a fenestrated bipolar grasper (arm 1) and an atraumatic bowel grasper (arm 4) (**Fig. 22**). A suction device placed through the gel port can be used to push gently down on the portal vein to keep it from harm's way, with a proficient assistant on the patient's right. Once the tunnel is developed, the pancreas is divided using robotic energized scissors or a hook cautery (**Fig. 23**).

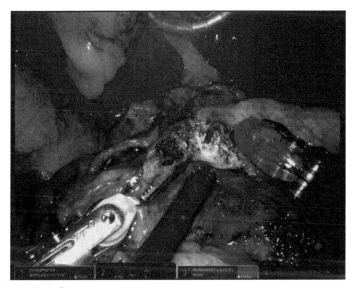

Fig. 23. Transecting the pancreas.

Step 5. Division of the Duodenal Mesentery/Removal of the Pancreatic Head

Robotic arm 1: fenestrated bipolar device.
  Robotic arm 2: camera.
  Robotic arm 3: vessel sealer (alternating with hook cautery), scissors, hook cautery.
  Robotic arm 4: atraumatic bowel grasper.
  Division of the uncinate process/duodenal mesentery begins caudally at the site of the jejunal division and proceeds cephalad until the pancreas and duodenum are freed (ie, until the common hepatic artery is reached). The bedside surgeon may provide a dynamic gentle lateral retraction of the specimen to the patient's right using a laparoscopic atraumatic bowel grasper. The laparoscopic suctioning device, through the Advanced Access Gelpoint, may facilitate this dissection as well by providing some tissue retraction as needed. The lymphatic basin is included with the specimen.
  The dissection continues along the lateral and posterior aspect of the portal vein to the common hepatic duct, which is transected. The SMA must be carefully identified and protected from any injury as the dissection is carried along it (**Fig. 24**). The SMA is skeletonized along its ventral, lateral, and dorsal surface.
  Once the dissection of the specimen from the SMV, SMA, and the portal vein attachments is complete, the distal common bile duct is identified as it enters the head of the pancreas. The distal common bile duct is identified and separated away from the portal vein by developing an avascular plane between them. The common bile duct lymph nodes, which are located along the right posterolateral aspect of the duct, are carefully taken with the specimen with hook cautery. The hepatic duct is divided with either robotic hook cautery or scissors (**Fig. 25**). The bile duct lumen is identified, and the bile effluent is suctioned off. If present, a bile duct stent is removed with the specimen.

Step 6. Cholecystectomy

Robotic arm 1: fenestrated bipolar device (alternating with a vessel sealer).
  Robotic arm 2: camera.
  Robotic arm 3: hook cautery.
  Robotic arm 4: atraumatic bowel grasper.
  A cholecystectomy is undertaken next; this is often an opportunity for a younger, more inexperienced surgeon to participate and gain robotic experience. The

A　　　　　　　　**B**

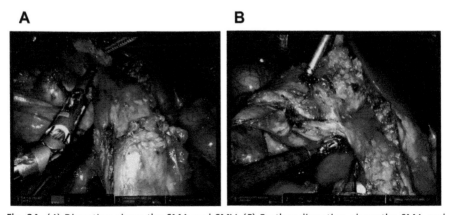

Fig. 24. (*A*) Dissecting along the SMA and SMV. (*B*) Further dissecting along the SMA and SMV.

A   B

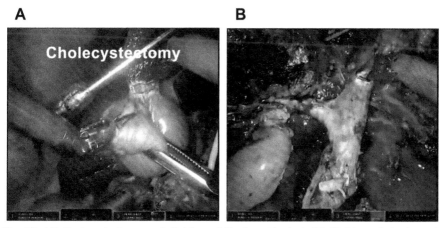

Fig. 25. (*A*) Cholecystectomy and division of the hepatic duct. (*B*) Division of the hepatic duct.

gallbladder and the pancreaticoduodenectomy specimen are then placed into a laparoscopic Endo Catch Bag (Applied Medical, Rancho Santo Margarita, CA) and removed via the Advanced Access Gelpoint (**Fig. 26**). Water-soluble gel applied in the gel port and on the extraction bag helps slip the specimen out through the gel port. With lubrication, it is possible to deliver a specimen the size of a cantaloupe out through an incision the size of an egg.

Reconstruction
All sutures used in the reconstruction (ie, hepaticojejunostomy, pancreaticojejunostomy, and duodenojejunostomy) are introduced into the peritoneal cavity through the Advanced Access Gelpoint.

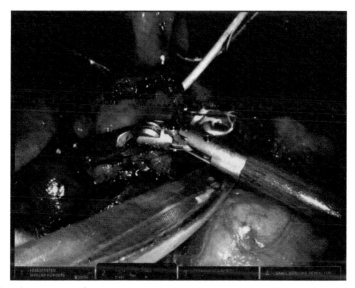

Fig. 26. Specimen removal.

Step 7. Construction of the Hepaticojejunostomy

Robotic arm 1: needle driver.
  Robotic arm 2: camera.
  Robotic arm 3: needle driver/scissors.
  Robotic arm 4: atraumatic bowel grasper.

A suitable length of proximal jejunum is brought under the root of the mesentery and advanced cephalad toward the porta hepatis and the cut edge of the pancreas. The laparoscopic liver retractor should be positioned so as to easily visualize the hepatic duct lumen. The proximal jejunal limb is held in position using an atraumatic bowel grasper in robotic arm 4, which should grasp the bowel limb proximal to the anastomosis. Constructing the hepaticojejunostomy before the pancreaticojejunostomy is our strong preference.

The cut end of the bile duct is further opened along the ventral surface of the bile duct if the duct is small (<1 cm) so as to increase the cross-sectional area of the bile duct anastomosis, thus decreasing the odds of a clinically apparent stricture. Construction of a single-layer anastomosis is started at the 9 o'clock position (looking at the end of the bile duct) using a 3-0 V-Loc (Medtronic, Minneapolis, MN) suture in a running fashion. The stitch is run dorsally toward the 3 o'clock position (going inside out on the duct and outside in on the jejunum) and kept tight after each needle pass. Another V-Loc suture (that starts at the 9 o'clock position) is used to construct the ventral aspect of the anastomosis, going outside in on the duct and inside out on the jejunum. The suture ends are tied on the outside of the anastomosis at the 3 o'clock position after ensuring that the sutures are snug. The anastomosis is inspected with additional sutures placed as needed (**Fig. 27**).

Step 8. Construction of the Pancreaticojejunostomy

Robotic arm 1: needle driver.
  Robotic arm 2: camera.
  Robotic arm 3: needle driver.
  Robotic arm 4: atraumatic bowel grasper.

The pancreaticojejunostomy is constructed using a 2-layer anastomosis with 3-0 V-Loc sutures. The posterior layer is undertaken by bringing the pancreatic parenchyma and posterior pancreatic capsule to the seromuscular layer of the jejunum in a running fashion. The pancreatic duct is then identified. The duct is generally posterior, so do not include it in the posterior layer of the anastomosis; this may require some of the sutures being placed in a transverse fashion. The pancreatic duct-to-jejunum anastomosis is undertaken after making a small jejunotomy by placing interrupted sutures at the 6, 9, 3, and 12 o'clock positions (looking at the pancreas) using 3-0 or 4-0 V-Loc sutures or 5-0 polypropylene sutures. All the suture ends are tied on the exterior circumference of the pancreatic duct anastomosis (ie, outside the lumen). The anterior layer of the pancreaticojejunostomy is constructed by bringing the anterior capsule of the pancreas to the seromuscular layer of the jejunum in a running fashion. The 2 sutures of the 'outer layer of the 2-layer anastomosis are tied together to complete the pancreaticojejunal anastomosis (**Fig. 28**).

Step 9. Reconstruction of the Ligamentum of Treitz

Robotic arm 1: needle driver (alternating with an atraumatic bowel grasper).
  Robotic arm 2: camera.
  Robotic arm 3: needle driver or fenestrated grasper or atraumatic bowel grasper (depending on the need for better exposure).

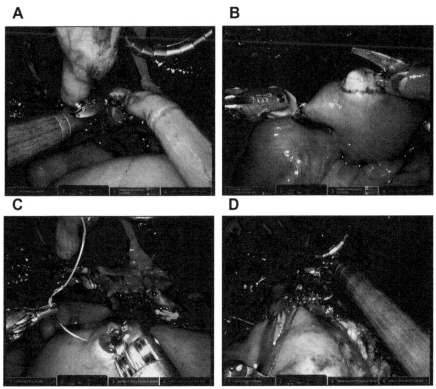

Fig. 27. Construction of hepaticojejunostomy. (*A*) Preparing the duct. (*B*) Opening the jejunum. (*C*) The anastomosis is begun at 9 o'clock. (*D*) The completed anastomosis.

Robotic arm 4: atraumatic bowel grasper.

The transverse colon is elevated ventrally and cephalad with atraumatic bowel graspers (one through the gel port) exposing the location of the divided ligament of Treitz. The jejunal limb coming down from the bile duct is identified and secured to defect under the root of the mesentery with a 3-0 V-Loc suture (**Fig. 29**). The goal of reconstructing the ligament of Treitz is to avoid potential internal herniation under the root of mesentery. Careful attention must be paid not to include any mesenteric vessel branches during placement of the sutures. It is also important to avoid excessive distal traction on the jejunal limb, which can promote mechanical tension between the hepaticojejunostomy and pancreaticojejunostomy. The jejunum for the duodenojejunostomy is identified and brought ventral to the colon as it is released; the jejunum is then brought to the duodenal remnant.

Step 10. Construction of the Duodenojejunostomy

The duodenojejunostomy is constructed using a single-layer running anastomosis with two 3-0 V-Loc sutures in a fashion like the construction of the hepaticojejunostomy. Construction is started at the 9 o'clock position (looking at the cut end of the duodenum) using a 3-0 V-Loc suture in a running fashion. The suture passes dorsally going inside out on the duodenum and outside in on the jejunum to the 3 o'clock position and must be kept tight after each needle pass. Another V-Loc suture, beginning

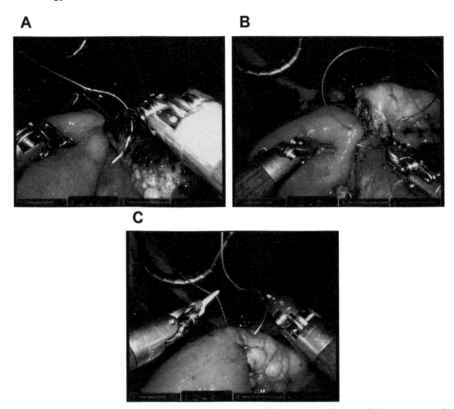

Fig. 28. Construction of the pancreaticojejunostomy. (*A*) The dorsal layer of the anastomosis has begun. (*B*) The dorsal layer is complete. (*C*) The portion of the anastomosis from the duct to (small hole in the) jejunum has been completed and the ventral second layer of the anastomosis is being completed.

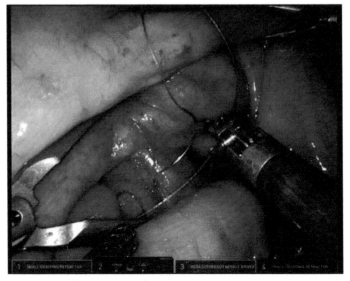

Fig. 29. Reconstructing the ligament of Treitz.

again at the 9 o'clock position, is used to construct the ventral aspect of the anastomosis, going outside in on the duodenum and inside out on the jejunum. Using a Gambee technique may aid in making a nice anastomosis. The suture ends are across from each other and are tied at the 3 o'clock position after ensuring that the sutures are tight. The afferent and efferent limbs are anchored to the distal stomach to avoid tension or twisting of the duodenojejunostomy (**Fig. 30**).

Step 11. Placement of Drain and Closure

A closed suction 10-French JP drain is routinely placed over the pancreaticojejunostomy through the foramen of Winslow to drain the hepaticojejunostomy. The JP drain is brought out in the right upper quadrant through the site of the 5-mm AirSeal Access Port incision.

To help decrease postoperative pain, the diaphragm is irrigated bilaterally and liberally with a solution of 7.5 mL of 0.25% Marcaine in 250 mL of normal saline. All incisions are closed along anatomic layers using absorbable monofilament sutures for fascial closure and then interrupted 3-0 absorbable sutures and Steri-Strips. To further aid in postoperative pain control, we routinely inject all incisions with a solution of 20 mL of Exparel (Pacira Pharmaceuticals, Parsippany, NJ) in 30 mL of normal saline before closure. Sterile 1.5 × 6 silver dressings (Therabond 3D, Alliqua Biomedical,

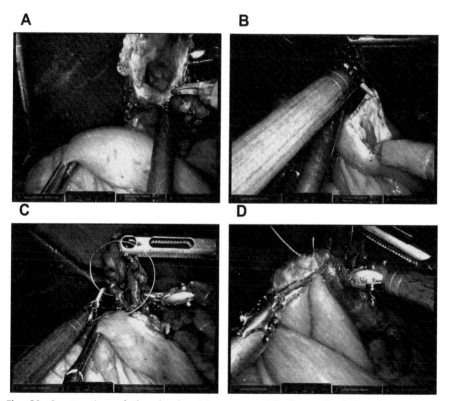

Fig. 30. Construction of the duodenojejunostomy. (*A*) The end of the duodenum is apparent. (*B*) The jejunum is being opened in preparation for the anastomosis. (*C*) As with the biliary anastomosis, this anastomosis begins at 9 o'clock. (*D*) The ventral layer of the 1-layer anastomosis is being completed.

Langhorne, PA) are applied to all incisions followed by sterile 2×2 gauze. All dressings are then covered with Tegaderm (3M, St Paul, MN) transparent dressings. These watertight dressings allow patients to shower at home after discharge. The dressings are removed 5 to 7 days postoperatively during clinic follow-up.

OTHER ASPECTS OF CARE

Judicious intraoperative fluid management and resuscitation is emphasized through our ERAS protocol. We follow perioperative goal-directed fluid therapy principles, guided by the ClearSight EV1000 System (Edwards Lifesciences, Irvine, CA). Using this system, hemodynamic metrics (eg, cardiac output, stroke volume, stroke volume variation) are continuously monitored within a strict protocol to allow precise volume administration. Percentage of stroke volume variations is followed to estimate fluid status and used to determine whether additional IV fluids are needed.

POSTOPERATIVE CARE

- POD 1: complete blood count and comprehensive metabolic panel daily.
- POD 1 to 2: Foley out, nasogastric tube out, start clear liquid diet.
- POD 3: intraperitoneal drain amylase levels. Drain removed if within normal limits. Progression of diet.
- Physical therapy: twice a day.
- Pain control: IV Tylenol (1000 mg every 6 hours for 3 days) in addition to IV ketorolac (15 mg every 6 hours for 3 days), oral gabapentin and oral celecoxib. Breakthrough pain is managed with IV hydromorphone (0.5–:1.0 mg while patients are still unable to tolerate a diet).
- Patients are encouraged to chew gum during recovery, beginning the day of their operation, to help stimulate gut function/motility.

Use of the robot does not change the nature of pancreatic surgery, only the approach and the morbidity associated with it. The robotic platform does not change the indications for operations, the goals of the operations, and the general conduct of the operations to be undertaken. The robotic platform does not change or alter the complications that can occur after pancreatic operations or the postoperative care, in general. To appropriately use the robotic platform requires the same skill and judgment that is required when pancreatic operations are undertaken as open or laparoscopic operations. Compassion, skill, competence, and professionalism will always be attributes of proficient surgeons; the robotic platform facilitates and, in our opinion, reduces morbidity of pancreatic surgery.

DISCLOSURES/CONFLICTS OF INTEREST

The authors A.S. Rosemurgy and S. Ross are consultants and proctors for Medtronicplc, (Minneapolis, MN) and Intuitive Surgical Inc (Sunnyvale, CA). K. Luberice, H. Browning, and I. Sucandy have no disclosures/conflicts of interest.

REFERENCES

1. Zureikat AH, Moser AJ, Boone BA, et al. 250 robotic pancreatic resections: safety and feasibility. Ann Surg 2013;258(4):554.
2. McGuigan A, Kelly P, Turkington RC, et al. Pancreatic cancer: A review of clinical diagnosis, epidemiology, treatment and outcomes. World J Gastroenterol 2018; 24(43):4846.

3. Ma C, Gocke CD, Hruban RH, et al. Mutational spectrum of intraepithelial neoplasia in pancreatic heterotopia. Hum Pathol 2016;48:117–21.
4. Magge DR, Zenati MS, Hamad A, et al. Comprehensive comparative analysis of cost-effectiveness and perioperative outcomes between open, laparoscopic, and robotic distal pancreatectomy. HPB (Oxford) 2018;20(12):1172–80.
5. American Cancer Society. Cancer facts & figures 2019. 2019. Available at: https://www.cancer.org/content/dam/cancer-org/research/cancer-facts-and-statistics/annual-cancer-facts-and-figures/2019/cancer-facts-and-figures-2019.pdf . Accessed September 19, 2019.
6. Ilic M, Ilic I. Epidemiology of pancreatic cancer. World J Gastroenterol 2016; 22(44):9694.
7. Higuera O, Ghanem I, Nasimi R, et al. Management of pancreatic cancer in the elderly. World J Gastroenterol 2016;22(2):764.
8. Fisher WE, Andersen DK, Windsor JA, et al. Pancreas. In: Brunicardi FC, Andersen DK, Billiar TR, et al, editors. Schwartz's principles of surgery, 11e. 11th edition. New York: McGraw-Hill Education; 2019. p. 1401–8.
9. Toomey P, Hernandez J, Golkar F, et al. Pancreatic adenocarcinoma: complete tumor extirpation improves survival benefit despite larger tumors for patients who undergo distal pancreatectomy and splenectomy. J Gastrointest Surg 2012;16(2):376–81.
10. Reames BN, Blair AB, Krell RW, et al. Management of locally advanced pancreatic cancer: results of an international survey of current practice. Ann Surg 2019. [Epub ahead of print].
11. van Veldhuisen E, van den Oord C, Brada LJ, et al. Locally advanced pancreatic cancer: Work-up, staging, and local intervention strategies. Cancers 2019; 11(7):976.
12. Kim Y, Kim SC, Song KB, et al. Improved survival after palliative resection of unsuspected stage IV pancreatic ductal adenocarcinoma. HPB 2016;18(4):325–31.
13. Bisht S, Brossart P, Feldmann G. Current therapeutic options for pancreatic ductal adenocarcinoma. Oncol Res Treat 2018;41(10):590–4.
14. Meng Q, Shi S, Liang C, et al. Diagnostic accuracy of a CA125-based biomarker panel in patients with pancreatic cancer: a systematic review and meta-analysis. J Cancer 2017;8(17):3615.
15. Gold G, Goh SK, Christophi C, et al. Dilemmas and limitations interpreting carbohydrate antigen 19-9 elevation after curative pancreatic surgery: A case report. Int J Surg case Rep 2019;54:20–2.
16. Tempero MA, Behrman S, Ben-Josef E, et al. Pancreatic adenocarcinoma: clinical practice guidelines in oncology. J Natl Compr Cancer Netw 2005;3(5):598–626.
17. Soufi M, Yip-Schneider MT, Carr RA, et al. Multifocal High-Grade Pancreatic Precursor Lesions: A Case Series and Management Recommendations. J Pancreat Cancer 2019;5(1):8–11.
18. Dietrich CF. The resectable pancreatic ductal adenocarcinoma: To FNA or not to FNA? A diagnostic dilemma, introduction. Endoscopic Ultrasound 2017;6(Suppl 3):S69.
19. Dietrich CF, Sahai AV, D'Onofrio M, et al. Differential diagnosis of small solid pancreatic lesions. Gastrointest Endosc 2016;84(6):933–40.
20. Burk KS, Knipp D, Sahani DV. Cystic pancreatic tumors. Magn Reson Imaging Clin 2018;26(3):405–20.
21. Chu LC, Singhi AD, Haroun RR, et al. The many faces of pancreatic serous cystadenoma: radiologic and pathologic correlation. Diagn Interv Imaging 2017; 98(3):191–202.

22. Munigala S, Javia SB, Agarwal B. Etiologic Distribution of Pancreatic Cystic Lesions Identified on Computed Tomography/Magnetic Resonance Imaging. Pancreas 2019;48(8):1092–7.

23. Tariq MU, Ahmad Z, Abdul-Ghafar J, et al. Serous cystadenoma of pancreas: A clinicopathologic experience of 23 cases from a major tertiary care center. Rare Tumors 2018;10. 2036361318809183.

24. Javia S, Munigala S, Guha S, et al. EUS morphology is reliable in selecting patients with mucinous pancreatic cyst (s) most likely to benefit from surgical resection. Gastroenterol Res Pract 2017;2017:9863952.

25. Yang J, Guo X, Ou X, et al. Discrimination of pancreatic serous cystadenomas from mucinous cystadenomas with CT textural features: based on machine learning. Front Oncol 2019;9:494.

26. Gurzu S, Bara T, Sincu M, et al. Solid pseudopapillary neoplasm of pancreas: Two case reports. Medicine 2019;98(29):e16455.

27. Hipp J, Mohamed S, Pott J, et al. Management and outcomes of intraductal papillary mucinous neoplasms. BJS Open 2019;3(4):490–9.

28. Del Chiaro M, Beckman R, Ateeb Z, et al. Main duct dilatation is the best predictor of high-grade dysplasia or invasion in intraductal papillary mucinous neoplasms of the pancreas. Ann Surg 2019. [Epub ahead of print].

29. Buscail E, Cauvin T, Fernandez B, et al. Intraductal papillary mucinous neoplasms of the pancreas and European guidelines: importance of the surgery type in the decision-making process. BMC Surg 2019;19(1):1–10.

30. Murakami Y, Uemura K, Sudo T, et al. Invasive intraductal papillary-mucinous neoplasm of the pancreas: Comparison with pancreatic ductal adenocarcinoma. J Surg Oncol 2009;100(1):13–8.

31. Izawa T, Obara T, Tanno S, et al. Clonality and field cancerization in intraductal papillary-mucinous tumors of the pancreas. Cancer 2001;92(7):1807–17.

32. Tanno S, Obara T, Koizumi K, et al. Risk of additional pancreatic cancer in patients with branch duct intraductal papillary-mucinous neoplasm. Clin J Gastroenterol 2009;2(6):365–70.

33. Cao F, Li J, Li A, et al. Prognostic significance of positive peritoneal cytology in resectable pancreatic cancer: a systemic review and meta-analysis. Oncotarget 2017;8(9):15004.

34. Rosemurgy A, Ross S, Bourdeau T, et al. Robotic pancreaticoduodenectomy is the future: here and now. J Am Coll Surg 2019;228(4):613–24.

35. Ryan CE, Ross SB, Sukharamwala PB, et al. Distal pancreatectomy and splenectomy: a robotic or LESS approach. JSLS 2015;19(1). e2014.00246.

36. Ramera M, Damoli I, Giardino A, et al. Robotic pancreatectomies. Robotic Surg Res Rev 2016;3:29.

37. Juo YY, King JC. Robotic-assisted spleen preserving distal pancreatectomy: a technical review. J Visualized Surg 2017;3:139.

38. Klaiber U, Mihaljevic A, Hackert T. Radical pancreatic cancer surgery—with arterial resection. Transl Gastroenterol Hepatol 2019;4:8.

39. Klompmaker S, Boggi U, Hackert T, et al. Distal pancreatectomy with celiac axis resection (DP-CAR) for pancreatic cancer. How I do it. J Gastrointest Surg 2018; 22(10):1804–10.

Robotic Colorectal Surgery

Poppy Addison, MD[a], Jennifer L. Agnew, MD[a], Joseph Martz, MD[a,b,*]

KEYWORDS

- Robotic colon surgery • Intracorporeal anastomosis • Robotic rectal surgery
- Rectal cancer

KEY POINTS

- Robotic colon surgery has clinically similar short-term and long-term outcomes for patients but may decrease conversion rates, allow off-midline incisions via intracorporeal anastomoses, and improve technical ease for surgeons.
- Robotic surgery can be a helpful adjunct during pelvic surgery, given the confines of the bony pelvis. Its use has been described in procedures for inflammatory bowel disease, pelvic organ prolapse, and rectal cancer.
- The laparoscopic approach to rectal cancer may offer limitations in the pathologic adequacy of the resection. The robotic technique offers enhancement in the grade of the mesorectal resection and circumferential resection margin.

INTRODUCTION

After its early success in biliary surgery, colon and rectal surgeons began applying the laparoscopic approach to provide patients with the enhanced benefits of minimally invasive surgery. Although this approach improved recovery time and postoperative pain, the difficult learning curve and intrinsic limitations in the equipment left room for improvement. The introduction of robotic devices into clinical practice sought to improve these limitations with a surgeon-controlled 3-dimensional view, increased dexterity, and scaled movement. This article reviews how successfully the robotic approach improves on laparoscopic colon and rectal surgery and addresses whether this impacts clinical outcomes.

COLON: LAPAROSCOPIC

Given the ultimate goal of oncologic surgery to improve survival, colectomy for cancer should resect the primary tumor with adequate margins and number of lymph nodes.

[a] Department of Surgery, Zucker School of Medicine at Hofstra/Northwell, Lenox Hill Hospital, 100 East 77th Street, New York, NY 10075, USA; [b] Division of Colon and Rectal Surgery, Western Region Northwell/Lenox Hill Hospital, New York, NY, USA
* Corresponding author. Department of Surgery, Lenox Hill Hospital, 100 East 77th Street, New York, NY 10075.
E-mail addresses: JMARTZ@CHPNET.ORG; JMartz@northwell.edu

Surg Clin N Am 100 (2020) 337–360
https://doi.org/10.1016/j.suc.2019.12.012
0039-6109/20/© 2020 Elsevier Inc. All rights reserved.

After the first laparoscopic colon resections in 1991 by Cooperman and colleagues,[1] Jacobs and colleagues,[2] and Fowler and White[3] proved that a laparoscopic approach is technically feasible, the question became if this approach is safe for patients. Although there were initial concerns based around the risk of port-site metastasis or exfoliation of tumor cells from manipulation with laparoscopic instrument,[4,5] large multi-institutional trials demonstrated similar long-term oncologic outcomes for open and laparoscopic approaches (**Table 1**). The Clinical Outcomes of Surgical Therapy (COST) Study Group conducted a multi-institutional noninferiority randomized controlled trial from 1994 to 2001 to evaluate the safety of laparoscopic colectomy for colon cancer. The results of this study identified that a laparoscopic approach was not associated with a significant increase in complications, including recurrence rate.[6] Shortly after the COST trial, the Medical Research Council Conventional versus Laparoscopic-Assisted Surgery In Colorectal Cancer (MRC CLASICC) trial recruited patients from 1996 to 2002 with either colon or rectal cancer and randomized their treatment to laparoscopic or open surgery. This group concluded that in the short-term and at 3-year and 5-year follow-ups, there were no significant differences between the 2 groups regarding oncologic outcomes, including overall survival, disease-free survival, and local and distant recurrence.[7–9] Finally, the COlon cancer Laparoscopic or Open Resection (COLOR) trial randomized European patients with nonmetastatic colon cancer from 1997 to 2003 to either laparoscopic or open surgery and found comparable oncologic outcomes to the CLASICC trial at 3-year, 5-year, and 10-year follow-ups.[10–14]

Several randomized controlled trials and a meta-analysis including studies up to 2002 demonstrated decreased time to flatus, postoperative pain, time to flatus, and hospital length of stay in patients who underwent a laparoscopic versus open colectomy.[15–19] Despite the benefits, adoption of laparoscopy has been slow, likely due to intrinsic limitations in the equipment. The single-camera laparoscope reduces 3-dimensional anatomy to a 2-dimensional plane, decreasing depth perception, and its view is often limited by condensation and assistant control. The nonarticulated, rigid instruments have only 4° of freedom versus 7 in the wrist, and placement through a trocar forces nonintuitive movement via the fulcrum effect, decreasing hand-eye coordination. With these limitations, laparoscopic colectomies are technically complex and mentally taxing, with a learning curve of 55 cases for right-sided and 62 cases for left-sided resections based on risk-adjusted conversion to open rates.[20] The Australian Laparoscopic Colon Cancer Surgical trial (ALCCaS) conducted between 1998 and 2005 in Australia and New Zealand compared laparoscopic versus open colectomy in patients with colon cancer, finding a 14.6% conversion rate, largely for inability to visualize critical structures (4.8%) or advanced disease (4.1%).[21–23] Conversion from laparoscopic to open adversely impacts patients, with increased morbidity, mortality, blood transfusion requirements, and length of stay.[24]

COLON: ROBOTIC

In an effort to overcome the intrinsic limitations of laparoscopic equipment, robotic-assisted surgical devices were designed to combine the benefits of open and laparoscopic surgery to allow natural wristed movements within a narrow field and provide a surgeon-controlled 3-dimensional field. Unfortunately, the literature is sparse for long-term safety comparisons. A Dutch group performed a nonrandomized prospective study comparing 378 patients undergoing robotic or laparoscopic resection for stage I-III colorectal cancer with a 15-month median follow-up, finding no statistically significant difference between the robotic and laparoscopic groups for radical margins,

Table 1
Summary of characteristics of landmark studies

Study Name	First Author, Year	Design	Sample Size	Comparison	Endpoints	Follow-up	Conclusion
COST trial	Weeks et al,[97] 2002 The Clinical Outcomes of Surgical Therapy Study Group,[6]2004	RCT	576 872	Laparoscopic vs open for colon cancer	Quality of life Disease-free survival	3 y	Laparoscopic noninferior to open
CLASICC trial	Jayne et al,[7] 2007 Jayne et al,[8] 2010 Green et al,[9] 2013	RCT	794	Laparoscopic vs open for colon cancer	Overall survival, disease-free survival, local recurrence	5 y	No difference in endpoints between laparoscopic and open
COLOR trial	Hazebroek et al,[11] 2002 Buunen et al,[12] 2009 Deijen et al,[14] 2017	RCT	859 1248 329 (Dutch only)	Laparoscopic vs open for colon cancer	Disease-free survival	5 y 10 y (Dutch only)	Unable to conclude noninferior Small clinical difference between groups
ALCCaS trial	Hewett et al,[21] 2008 Bagshaw et al,[22] 2012 McCombie et al,[23] 2018	RCT	601 587 592	Laparoscopic vs open for colon cancer	Overall survival Disease-free survival Quality of life	3 y 5 y	Laparoscopic noninferior to open

Abbreviation: RCT, randomized controlled trial.
Data from Refs [6–9,11,12,14,21–23,97]

number of nodes, or locoregional recurrence rates.[25] A Korean group compared open, laparoscopic, and robotic approaches for right-sided colon cancer, finding no difference in the number of nodes or 5-year disease-free survival.[26] Although these preliminary studies suggest that the robotic approach may have comparable oncologic outcomes, there exists a clear need for large, prospective randomized controlled trials before any definitive conclusions can be made.

Given that rigid laparoscopic instruments make intracorporeal anastomoses difficult and time-consuming, more commonly the bowel is exteriorized through a mini-laparotomy excision to perform an extracorporeal anastomosis. Although this may be easier to perform,[27] it requires more mobilization of bowel, a larger incision, and theoretically increases the risk of mesenteric twisting. In 2017, van Oostendorp and colleagues[28] performed a systematic review comparing intracorporeal versus extracorporeal anastomoses in laparoscopic right hemicolectomies, including 1 randomized control trial and 11 retrospective reviews, and found intracorporeal anastomosis was correlated with decreased surgical site infection and decreased overall short-term morbidity, which was defined individually for each study included. The only prospective trial conducted with 80 patients found laparoscopic intracorporeal anastomosis added 30 minutes to the operative time and shortened the incision by approximately 2 cm; otherwise, there were no significant differences in outcomes between the 2 groups.[29] Compared with laparoscopic extracorporeal anastomosis, robotic intracorporeal anastomosis was associated with decreased intraoperative blood loss, longer specimen lengths, and increased operative times.[30]

An intracorporeal anastomosis allows the incision to be shifted off-midline, reducing the rate of incisional hernias. With midline incisions and extracorporeal anastomoses, laparoscopic and robotic approaches both have an incisional hernia rate of approximately 20% with an average follow-up of 910 and 360 days, respectively[31]; however, decreased hernia rates with an off-midline incision have been well-established in the literature for laparoscopy. A retrospective review with an average follow-up of 3.5 years found hernias developed after 8.9% of midline incisions versus 2.3% for off-midline and 3.8% for Pfannenstiel incisions.[32] After 30 months of follow-up, 4% of patients undergoing laparoscopic extracorporeal anastomosis experienced an incisional hernia versus 0% of robotic intracorporeal anastomoses.[30]

Although the robotic approach may improve on the limitations intrinsic to the laparoscopic equipment, the robot has several important limitations. The upfront cost of a robot ranges from $1.0 million to $2.5 million, not including the cost for surgeon and operating room staff training and lost revenue while implementing a new robotic program. For robotic rectal dissections for a single surgeon, there were no differences in the first 43 cases compared with the next 42, suggesting that robotic costs may be fixed and not improved as surgeons progress through the learning curve.[33] When comparing laparoscopic versus robotic colorectal surgeries, the literature varies significantly. In one retrospective review, there were no differences in operating room time, hospital length of stay, or overall hospital cost.[34] In another, robotic cases were approximately $17,000 versus $15,000[35]; however, the difference may lie in including cases converted to open. Robotic cases required conversion to open half the time that laparoscopic cases did, 15% versus 7%, and including the cost of conversion decreased the difference between robotic and laparoscopic cases from approximately $2000 to $1000.[35] A recent large National Surgical Quality Improvement Program (NSQIP) review found a conversion rate of 2.4% versus 3.4% for robotic versus laparoscopic and a hospital length of stay of 4.5 versus 5.1 days, respectively.[36] The cost of purchasing and implementing a new robot may be offset by decreased conversion costs and decreased length of stay. Increased operative time has been attributed to the time required for docking and undocking, which can be prolonged in colon surgery, as accessing all abdominal quadrants can require redocking in the middle of a case. Longer operative times increases room time and decreases the number of cases a single surgeon can perform in a day.

Given the paucity of randomized controlled trials comparing the robotic approach with laparoscopic or open, the highest levels of evidence available are retrospective multi-institutional studies based on a regional or national database (**Table 2**). Bhama and colleagues[37] conducted a review of the 2013 American College of Surgeons NSQIP database with 11,477 patients undergoing laparoscopic or robotic colorectal surgeries. In this study, robotic operations had a longer operative time and a statistically significant decreased length of stay (4.3 days compared with 5.3) and decreased conversion rates. Subsequent reviews of the NSQIP and the Michigan Surgical Quality Collaborative databases have found similar results.[36,38,39] These large sample sizes afford adequate statistical power to find small differences between groups that may not be clinically significant. Given the small effect sizes in these studies, robotic surgery should be considered to have clinically equivalent outcomes compared with laparoscopic.

RECTUM

As robotic surgery has been incorporated into clinical practice, its application to surgery of the rectum has continued to evolve for both benign and malignant pathologies. The robotic platform and instrumentation have unique potential for rectal surgery, given the anatomic considerations and constraints of the pelvis.

Anatomy of the Rectum

From a surgical standpoint, the rectum is generally considered to begin at the level of the sacral promontory, descends through the bony confines of the pelvis, and exits through the levator ani muscles to become the anal canal. The anatomic relation of the rectum to nearby organs (gynecologic and urologic), nerves (sacral nerve plexus), and vasculature (median sacral and iliac vessels) must always be carefully respected during dissection. As a fixed organ within the confines of a bony compartment, the surgical field can be limited both visually and spatially during rectal dissection, as is particularly evident in an obese or male patient with a narrow pelvis. The technological advantages of the robot may help overcome some of these limitations and can serve as a useful tool to aid in pelvic dissection.

Pelvic Organ Prolapse

Robotic surgery has been shown to be a safe and effective technique that can be used in the surgical correction of pelvic organ prolapse (**Table 3**). Mäkelä-Kaikkonen and colleagues[40] performed a randomized controlled trial comparing robotic and laparoscopic ventral rectopexy for rectal prolapse and enterocele that demonstrated similar operative times between technical approaches. Retrospective reviews of robotic rectopexy procedures performed by Haahr and colleagues[41] and Inaba and colleagues[42] found the technique also to be safe, with acceptable functional outcomes and recurrence rates, as well as low short-term morbidity and mortality. Several meta-analyses have been performed comparing laparoscopic and robotic techniques for ventral mesh rectopexy. Analysis by Ramage and colleagues[43] revealed no significant difference in conversion rates between laparoscopic and robotic rectopexy, with similar recurrence rates of prolapse and comparable functional outcomes postoperatively. Similarly, recurrence rates of prolapse, as well as conversion and reoperation rates,

Table 2
Summary of studies comparing laparoscopic and robotic colon surgery

First Author, Year	Design	Sample Size	Endpoints	Follow-up (Median)	Conclusion
Bhama et al,[37] 2016	Retrospective	11,477	30-d outcomes	30 d	Longer operative times, decreased length of stay, and decreased conversion rate for robotic
Bhama et al[37] 2016	Retrospective	4796	Conversion	n/a	Lower conversion rate for robotic
Kang et al,[26] 2016	Retrospective	96 33 open, 43 laparoscopic, 20 robot	Overall survival Disease-free survival Cost	40 mo	Similar outcomes for robotic vs laparoscopic
Tam et al,[39] 2016	Retrospective	2735	Conversion Length of stay	n/a	Lower conversion rate and shorter length of stay for robotic
Widmar et al,[31] 2016	Retrospective	276	Incisional hernia	1 y (robot)	Similar incisional hernia rate
Vasudevan et al,[34] 2016	Retrospective	227	Short-term clinical outcomes Cost	90 d	Similar outcomes
Cleary et al,[35] 2018	Retrospective	2940 1061 open, 1 604 lap, 275 robot	Cost Conversion rate	n/a	Higher cost, decreased conversion rate with robotic
Harr et al,[36] 2018	Retrospective	29,172	30-d outcomes	30 d	Fewer conversions, shorter length of stay with robotic
Law et al,[98] 2018	Retrospective	238	Mental and physical workload	n/a	Less mental demand, physical demand and effort in robot group
Lujan et al,[30] 2018	Retrospective	224	Short-term clinical outcomes Incisional hernia	30 mo (robot)	Less blood loss, shorter incisions, longer specimen in the robotic group
Armijo et al,[99] 2019	Retrospective	28	Physical fatigue	n/a	Similar physical fatigue
Polat et al,[25] 2019	Retrospective	378	Radical margins, number of retrieved lymph nodes, locoregional recurrence	15 mo	No difference in oncologic outcomes

Data from Refs [25,26,30,31,34,35,36,37,39,98,99]

Table 3
Robotic pelvic floor studies

First Author, Year	Design	Sample Size	Comparison	Endpoints	Follow-up	Conclusion
Perrenot,[100] 2013	Prospectively collected data of consecutive cases, follow-up questionnaire	77 robotic rectopexy	None	Long-term functional and anatomic results, evaluation of learning curve	52.5 mo (mean)	Acceptable long-term results Learning curve completed after 18 patients
Germain,[101] 2013	Retrospective review	77 robotic rectopexy (18 elderly, 59 younger)	Elderly (age >75 y) vs younger patients	Perioperative and long-term clinical results and function	51.8 mo (median)	No difference in operative time, conversion, morbidity, or length of stay, functional outcomes, recurrence, or satisfaction
Haahr et al,[41] 2014	Retrospective review of consecutive cases	24 robotic-assisted rectopexy (18 with long-term follow-up)	None	Perioperative parameters, postoperative morbidity, long-term recurrence, incontinence, and satisfaction	10 mo (average)	Acceptable functional outcomes and recurrence rates
Rondelli et al,[44] 2014	Systematic review and meta-analysis	6 studies, 340 patients total	Robotic-assisted and laparoscopic rectopexy	Recurrence rate, conversion rate, operative time, intraoperative blood loss, postoperative complications, reoperation rate, length of stay	N/a	Similar recurrence, conversion and reoperation rates Decreased intraoperative blood loss, postoperative complications, and length of stay in robotic group Longer operative time in robotic group

(continued on next page)

Table 3
(continued)

First Author, Year	Design	Sample Size	Comparison	Endpoints	Follow-up	Conclusion
Mäkelä-Kaikkonen et al,[40] 2016	Prospective randomized	16 robotic ventral mesh rectopexy, 14 laparoscopic ventral mesh rectopexy	Robot-assisted and laparoscopic ventral rectopexy procedures	Perioperative parameters, complications, restoration of anatomy (assessed by dynamic MR defecography)	3 mo	Similar operative time, similar length of stay, similar anatomic correction of pathology
Ramage et al,[43] 2015	Meta-analysis	5 prospective, nonrandomized studies, 244 patients total (101 robotic, 143 laparoscopic)	Robotic and laparoscopic ventral mesh rectopexy	Operative time, conversion rate, length of stay, postoperative complications, recurrence rates, functional results	N/a	Longer operative time, trend toward reduced length of stay, trend toward reduced complications for robotic Conversion rate, recurrence rate, and functional results similar between groups
Hiller,[102] 2016	Retrospective review	4 pediatric patients for robotic rectopexy	None	Conversion, length of stay, recurrence	11.5 mo (average)	No recurrence
van Iersel et al,[45] 2016	Prospective, observational cohort	51 robotic-assisted sacrocolporectopexy	None	Safety, quality of life, functional and sexual outcomes	12.5 mo (median)	Improved functional outcomes, quality of life, and sexual function after intervention
Inaba et al,[42] 2017	Retrospective review	24 robotic ventral mesh rectopexy	None	Perioperative parameters, conversion, postoperative complication, recurrence, incontinence, mortality	3.8 mo (median)	Low short-term morbidity and mortality

Data from Refs[40–45,100–102]

were noted to be comparable between laparoscopic and robotic rectopexies in an analysis performed by Rondelli and colleagues.[44]

Gynecologists were early adopters of robotic surgical techniques for pelvic surgery. Application of robotic surgery for rectal prolapse may be advantageous, particularly in cases of multicompartment pelvic organ prolapse that may be addressed through combined surgical procedures with gynecology colleagues. A prospective cohort study by van Iersel and colleagues[45] showed that robotic-assisted sacrocolporecto-pexy can be performed safely, with acceptable functional outcomes, quality of life, and sexual function at the study's median follow-up of 12.5 months.

Inflammatory Bowel Disease

Robotic surgery has been described previously for use in patients with medically re-fractory ulcerative colitis or neoplasia associated with chronic inflammatory bowel dis-ease (IBD) (**Table 4**). Throughout the past decade, robotic techniques have been described to complete robotic-assisted restorative proctectomy with restorative ileal pouch anal anastomosis (IPAA).[46–48] Robotic proctectomy for IBD has been found to be safe, with comparable perioperative outcomes when compared with laparoscopic proctectomy. In a case-matched study, robotic and laparoscopic proctectomy for IBD yielded similar short-term functional results without a significant difference between complication rates.[49] Similarly, in a case-matched comparison of robotic and laparo-scopic proctectomy performed at the Cleveland Clinic for IBD, no difference was seen in postoperative complications, IPAA outcomes, or quality-of-life outcomes.[50] In the largest reported series to date, Hamzaoglu and colleagues[51] demonstrated restorative proctocolectomy via a totally robotic approach is both safe and feasible, noting acceptable short-term perioperative outcomes.

Further studies have recently shown that the robotic approach during proctectomy and IPAA offer significant advantages when compared with the laparoscopic tech-nique. Lightner and colleagues[52] noted when compared with laparoscopy, the robotic platform allows for improved visibility when constructing an intracorporeal minimally invasive anastomosis. In addition, improved maneuverability was also noted due to multiple degrees of freedom of the robotic instruments, allowing better navigation of difficult angles created by the distal bony pelvis.

Robotic techniques have been described not only for initial construction of an IPAA, but also for reoperative pouch surgery in specialized cases. For example, Ragupathi and colleagues[53] described the use of robotic surgery to perform a minimally invasive rectopexy of recurrent pouch prolapse, thus salvaging the patient's pouch. Novel ap-proaches such as this can be considered, but should be individualized with respect to the patient's pathology and the surgeon's experience.

Rectal Cancer

Regardless of the surgical technique used, the oncologic principles associated with total mesorectal excision (TME) must be maintained. When performing a proctec-tomy for rectal cancer, one must include removal of the blood supply and lymphatics with appropriate mesorectal excision with radial clearance. Precise, sharp dissection of an intact TME will allow for autonomic nerve preservation, complete he-mostasis, and locoregional control of disease in the pelvis.[54,55] A major decision point in rectal resection is whether sphincter preservation can be achieved without compromising oncological resection principles.[56] With advances in technology and technique, sphincter-preserving procedures are becoming more prevalent in the era of minimally invasive surgery.

Table 4
Robotic inflammatory bowel disease studies

First Author, Year	Design	Sample Size	Comparison	Endpoints	Follow-up	Conclusion
Pedraza et al,[46] 2011	Retrospective review of consecutive cases	5 robotic-assisted restorative proctectomy with IPAA	None	Perioperative parameters, intraoperative parameters, postoperative outcomes	N/a	No complications, no conversions
McLemore et al,[48] 2012	Retrospective review, case series	3 robotic-assisted proctectomy with IPAA	None	Operative time, functional outcomes	N/a	Acceptable functional outcomes
Miller et al,[49] 2012	Case-matched comparison	17 robotic, 17 laparoscopic	Robotic and laparoscopic proctectomy	Short-term and functional outcomes	N/a	Robotic is comparable to laparoscopic with regard to perioperative outcomes, complications, and short-term functional results
Rencuzogullari et al,[50] 2016	Case-matched comparison	21 robotic, 21 laparoscopic	Robotic and laparoscopic proctectomy	Perioperative parameter, conversion rate, complication rate	N/a	Longer operative time and estimated blood loss in robotic Conversion, length of stay, and complication rate were similar
Hamzaoglu et al,[51] 2019	Retrospective review	10 totally robotic restorative proctocolectomy	None	Perioperative parameters, and short-term outcomes	30 d	No conversion, no mortality, acceptable short-term outcomes

Abbreviation: IPAA, ileal pouch and anastomosis.
Data from Refs[46,48–51]

Desire to preserve the sphincter complex and maintain intestinal continuity during rectal resection has further highlighted the need for technical precision. For example, robotic surgical techniques have been described to complete partial intersphincteric resection (ISR) for very low rectal cancer,[57] whereas a Korean study has demonstrated that robotic ISR can be performed with oncological safety.[58] Minimally invasive transanal approaches have been described to resect distal rectal tumors in close proximity to the anus. Atallah and colleagues[59] first described the use of robotic instruments to perform transanal excision of a rectal neoplasm. Early studies have reported that transanal TME can be performed with similar oncologic and perioperative outcomes compared with laparoscopic TME,[60,61] whereas Gómez-Ruiz and colleagues[62] reported that the robotic platform can be used to perform the perineal approach for transanal TME.

As minimally invasive techniques evolved, concern arose regarding if the quality of TME will be comparable to the gold-standard open resection (see **Table 6**). The COR-EAN trial provided a randomized comparison of open versus laparoscopic surgery for mid to low rectal cancer after neoadjuvant chemoradiotherapy. This study revealed no difference in the rate of circumferential resection margin (CRM) positivity, similar rates of completeness of mesorectal resection, and no difference in 3-year disease-free survival between open and laparoscopic resection groups.[63,64] The European COLOR II trial involved a randomized, international, multicenter study comparing the outcomes of laparoscopic and conventional resection of rectal carcinoma. The laparoscopic group resulted in similar safety, resection margins, and completeness of resection to that of open surgery. The 3-year locoregional recurrence and survival rates were also comparable between surgical approaches.[65–67] These studies pioneered the consideration for safety of use of minimally invasive techniques for rectal cancer resection.

The greatest potential benefit of the robotic approach when compared with laparoscopic or open techniques exists for low to mid rectal lesions deep in the pelvis (**Table 5**). Robotic TME has been shown to be safe and feasible compared with open procedure, with comparable perioperative and pathologic outcomes. However, the robotic approach was associated with longer operative times in early studies.[68–71] Robotic proctectomy has been associated with lower conversion rates compared with laparoscopic resection. Choi and colleagues[72] in a series of 50 patients undergoing a standardized step-by-step approach, demonstrated reproducibility of technique, with a positive CRM in only 1 (2%) of 50 patients. Baik and colleagues[73] reported a series of robotic versus laparoscopic low anterior resection (LAR) for rectal cancer. This study found that operative times were similar, there was no difference in leak rate and complication rate, there was a reduced risk of conversion, and that the quality of TME specimen was acceptable in both groups, with more complete specimens in the robotic group. Patriti and colleagues[74] in a case-matched cohort study of robotic versus laparoscopic LAR found that robotic technique resulted in shorter operative times with comparable postoperative morbidity. The conversion rate was significantly lower for the robotic group compared with the laparoscopic group. Overall survival and disease-free survival were comparable between groups, with a trend toward better disease-free survival in the robotic group.

Few studies are available analyzing the long-term oncological follow-up of robotic rectal cancer surgical resections (see **Table 5**). Baek and colleagues[75] provided analysis of oncologic outcomes after robotic rectal surgery. They reported a median number of harvested lymph nodes of 14.5, a median distal resection margin (DRM) of tumor of 3.4 cm, negative CRM in all specimens, and no port-site recurrences. At mean follow-up of 20.2 months (range: 1.7–52.5), none of the patients developed isolated local recurrence. The 3-year overall survival and disease-free survival were 96.2% and 73.7%, respectively.

Table 5
Robotic rectal cancer studies

First Author, Year	Design	Sample Size	Comparison	Endpoints	Follow-up	Conclusion
Baik et al,[73] 2009	Prospective comparison	113 total (56 robotic, 57 laparoscopic)	Robotic vs laparoscopic LAR	Perioperative clinical results, complications, pathologic details	N/a	Similar operative time and pathologic parameters Reduced complication rate in robotic
Choi et al,[72] 2009	Prospectively collected data of consecutive cases	50 robotic rectal cancer resection	None	Operative time, CRM, lymph node harvest, length of stay, anastomotic leak rate	N/a	Acceptable short-term outcomes
Patriti et al,[74] 2009	Case-matched	66 patients (29 robotic, 37 laparoscopic)	Robotic vs laparoscopic rectal resection	Perioperative parameters, morbidity, survival data	12 mo	Shorter operative time, lower conversion rate for robotic Comparable morbidity, overall survival and disease-free survival
Baek et al,[75] 2010	Retrospective review of consecutive cases	64 robotic TME	None	Perioperative parameters, pathologic data, local recurrence, and survival	3 y	Safe and effective in terms of recurrence and survival rates
deSouza et al,[71] 2011	Retrospective	36 robotic, 46 open	Open vs robotic TME	Demographics, perioperative outcomes, pathology	N/a	Comparable perioperative and pathologic outcomes Longer operative time in robotic group
Memon et al,[69] 2012	Meta-analysis	7 studies (353 robotic, 401 laparoscopic)	Robotic vs laparoscopic proctectomy	Conversion rates, operation times, length of stay, complications, oncologic outcomes (CRM, lymph node harvest, DRM)	N/a	Decreased conversion rate in robotic Equivalent oncologic outcomes

Study	Type	Sample	Comparison	Outcomes		Conclusion
Xiong et al,[70] 2015	Meta-analysis	8 studies 1229 patients total (554 robotic, 675 laparoscopic)	Robotic vs laparoscopic TME	Operative and recovery outcomes, early postoperative morbidity, oncological parameters	N/a	Equivalent or preferable robotic short-term oncological and functional outcomes
Rouanet et al,[81] 2018	Retrospective cohort	200 laparoscopic 200 robotic	Robotic vs laparoscopic TME for sphincter-saving surgery	Conversion to open or transanal approaches, operative time, postoperative morbidity, CRM, DRM, quality of life, genitourinary function, oncological outcomes	N/a	Robotic TME is less likely to convert to open Equivalent operative times, pathologic criteria
Jones et al,[82] 2018	Systematic review	1 RCT, 27 comparative studies	Robotic vs laparoscopic TME	Operative, postoperative and oncological outcomes	N/a	Robotic TME had longer operative time, earlier return of bowel function, lower risk of conversion, shorter hospitalization Equivalent blood loss, morbidity, mortality, reoperation risk, recurrence, lymph node harvest, CRM, DRM

Abbreviations: CRM, circumferential resection margin; DRM, distal resection margin; LAR, laparoscopic low anterior resection; RCT, randomized controlled trial; TME, total mesorectal incision.
Data from Refs[69–75,81,82].

Several multicenter randomized trials have recently investigated reproducibility and applicability of minimally invasive techniques to oncologic dissection for rectal cancer (**Table 6**). The Australasian Laparoscopic Cancer of the Rectum (ALaCaRT) trial randomized patients with rectal cancer to compare laparoscopic and open resection and reported results that revealed a lack of noninferiority of laparoscopic resection over the gold-standard open resections.[76] The American College of Surgeons Oncology Group (ACOSOG)-Z6051 trial involved a multicenter, noninferiority randomized trial to compare laparoscopic versus open rectal cancer surgery. Fleshman and colleagues[77] concluded that laparoscopic surgery for patients with stage II or III rectal cancer failed to demonstrate noninferiority for pathologic outcomes when compared with open resection, therefore questioning the use of laparoscopy in this patient population. Subsequent 2-year follow-up disease-free survival and recurrence data revealed no statistically significant difference between rates in the laparoscopic resection group when compared with traditional open resections.[78]

The Robotic versus Laparoscopic Resection for Rectal Cancer (ROLARR) trial investigated the safety, efficacy, and outcomes of robotic versus laparoscopic rectal cancer surgery (see **Table 6**). This international, multicenter, prospective, randomized controlled trial compared the 2 minimally invasive approaches for risk of conversion to open procedure, with secondary end points that included intraoperative and postoperative complications, as well as pathologic, functional, and short-term oncologic outcomes. The initial study results found that the robotic approach did not significantly reduce the risk of conversion to open procedure when compared with laparoscopic resection, suggesting that robotic-assisted surgery, performed by surgeons with varying degrees of experience, did not offer an advantage over laparoscopy. Subgroup analysis in male patients suggested a benefit of robotic surgery over laparoscopic surgery with regard to conversion rates, although due to insufficient numbers of patients per group, statistical significance could not be concluded.[79] Corrigan and colleagues[80] analyzed the ROLARR trials initial results, using multilevel logistic regression to adjust for varying experience levels of the operating robotic surgeon. This study concluded that the participating surgeons in ROLARR were experts in laparoscopic surgery, whereas some of these surgeons were still in the learning-curve phase of robotic surgery, suggesting that this factor may have confounded the concluded results of the ROLARR trial.

In response to the ROLARR trial, Rouanet and colleagues[81] performed a prospectively registered, retrospective single-center cohort study comparing robotic and laparoscopic TME, using similar primary and secondary end points as examined in ROLARR. In their experience, robotic TME was less likely to be converted to open when compared with laparoscopic surgery, with equivalent operative times and pathologic outcomes between the 2 cohorts. Following the ROLARR trial publication, Jones and colleagues[82] subsequently performed a systematic review to compare outcomes in patients undergoing TME robotically versus laparoscopically. Meta-analysis of 547 patients from 28 studies revealed comparable oncologic and perioperative outcomes between minimally invasive approaches, concluding that robotic rectal cancer resection is not superior to laparoscopic resection, but is an oncologically safe and feasible approach associated with reduced rates of conversion.

The benefits of a minimally invasive surgical approach to rectal cancer have included less blood loss, earlier return of bowel function, and shortened length of hospital stay.[63,65,83] In multiple randomized controlled trials, including the COLOR II and COREAN trials, the oncological safety and feasibility of the laparoscopic technique were established. There was no difference in pathologic outcomes, overall survival, and disease-free survival between these approaches.[84–87] Yet, despite

Table 6
Landmark minimally invasive rectal cancer studies

Study Name	First Author, Year	Design	Sample Size	Comparison	Endpoints	Follow-up	Conclusion
COREAN	Kang et al,[63] 2010 Jeong et al,[64] 2014	Randomized controlled trial	340 total patients (170 laparoscopic, 170 open)	Open vs laparoscopic surgery for mid and low rectal cancer after neoadjuvant chemoradiation	Involvement of CRM, macroscopic quality of TME, lymph node harvest, recovery of bowel function, perioperative morbidity, postoperative pain, quality of life	3-y disease-free survival	Quality of oncological resection was equivalent Improved short-term outcomes in robotic group Similar disease-free survival
COLOR II	van der Pas et al,[65] 2013 Andersson et al,[66] 2014 Bonjer et al,[67] 2015	Randomized	739 laparoscopic, 364 open 385 patients 1044 patients (699 laparoscopic, 345 open)	Open vs laparoscopic rectal cancer resection	Short-term outcomes: operative findings, complications, mortality, pathology parameters Genitourinary function Locoregional recurrence, disease-free and overall survival	24 mo 3 y	Similar safety, resection margins, and completeness of resection Improved recovery after laparoscopy No change in genitourinary functional outcomes Similar locoregional recurrence and disease-free survival
ALaCaRT	Stevenson et al,[76] 2015	Randomized	237 open, 238 robotic	Open vs laparoscopic rectal resection	Oncologic parameters (completeness of TME CRM, DRM)	N/a	Noninferiority of laparoscopic surgery compared with open surgery was not established

(continued on next page)

Table 6
(continued)

Study Name	First Author, Year	Design	Sample Size	Comparison	Endpoints	Follow-up	Conclusion
ACOSOG Z6051	Fleshman et al,[77] 2015 Fleshman et al,[78] 2019	Randomized	240 laparoscopic, 222 open	Open vs laparoscopic rectal cancer resection after neoadjuvant therapy	CRM, DRM, completeness of TME Disease-free survival and recurrence	47.9 mo (median)	Use of laparoscopy compared with open failed to meet criterion for noninferiority Similar disease-free survival and recurrence rates
ROLARR	Jayne et al,[79] 2017	Randomized controlled trial	471 patients (237 robotic, 234 laparoscopic)	Robotic-assisted vs laparoscopic rectal cancer resection	Conversion to open, intraoperative and postoperative complications, CRM, pathologic outcomes, quality of life, genitourinary function	30 d, 6 mo	Robotic surgery did not significantly reduce risk of conversion to open

Abbreviations: CRM, circumferential resection margin; DRM, distal resection margin; TME, total mesorectal incision.
Data from Refs [63–67,76–79].

this evidence, much concern has been brought to light after the recent findings of the ACOSOG Z6051 and ALaCaRT trials regarding the efficacy of the laparoscopic approach.[76,77] The failure to prove noninferiority in these studies was related to the pathologic composite scoring consisting of the DRM, CRM, and the pathologic quality of the mesorectum. It has been well-established that the quality of the mesorectum and the ability to obtain a negative CRM are associated with lower local and distal recurrence rates and improved long-term survival.[88–92] Quirke and colleagues[88] identified that the ability to achieve a complete mesorectal excision translated into a 4% 3-year local recurrence rate and increased to 7% for a near complete and 13% for an incomplete excision. In a recent meta-analysis performed after the ALaCaRT and ACOSOG trials, the risk of obtaining a noncomplete mesorectal excision is significantly increased in patients undergoing a laparoscopic TME.[93] Although no differences were identified in the rate of a positive CRM, there was a significant difference in the grade of mesorectal excision. In these studies, noncomplete mesorectal excision (nearly complete and incomplete) was reported in 12.3% of patients undergoing a laparoscopic TME and 10.5% of patients undergoing an open TME ($P = .02$). There were no identifiable differences in the DRM, number of lymph nodes, and mean distance to the radial margin.[94] The ALaCaRT and ACOSOG trials that have raised similar concerns regarding the oncological difference between laparoscopic and open TME.[76,77] In the ALaCaRT trial, TME completeness was 92% for the open group and 87% for the laparoscopic TME group. In the ACOSOG Z6051 trial, complete TME was 95% for the open group and 92% for the laparoscopic group. These results were further studied in a recent meta-analysis. Creavin and colleagues[95] included the most recent 4 randomized controlled trials, which included 2319 patients. The mesorectum was noted to be intact in 83.6% of patients undergoing laparoscopic TME compared with 87.1% of patients undergoing an open resection ($P = .001$). Superficial defects in the mesorectum were identified more frequently in the laparoscopic group. However, there was no difference in the 2 groups in relation to deep defects, CRM positivity, DRM, and number of obtained lymph nodes. The investigators hypothesized that the increased incidence of superficial defects in the laparoscopic group were secondary to grasping injuries or traction tears from the laparoscopic instruments. The robotic approach to TME is focused on addressing the limitations of transabdominal laparoscopic surgery in the narrow confines of the pelvis. Studies addressing this potential advantage have had mixed results. Hoshino and colleagues,[94] in a meta-analysis, identified a significantly lower incidence of a positive CRM in 2 reviews and not significantly different in 9 reviews. There was no identifiable significant difference for DRM, local recurrence, disease-free survival, and overall survival. The issue regarding the completeness of the TME has been further studied in a meta-analysis by Milone and colleagues[96] in 2019. Twelve articles were included in the analysis involving 1520 procedures. Complete TME showed a statistically significant difference in favor of robotic surgery (odds ratio 1.83, 95% confidence interval 1.08–3.10, $P = .03$). These investigators concluded the "results are encouraging to consider the robotic approach to rectal resection is the better way to obtain a complete TME resection." The value of the robot in obtaining an oncologically equivalent result to open surgery with specific concern to the quality of the mesorectal resection is paramount to the benefits of the robotic approach.

DISCLOSURE

None.

REFERENCES

1. Cooperman A, Katz V, Zimmon D, et al. Laparoscopic colon resection: a case report. J Laparoendosc Surg 1991;1(4):221–4.
2. Jacobs M, Verdeja J, Goldstein H. Minimally invasive colon resection (laparoscopic colectomy). Surg Laparosc Endosc 1991;1(3):144–50.
3. Fowler D, White S. Laparoscopy-assisted sigmoid resection. Surg Laparosc Endosc 1991;1(3):183–8.
4. Alexander RJT, Jaques BC, Mitchell KG. Laparoscopically assisted colectomy and wound recurrence. Lancet 1993;341(8839):249–50.
5. O'Rourke N, Price PM, Kelly S, et al. Tumour inoculation during laparoscopy. Lancet 1993;342(8867):368–9.
6. The Clinical Outcomes of Surgical Therapy Study Group. A comparison of laparoscopically assisted and open colectomy for colon cancer. N Engl J Med 2004;350(20):2050–9.
7. Jayne DG, Guillou PJ, Thorpe H, et al. Randomized trial of laparoscopic-assisted resection of colorectal carcinoma: 3-year results of the UK MRC CLASICC Trial Group. J Clin Oncol 2007;25(21):3061–8.
8. Jayne DG, Thorpe HC, Copeland J, et al. Five-year follow-up of the Medical Research Council CLASICC trial of laparoscopically assisted versus open surgery for colorectal cancer. Br J Surg 2010;97(11):1638–45.
9. Green BL, Marshall HC, Collinson F, et al. Long-term follow-up of the Medical Research Council CLASICC trial of conventional versus laparoscopically assisted resection in colorectal cancer. Br J Surg 2013;100(1):75–82.
10. Color Study Group. COLOR: a randomized clinical trial comparing laparoscopic and open resection for colon cancer. Dig Surg 2000;17(6):617–22.
11. Hazebroek EJ, The Color Study Group. COLOR. Surg Endosc 2002;16(6):949–53.
12. Colon Cancer Laparoscopic or Open Resection Study Group, Buunen M, Veldkamp R, Hop WC, et al. Survival after laparoscopic surgery versus open surgery for colon cancer: long-term outcome of a randomised clinical trial. Lancet Oncol 2009;10(1):44–52.
13. Veldkamp R, Kuhry E, Hop W, et al. Laparoscopic surgery versus open surgery for colon cancer: short-term outcomes of a randomised trial. Lancet Oncol 2005;6(7):477–84.
14. Deijen CL, Vasmel JE, de Lange-de Klerk ESM, et al. Ten-year outcomes of a randomised trial of laparoscopic versus open surgery for colon cancer. Surg Endosc 2017;31(6):2607–15.
15. Braga M, Vignali A, Gianotti L, et al. Laparoscopic versus open colorectal surgery: a randomized trial on short-term outcome. Ann Surg 2002;236(6):759–67.
16. Lacy AM, García-Valdecasas JC, Delgado S, et al. Laparoscopy-assisted colectomy versus open colectomy for treatment of non-metastatic colon cancer: a randomised trial. Lancet 2002;359(9325):2224–9.
17. Liang J-T, Huang K-C, Lai H-S, et al. Oncologic results of laparoscopic versus conventional open surgery for stage II or III left-sided colon cancers: a randomized controlled trial. Ann Surg Oncol 2007;14(1):109–17.
18. Braga M, Frasson M, Zuliani W, et al. Randomized clinical trial of laparoscopic versus open left colonic resection. Br J Surg 2010;97(8):1180–6.
19. Abraham NS, Young JM, Solomon MJ. Meta-analysis of short-term outcomes after laparoscopic resection for colorectal cancer. Br J Surg 2004;91(9):1111–24.

20. Tekkis PP, Senagore AJ, Delaney CP, et al. Evaluation of the learning curve in laparoscopic colorectal surgery: comparison of right-sided and left-sided resections. Ann Surg 2005;242(1):83–91.

21. Hewett PJ, Allardyce RA, Bagshaw PF, et al. Short-term outcomes of the australasian randomized clinical study comparing laparoscopic and conventional open surgical treatments for colon cancer: the ALCCaS trial. Ann Surg 2008;248(5): 728–38.

22. Bagshaw PF, Allardyce RA, Frampton CM, et al, Australasian Laparoscopic Colon Cancer Study Group. Long-term outcomes of the Australasian randomized clinical trial comparing laparoscopic and conventional open surgical treatments for colon cancer: the Australasian Laparoscopic Colon Cancer Study trial. Ann Surg 2012;256(6):915–9.

23. McCombie AM, Frizelle F, Bagshaw PF, et al. The ALCCaS trial: a randomized controlled trial comparing quality of life following laparoscopic versus open colectomy for colon cancer. Dis Colon Rectum 2018;61(10):1156–62.

24. Marusch F, Gastinger I, Schneider C, et al. Importance of conversion for results obtained with laparoscopic colorectal surgery. Dis Colon Rectum 2001;44(2): 207–14.

25. Polat F, Willems LH, Dogan K, et al. The oncological and surgical safety of robot-assisted surgery in colorectal cancer: outcomes of a longitudinal prospective cohort study. Surg Endosc 2019;33(11):3644–55.

26. Kang J, Park YA, Baik SH, et al. A comparison of open, laparoscopic, and robotic surgery in the treatment of right-sided colon cancer. Surg Laparosc Endosc Percutan Tech 2016;26(6):497–502.

27. Reitz ACW, Lin E, Rosen SA. A single surgeon's experience transitioning to robotic-assisted right colectomy with intracorporeal anastomosis. Surg Endosc 2018;32(8):3525–32.

28. van Oostendorp S, Elfrink A, Borstlap W, et al. Intracorporeal versus extracorporeal anastomosis in right hemicolectomy: a systematic review and meta-analysis. Surg Endosc 2017;31(1):64–77.

29. Magistro C, Lernia SD, Ferrari G, et al. Totally laparoscopic versus laparoscopic-assisted right colectomy for colon cancer: is there any advantage in short-term outcomes? A prospective comparative assessment in our center. Surg Endosc 2013;27(7):2613–8.

30. Lujan HJ, Plasencia G, Rivera BX, et al. Advantages of robotic right colectomy with intracorporeal anastomosis. Surg Laparosc Endosc Percutan Tech 2018; 28(1):36–41

31. Widmar M, Keskin M, Beltran P, et al. Incisional hernias after laparoscopic and robotic right colectomy. Hernia 2016;20(5):723–8.

32. Samia H, Lawrence J, Nobel T, et al. Extraction site location and incisional hernias after laparoscopic colorectal surgery: should we be avoiding the midline? Am J Surg 2013;205(3):264–8.

33. Byrn JC, Hrabe JE, Charlton ME. An initial experience with 85 consecutive robotic-assisted rectal dissections: improved operating times and lower costs with experience. Surg Endosc 2014;28(11):3101–7.

34. Vasudevan V, Reusche R, Wallace H, et al. Clinical outcomes and cost–benefit analysis comparing laparoscopic and robotic colorectal surgeries. Surg Endosc 2016;30(12):5490–3.

35. Cleary RK, Mullard AJ, Ferraro J, et al. The cost of conversion in robotic and laparoscopic colorectal surgery. Surg Endosc 2018;32(3):1515–24.

36. Harr JN, Haskins IN, Amdur RL, et al. The effect of obesity on laparoscopic and robotic-assisted colorectal surgery outcomes: an ACS-NSQIP database analysis. J Robot Surg 2018;12(2):317–23.

37. Bhama AR, Obias V, Welch KB, et al. A comparison of laparoscopic and robotic colorectal surgery outcomes using the American College of Surgeons National Surgical Quality Improvement Program (ACS NSQIP) database. Surg Endosc 2016;30(4):1576–84.

38. Bhama AR, Wafa AM, Ferraro J, et al. Comparison of risk factors for unplanned conversion from laparoscopic and robotic to open colorectal surgery using the Michigan Surgical Quality Collaborative (MSQC) database. J Gastrointest Surg 2016;20(6):1223–30.

39. Tam MS, Kaoutzanis C, Mullard AJ, et al. A population-based study comparing laparoscopic and robotic outcomes in colorectal surgery. Surg Endosc 2016; 30(2):455–63.

40. Mäkelä-Kaikkonen J, Rautio T, Pääkkö E, et al. Robot-assisted vs laparoscopic ventral rectopexy for external or internal rectal prolapse and enterocele: a randomized controlled trial. Colorectal Dis 2016;18(10):1010–5.

41. Haahr C, Jakobsen H, Gögenur I. Robot-assisted rectopexy is a safe and feasible option for treatment of rectal prolapse. Dan Med J 2014;61(5):A4842.

42. Inaba CS, Sujatha-Bhaskar S, Koh CY, et al. Robotic ventral mesh rectopexy for rectal prolapse: a single-institution experience. Tech Coloproctol 2017;21(8): 667–71.

43. Ramage L, Georgiou P, Tekkis P, et al. Is robotic ventral mesh rectopexy better than laparoscopy in the treatment of rectal prolapse and obstructed defecation? A meta-analysis. Tech Coloproctol 2015;19(7):381–9.

44. Rondelli F, Bugiantella W, Villa F, et al. Robot-assisted or conventional laparoscopic rectopexy for rectal prolapse? Systematic review and meta-analysis. Int J Surg 2014;12:S153–9.

45. van Iersel JJ, de Witte CJ, Verheijen PM, et al. Robot-assisted sacrocolporectopexy for multicompartment prolapse of the pelvic floor: a prospective cohort study evaluating functional and sexual outcome. Dis Colon Rectum 2016; 59(10):968–74.

46. Pedraza R, Patel CB, Ramos-Valadez DI, et al. Robotic-assisted laparoscopic surgery for restorative proctocolectomy with ileal J pouch-anal anastomosis. Minim Invasive Ther Allied Technol 2011;20(4):234–9.

47. Anzai H, Ishihara S, Kiyomatsu T, et al. Robot-assisted restorative proctocolectomy and ileal pouch–anal anastomosis for ulcerative colitis. Videoscopy 2017;27(4). Available at: https://www.liebertpub.com/doi/10.1089/vor.2016.0383. Accessed January 23, 2020.

48. McLemore EC, Cullen J, Horgan S, et al. Robotic-assisted laparoscopic stage II restorative proctectomy for toxic ulcerative colitis. Int J Med Robot 2012;8(2): 178–83.

49. Miller AT, Berian JR, Rubin M, et al. Robotic-assisted proctectomy for inflammatory bowel disease: a case-matched comparison of laparoscopic and robotic technique. J Gastrointest Surg 2012;16(3):587–94.

50. Rencuzogullari A, Gorgun E, Costedio M, et al. Case-matched comparison of robotic versus laparoscopic proctectomy for inflammatory bowel disease. Surg Laparosc Endosc Percutan Tech 2016;26(3):e37–40.

51. Hamzaoglu I, Baca B, Esen E, et al. Short-term results after totally robotic restorative total proctocolectomy with ileal pouch anal anastomosis for ulcerative colitis. Surg Laparosc Endosc Percutan Tech 2019;30(1):40–4.

52. Lightner AL, Kelley SR, Larson DW. Robotic platform for an IPAA. Dis Colon Rectum 2018;61(7).

53. Ragupathi M, Patel CB, Ramos-Valadez DI, et al. Robotic-assisted laparoscopic "salvage" rectopexy for recurrent ileoanal J-pouch prolapse. Gastroenterol Res Pract 2010;2010:4.

54. Beck D, Nasseri Y, Hull T, et al. The ASCRS manual of colon and rectal surgery. Berlin, Germany: Springer; 2014.

55. Heald RJ, Husband EM, Ryall RDH. The mesorectum in rectal cancer surgery—the clue to pelvic recurrence? Br J Surg 1982;69(10):613–6.

56. Corman ML. Principles of surgical technique in the treatment of carcinoma of the large bowel. World J Surg 1991;15(5):592–6.

57. Gorgun E, Benlice C. Robotic partial intersphincteric resection with colonic J-pouch anal anastomosis for a very low rectal cancer. Tech Coloproctol 2016;20(10):725.

58. Park SY, Choi G-S, Park JS, et al. Short-term clinical outcome of robot-assisted intersphincteric resection for low rectal cancer: a retrospective comparison with conventional laparoscopy. Surg Endosc 2013;27(1):48–55.

59. Atallah S, Parra-Davila E, deBeche-Adams T, et al. Excision of a rectal neoplasm using robotic transanal surgery (RTS): a description of the technique. Tech Coloproctol 2012;16(5):389–92.

60. Ma B, Gao P, Song Y, et al. Transanal total mesorectal excision (taTME) for rectal cancer: a systematic review and meta-analysis of oncological and perioperative outcomes compared with laparoscopic total mesorectal excision. BMC Cancer 2016;16:380.

61. Penna M, Hompes R, Arnold S, et al. Transanal total mesorectal excision: international registry results of the first 720 cases. Ann Surg 2017;266(1):111–7.

62. Gómez Ruiz M, Parra IM, Palazuelos CM, et al. Robotic-assisted laparoscopic transanal total mesorectal excision for rectal cancer: a prospective pilot study. Dis Colon Rectum 2015;58(1):145–53.

63. Kang S-B, Park JW, Jeong S-Y, et al. Open versus laparoscopic surgery for mid or low rectal cancer after neoadjuvant chemoradiotherapy (COREAN trial): short-term outcomes of an open-label randomised controlled trial. Lancet Oncol 2010;11(7):637–45.

64. Jeong S-Y, Park JW, Nam BH, et al. Open versus laparoscopic surgery for mid-rectal or low-rectal cancer after neoadjuvant chemoradiotherapy (COREAN trial): survival outcomes of an open-label, non-inferiority, randomised controlled trial. Lancet Oncol 2014;15(7):767–74.

65. van der Pas MHGM, Haglind E, Cuesta MA, et al. Laparoscopic versus open surgery for rectal cancer (COLOR II): short-term outcomes of a randomised, phase 3 trial. Lancet Oncol 2013;14(3):210–8.

66. Andersson J, Abis G, Gellerstedt M, et al. Patient-reported genitourinary dysfunction after laparoscopic and open rectal cancer surgery in a randomized trial (COLOR II). Br J Surg 2014;101(10):1272–9.

67. Bonjer HJ, Deijen CL, Abis GA, et al. A randomized trial of laparoscopic versus open surgery for rectal cancer. N Engl J Med 2015;372(14):1324–32.

68. Ballantyne GH. Robotic surgery, telerobotic surgery, telepresence, and telementoring. Surg Endosc 2002;16(10):1389–402.

69. Memon S, Heriot AG, Murphy DG, et al. Robotic versus laparoscopic proctectomy for rectal cancer: a meta-analysis. Ann Surg Oncol 2012;19(7):2095–101.

70. Xiong B, Ma L, Huang W, et al. Robotic versus laparoscopic total mesorectal excision for rectal cancer: a meta-analysis of eight studies. J Gastrointest Surg 2015;19(3):516–26.

71. deSouza AL, Prasad LM, Ricci J, et al. A comparison of open and robotic total mesorectal excision for rectal adenocarcinoma. Dis Colon Rectum 2011;54(3): 275–82.

72. Choi DJ, Kim SH, Lee PJM, et al. Single-stage totally robotic dissection for rectal cancer surgery: technique and short-term outcome in 50 consecutive patients. Dis Colon Rectum 2009;52(11):1824–30.

73. Baik SH, Kwon HY, Kim JS, et al. Robotic versus laparoscopic low anterior resection of rectal cancer: short-term outcome of a prospective comparative study. Ann Surg Oncol 2009;16(6):1480–7.

74. Patriti A, Ceccarelli G, Bartoli A, et al. Short- and medium-term outcome of robot-assisted and traditional laparoscopic rectal resection. JSLS 2009;13(2): 176–83.

75. Baek J-H, McKenzie S, Garcia-Aguilar J, et al. Oncologic outcomes of robotic-assisted total mesorectal excision for the treatment of rectal cancer. Ann Surg 2010;251(5):882–6.

76. Stevenson ARL, Solomon MJ, Lumley JW, et al. Effect of laparoscopic-assisted resection vs open resection on pathological outcomes in rectal cancer: the ALa-CaRT randomized clinical trial laparoscopic-assisted resection vs open resection for rectal cancer laparoscopic-assisted resection vs open resection for rectal cancer. JAMA 2015;314(13):1356–63.

77. Fleshman J, Branda M, Sargent DJ, et al. Effect of laparoscopic-assisted resection vs open resection of stage II or III rectal cancer on pathologic outcomes: the ACOSOG Z6051 randomized clinical trial. JAMA 2015;314(13):1346–55.

78. Fleshman J, Branda ME, Sargent DJ, et al. Disease-free survival and local recurrence for laparoscopic resection compared with open resection of stage II to III rectal cancer: follow-up results of the ACOSOG Z6051 randomized controlled trial. Ann Surg 2019;269(4):589–95.

79. Jayne D, Pigazzi A, Marshall H, et al. Effect of robotic-assisted vs conventional laparoscopic surgery on risk of conversion to open laparotomy among patients undergoing resection for rectal cancer: the ROLARR randomized clinical trial. JAMA 2017;318(16):1569–80.

80. Corrigan N, Marshall H, Croft J, et al. Exploring and adjusting for potential learning effects in ROLARR: a randomised controlled trial comparing robotic-assisted vs. standard laparoscopic surgery for rectal cancer resection. Trials 2018;19(1):339.

81. Rouanet P, Bertrand MM, Jarlier M, et al. Robotic versus laparoscopic total mesorectal excision for sphincter-saving surgery: results of a single-center series of 400 consecutive patients and perspectives. Ann Surg Oncol 2018;25(12): 3572–9.

82. Jones K, Qassem MG, Sains P, et al. Robotic total meso-rectal excision for rectal cancer: a systematic review following the publication of the ROLARR trial. World J Gastrointest Oncol 2018;10(11):449–64.

83. Guillou PJ, Quirke P, Thorpe H, et al. Short-term endpoints of conventional versus laparoscopic-assisted surgery in patients with colorectal cancer (MRC CLASICC trial): multicentre, randomised controlled trial. Lancet 2005; 365(9472):1718–26.

84. Zhao J-K, Chen N-Z, Zheng J-B, et al. Laparoscopic versus open surgery for rectal cancer: results of a systematic review and meta-analysis on clinical efficacy. Mol Clin Oncol 2014;2(6):1097–102.

85. Vennix S, Pelzers L, Bouvy N, et al. Laparoscopic versus open total mesorectal excision for rectal cancer. Cochrane Database Syst Rev 2014;(4):CD005200.

86. Xiong B, Ma L, Zhang C. Laparoscopic versus open total mesorectal excision for middle and low rectal cancer: a meta-analysis of results of randomized controlled trials. J Laparoendosc Adv Surg Tech A 2012;22(7): 674–84.

87. Arezzo A, Passera R, Salvai A, et al. Laparoscopy for rectal cancer is oncologically adequate: a systematic review and meta-analysis of the literature. Surg Endosc 2015;29(2):334–48.

88. Quirke P, Steele R, Monson J, et al. Effect of the plane of surgery achieved on local recurrence in patients with operable rectal cancer: a prospective study using data from the MRC CR07 and NCIC-CTG CO16 randomised clinical trial. Lancet 2009;373(9666):821–8.

89. Kusters M, Marijnen CAM, van de Velde CJH, et al. Patterns of local recurrence in rectal cancer; a study of the Dutch TME trial. Eur J Surg Oncol 2010;36(5): 470–6.

90. Nagtegaal ID, Quirke P. What is the role for the circumferential margin in the modern treatment of rectal cancer? J Clin Oncol 2008;26(2):303–12.

91. Birbeck KF, Macklin CP, Tiffin NJ, et al. Rates of circumferential resection margin involvement vary between surgeons and predict outcomes in rectal cancer surgery. Ann Surg 2002;235(4):449–57.

92. García-Granero E, Faiz O, Muñoz E, et al. Macroscopic assessment of mesorectal excision in rectal cancer. Cancer 2009;115(15):3400–11.

93. Martínez-Pérez A, Carra MC, Brunetti F, et al. Pathologic outcomes of laparoscopic vs open mesorectal excision for rectal cancer: a systematic review and meta-analysis. JAMA Surg 2017;152(4):e165665.

94. Hoshino N, Sakamoto T, Hida K, et al. Robotic versus laparoscopic surgery for rectal cancer: an overview of systematic reviews with quality assessment of current evidence. Surg Today 2019;49(7):556–70.

95. Creavin B, Kelly ME, Ryan E, et al. Meta-analysis of the impact of surgical approach on the grade of mesorectal excision in rectal cancer. Br J Surg 2017;104(12):1609–19.

96. Milone M, Manigrasso M, Velotti N, et al. Completeness of total mesorectum excision of laparoscopic versus robotic surgery: a review with a meta-analysis. Int J Colorectal Dis 2019;34(6):983–91.

97. Weeks JC, Nelson H, Gelber S, et al, Clinical Outcomes of Surgical Therapy (COST) Study Group. Short-term quality-of-life outcomes following laparoscopic-assisted colectomy vs open colectomy for colon cancer: a randomized trial. JAMA 2002;287(3):321–8.

98. Law KE, Lowndes BR, Kelley SR, et al. NASA-task load index differentiates surgical approach: opportunities for improvement in colon and rectal surgery. Ann Surg 2019. [Epub ahead of print].

99. Armijo PR, Huang C-K, High R, et al. Ergonomics of minimally invasive surgery: an analysis of muscle effort and fatigue in the operating room between laparoscopic and robotic surgery. Surg Endosc 2019;33(7):2323–31.

100. Perrenot C, Germain A, Scherrer M-L, et al. Long-term outcomes of robot-assisted laparoscopic rectopexy for rectal prolapse. Dis Colon Rectum 2013;56: 909–14.
101. Germain A, Perrenot C, Scherrer ML, et al. Long-term outcome of robotic-assisted laparoscopic rectopexy for full-thickness rectal prolapse in elderly patients. Colorectal Dis 2014;16(3):198–202.
102. Hiller D, Bohl J, Zeller K. Robotic Rectopexy for Rectal Prolapse in Pediatric Patients. Am Surg 2017;83(12):1386–9.

Urologic Robotic Surgery

David Mikhail, MD[a],*, Joseph Sarcona, MD[a], Mina Mekhail, BSc (Hons)[b],
Lee Richstone, MD[a,1]

KEYWORDS

- Robotic surgery • Robotic partial nephrectomy • Robotic prostatectomy
- Robotic cystectomy • Single-port robotic surgery • Robotic pyeloplasty
- Pediatric robotic surgery

KEY POINTS

- Urology has been at the forefront of modern robotic surgery since the 1990s. Currently, almost all urologic procedures are performed robotically.
- As technology improves and the community's experience expands, use of modern robotic surgery continues to become more efficient and cost effective.
- The learning curve continues to decrease for urologic robotic procedures. Simultaneously, post-operative outcomes continue to improve and most would agree have surpassed open surgical outcomes for most procedures.
- Robotics continue to evolve with the development of single-port robotic consoles – already being used by urologists for multiple procedures.
- Robotic surgery in urology is quickly becoming the gold standard in the United States and is expanding significantly throughout the developed world. The future is exciting.

INTRODUCTION AND HISTORY OF ROBOTICS IN UROLOGY

Urologists have always been leaders in advancing surgical technology, including endoscopic transurethral surgery, the use of lasers for various applications, and were early adopters and innovators of laparoscopy in the early 1990s.[1] Less than a decade later, urologists were the first to use the modern robotic surgical system, as Pasticier and colleagues[2] reported their experience of robotic-assisted laparoscopic radical proctectomy. Although this case series only included 5 patient participants, it was the first to show the feasibility and benefit of modern robotic systems with the da Vinci surgical system (Intuitive Surgical, Sunnyvale, CA). Variables such as surgeon ergonomics, improved instrument precision, operative time, and postoperative recovery were objectively improved.[2]

[a] Lenox Hill Hospital (Northwell Health), 170 E 77th Street, Suite B, New York, NY, 10075; [b] St. George's University, School of Medicine, PO Box 7, St George's, Grenada, West Indies
[1] Present address: 170 E 77th Street, Suite B, New York, NY, 10075.
* Corresponding author.
E-mail address: dmikhail2013@gmail.com

https://doi.org/10.1016/j.suc.2019.12.003
surgical.theclinics.com

The US Food and Drug Administration has approved 5 robotic systems to date: AESOP, Endoassist, Neuromate, Zeus, and da Vinci[3]; however, the term 'robotic surgery' became synonymous with the da Vinci Surgical System (Intuitive Surgical) soon after that seminal report was published. The system includes 3 components: a surgeon console (the control), patient cart, and vision cart.[4] Intuitive Surgical had patented EndoWrist Technology to the console, which provides 7° of freedom and 90° of articulation[4] per controller, mimicking the actual range of motion of the human wrist. The patient cart interacts with the patient, and the vision cart displays a real-time visualization of the procedure.[5] These 3 components work in unison to facilitate surgical procedures. In 2001, the first transatlantic surgery (remote laparoscopic cholecystectomy) was performed on a 68-year-old female patient in Stratsbourg, France, while the surgeons controlled the robot (Zeus, now owned by Intuitive Surgical) from New York, New York, with a delay of only 155 ms.[6]

A review of the da Vinci system's surgical resume displays the machine's versatility in urology, with notable applications beyond radical and simple prostatectomies, including radical and partial nephrectomy, living donor nephrectomy, pyeloplasty, pyelolithotomy, radical and simple cystectomy, adrenalectomy, diverticulotomy, spermatic cord denervation, sural nerve grafting, simple cystectomy, sacrocolpopexy, urolithiasis, fistula repair, ureteroureterostomy, ureterolysis, vasectomy reversal, varicoceletomy, and vasovasostomy.[7,8]

This review aims to highlight the current advances in robotic-assisted urologic surgery, present the challenges faced, and highlight the potential for future development.

CURRENT PRACTICES
Radical Prostatectomy

Prostate cancer is the most common nonskin cancer and the second leading cause of male cancer-related deaths in the United States. In 2014, it was estimated that 233,000 new cases would occur; it would be the cause of death for 29,480 men.[9] Modern treatment of prostate cancer with early detection through screening and improved treatment for later stage disease has resulted in a decreased mortality of 16% as of 2014. This equates to a 3% cause of death in the US male population.[9] More recently, controversy surrounding prostate-specific antigen screening and changes in US Preventive Services Task Force recommendations have led to decreased prostate-specific antigen testing and biopsy with a subsequent decline in incidence of localized prostate cancer. Some data has shown early signs of a shift toward a higher burden of disease at presentation.[10]

Although practice paradigms are changing with the modernization of active surveillance, surgery remains as the mainstay of treatment for localized prostate cancer. Studies such as the Scandinavian Prostate Cancer Study Group-4 (SPCG-4) trial and the Prostate Cancer Intervention versus Observation Trial (PIVOT) showed that, compared with observation, men who undergo radical prostatectomy have a significant improvement in overall survival (6.1% vs 68.9%; relative risk, 0.71; 95% confidence interval, 0.59–0.86; $P = .001$) and cancer-specific survival—especially in intermediate risk groups, as well as lower risk of local and systemic disease progression (40.9% vs 68.4%).[11-13] Meanwhile, the Prostate Testing for Cancer and Treatment (ProtecT) trial showed that low-risk disease reinforced that active surveillance can safely be used for well selected patients with low-risk prostate cancer.[14]

Since 2000, with the release of the da Vinci Surgical System, the majority of radical prostatectomies have been performed with robotic assistance. In 2016, a study of SEER-Medicare database showed that more than 70% radical prostatectomies were performed robotically that year, compared with only 14% in 2003.[15] Many studies have shown that cancer control outcomes are at least similar between robot-assisted laparoscopic prostatectomy (RALP) and open radical prostatectomy with possible improvement of RALP in decreased need for subsequent treatment.[16,17] The advantage of minimally invasive RALP is the decrease in transfusion rate and a 23-hour hospital stay, on average.[18]

Radiation and RALP have similar oncologic outcomes.[19] The goal of the RALP is to maintain potency and continence in cases where nerve sparing surgery is feasible. Open surgery studies showed that, in patients with good erectile function preoperatively and bilateral nerve-sparing RALP, erection maintenance approaches 60% to 70%.[20] A large Swedish study entitled LAParoscopic Prostatectomy Robot Open (LAPPRO) included 2625 men from 2008 to 2011 who were followed prospectively but not randomly as they underwent open radical prostatectomy versus RALP. Although there was no difference in continence rates, RALP had a small but statistically significant improvement in erection quality postoperatively (75% vs 70%; odds ratio, 0.81; 95% confidence interval 0.66–0.98).[21] Continence rates improve over the first year with continence rates of approximately 50% at 2 months after surgery with improvement to up to 80% by 12 months, which has been reported in many studies.[22]

Techniques used to attempt improvement of continence include perianastomotic stitches, such as the Rocco Stitch and Retzius-sparing techniques. Retrospective studies with approximately 140 patient have not been able to show an improvement of urinary continence with the Rocco stitch, which is placed posterior to the urethra, thus, providing a posterior reconstruction of the Denonvilliers' musculofascial plate.[23] Retzius-sparing RALP is a completely posterior approach that spares dropping the bladder from the space of Retzius. In 2019, a randomized parallel design study with a single surgeon looked at 102 consecutive RALPs, which were randomized to either Retzius-sparing RALP versus traditional, trans-Retzius RALP. It showed quicker return of continence with 90.5% (95% confidence interval, 78.5%–97.3%) of Retzius-sparing RALP patients continent versus 64.1% (95% confidence interval, 51.6%–76.4%) for trans-Retzius RALP.[24] This shows promising results for continence, although further studies analyzing oncologic outcomes are still needed. In summary, as robotic surgery continues to evolve in technology and efficiency, the radical prostatectomy is a prime example of robotic surgery taking over as the primary modality performed in developed countries.

Robotic Cystectomy

The hallmark of surgical treatment for muscle invasive urothelial cancer of the bladder has been radical cystectomy with pelvic lymph node dissection (PLND). Although major complications are infrequent (13%) in open radical cystectomy (ORC), overall complication rates are quite high (~60%). The most frequent complications being gastrointestinal (29%) or infectious (25%).[25] Traditional laparoscopic cystectomy was generally abandoned by the community, but robotic-assisted cystectomy has become relatively common in an attempt to decrease the morbidity of traditionally large open cystectomy incisions.

In 2003, Mani Menon described the development of a technique for performing robotic-assisted radical cystectomy in 17 patients from 2002 to 2003.[26] The cases were performed using the original da Vinci Surgical System (Intuitive Surgical). The urinary reconstruction portions of the case were performed extracorporeally with an average total time of 260 minutes for an ileal conduit and 308 minutes for an orthotopic neobladder.

As the technique was popularized, randomized studies showed noninferiority of robotic-assisted radical cystectomy to ORC. This finding has culminated in a Cochrane Review released in 2019 that included 5 randomized controlled trials, including the RAZOR trial, which included 541 patients, 270 ORC and 271 robotic-assisted radical cystectomy.[27] The Cochrane Review showed a similar time to recurrence, similar major complications (risk ratio, 1.06; 95% confidence interval, 0.76–1.48, for robotic-assisted radical cystectomy versus ORC) as primary outcomes. Secondary outcomes showed a very low certainty of evidence for comparing minor complications, a high likelihood of decreased blood transfusions (relative risk, 0.58; 95% confidence interval, 0.43–0.80; 2 trials) with the possibility of a minor decreased length of stay in the robotic-assisted radical cystectomy versus ORC groups (mean difference, −0.67; 95% confidence interval, −1.22 to −0.12).[28]

It is important to note that the randomized group studies included in the Cochrane Review contained mostly extracorporeal or unlisted urinary diversion techniques. This factor may or may not limit the improvement or detriment that fully intracorporeal robotic-assisted radical cystectomy may contribute compared with ORC. A retrospective study comparing intracorporeal with extracorporeal urinary diversion after robot-assisted radical cystectomy by the International Robotic Cystectomy Consortium showed no statistical difference between hospital length of stay, reoperation rates within 30 days, or in the 90-day complication rates. There was a significantly lower rate of gastrointestinal complications in the intracorporeal urinary division group (10% vs 23%; $P \leq .001$) as well as a decrease in postoperative complications (odds ratio, 0.68; 95% CI 0.50–0.94; $P = .02$).[29]

Technique

Surgical position and port placement Patients are positioned in low dorsal lithotomy with arms tucked bilaterally. The operating table is placed at a 30° Trendelenburg orientation for the cystectomy portion and can be flattened for the urinary diversion, if completed intracorporeally (either with the da Vinci Si robotic system with integrated bed or by undocking and redocking the robot). Foley is placed on the field. Either a 6- or 7-trocar configuration can be used with the assistant either on the left or right of the patient. The camera port is positioned approximately midline, 5 cm above the umbilicus. The robotic trocars are placed in a line 3 to 5 cm caudad to the camera port. The assistant has a port in line with the robotic trocars, opposite the fourth robotic arm. An additional 1 to 2 assistant ports are placed, one at the level of or just cephalad to the camera port and an optional third assistant port (15 mm) can be placed at the midline of the Pfannenstiel incision for assistance with intracorporeal diversion (**Fig. 1**). After insufflation, the PLND can occur before or after the cystectomy. Robotic-assisted PLND has been shown even as early as 2010 to have at least a 93% yield of that of open surgery.[30] See section on PLND for description.

Next steps and future directions Multiple studies are ongoing that are trying to fill the gap in literature comparing robotic-assisted radical cystectomy with intracorporeal urinary diversion with ORC, including a multicenter prospective randomized control trial in the English National Health Service[31] and the Regina Elena Cancer Institute in Italy (NCT03434132). These studies aim to show decrease rate of transfusion, decrease in hospital stay by adhering to Early Recovery after Surgery protocols associated with robotic-assisted surgery.

Other groups are looking to take minimally invasive surgery even further by describing robotic-assisted radical cystectomy through a single port using the da Vinci single port surgical system (Intuitive Surgical).[32]

Pelvic Lymphadenectomy

Prostatectomy and cystectomy both include some form of PLND, albeit with different evidence to support optimal extent of surgery and extent of oncologic improvement.

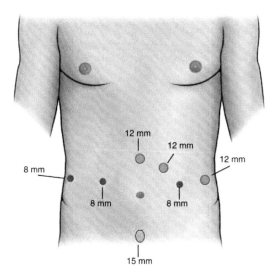

Fig. 1. Port site placement for robotic cystoprostatectomy with intracorporeal diversion. After insufflation, a 10- to 12-mm, bladed disposable trocar is placed superior to the umbilicus; the cephalad placement is important to reach the aortic bifurcation during extended lymphadenectomy and for intracorporeal bowel work. All remaining trocars are placed under direct vision. Left and right 8-mm robotic ports are placed 10 cm lateral to and 4 cm inferior to the camera port. A 12-mm trocar is placed for the bedside assistant port 2 fingerbreadths above the left anterior superior iliac spine; the fourth robotic arm is used with an 8-mm robotic trocar two fingerbreadths above the right anterior superior iliac spine. An additional 12-mm assistant trocar is placed midway between the camera port 8-mm robotic port on the ipsilateral side as the primary bedside assistant; this accommodates either a 10-mm LigaSure or a GIA stapling device to aid in transection of the bladder pedicles. Last, a 15-mm suprapubic trocar is used when performing intracorporeal urinary diversion, which aids in placement of the Endo GIA for side-to-side ileal anastomosis. (*From* Richstone L, Scherr DS. Robotic and laproscopic bladder surgery. In: Wein AJ, Kavoussi LR, Partin AW, Peters CA, eds. Campbell-Walsh Urology 11th ed. Philadelphia PA: Elsevier; 2016: 2254-2280; with permission.)

There is a lack of evidence regarding the therapeutic benefit of cancer-containing lymph node excision after metastatic radical prostatectomy. Some studies show improved biochemical relapse free survival with extended lymph node dissection,[33] but the CaPSURE study showed that these findings fail to reach significance when limited PLND are performed.[34] Memorial Sloan Kettering Cancer Center and European collaborations both created nomograms to predict the likelihood of having positive lymph nodes, allowing surgeons to better stratify and council patients.[35,36] These findings have led the American Urologic Association (AUA) to recommend PLND be considered for any localized prostate cancer and recommended for those with unfavorable intermediate-risk or high-risk, with appropriate counselling regarding common complications of lymphadenectomy and their treatment".[37]

Extended PLND, however, is a critical component of radical cystectomy - with oncologic outcomes found to correlate with extent of lymphadenectomy.[38] Although the extent of PLND has been debated, typical borders for PLND for radical cystectomy include the inferior mesenteric artery/aortic bifurcation proximally, pectineal ligament (or Cooper's ligament) inferiorly, genitofemoral nerve laterally, and sacral promontory medially. The nodes targeted include the presacral, hypogastric, external iliac, obturator, and common iliac lymph nodes (**Figs. 2** and **3**).

Benign Robotic-Assisted Lower Urinary Tract Surgery

Female pelvic organ prolapse

Female pelvic organ prolapse is a challenging disease process that has multifactorial cause leading to substantial quality of life detriment. Surgery for pelvic organ prolapse includes a number of transvaginal and abdominal approaches with various techniques using various amounts of biologic and synthetic materials to aid in structural integrity. Robotics have been used for abdominal sacrocolpopexy for apical prolapse and enterocele. Indication for abdominal sacrocolpopexy includes (1) failed previous vaginal repair, (2) isolated uterine prolapse and/or enterocele, and (3) younger women, especially with highly active lifestyles who are sexually active and opt-in for a more durable repair, despite its invasive nature. Although limited large studies exist, small studies and meta-analyses have shown anatomic success rates ranging from 60% to 100% with a mean of 93%, and subjective success ranging from 91% to 94%. Average mesh erosion rates were 5%.[39] Major complications of the procedure include significant bleeding from the presacral vessels and mesh erosion. Mesh erosion risk is increased with concurrent hysterectomy, although randomized studies have not confirmed this finding.[40]

Simple prostatectomy

Benign prostatic hyperplasia (BPH) is one of the hallmarks of urologic care. In epidemiologic studies, up to 88% of men in their 80s will have histologic BPH. With the increase of α-blocker therapy in the 1980s, surgical treatment rates for BPH have

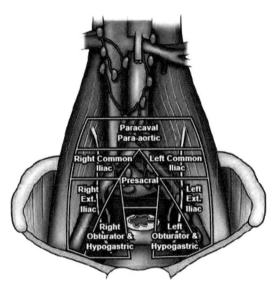

Fig. 2. Distributions of the 8 node packets from an extended pelvic and retroperitoneal lymph node dissection. Pelvic nodes, with some extension superiorly to the common iliacs and presacral regions, are taken for cystoprostatectomies. Paracaval and para-aortic nodes are involved mainly in retroperitoneal lymph node dissection for the treatment of testicular cancer. Ext., exterior. (*From* Navai N, Dinney, CPN. Transurethral and open surgery for bladder cancer. In: Wein AJ, Kavoussi LR, Partin AW, Peters CA, eds. Campbell-Walsh Urology 11th ed. Philadelphia PA: Elsevier; 2016: 2242-2253; with permission.)

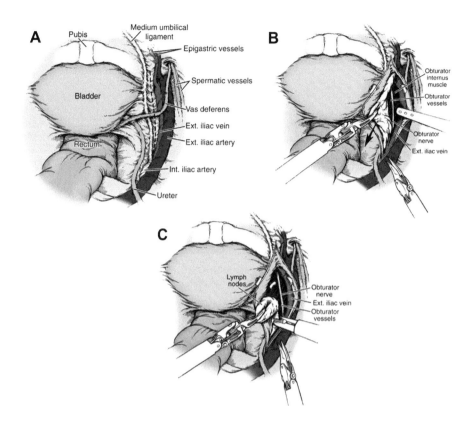

Fig. 3. Robotic-assisted PLND. (*A*) Initial transperitoneal view of the obturator fossa and relevant anatomy. The *dashed line* indicates the longitudinal incision that is made in the peritoneum lateral and parallel to the median umbilical ligament back toward the bifurcation of the iliac vessels in efforts to provide exposure to the obturator fossa and lymph nodes. Ext., exterior; Int., interior. (*B*) The vas deferens has been clipped and divided. With medial traction on the lymph node packet, the lateral extent of the dissection is defined using mainly blunt dissection. Ext., exterior. (*C*) Final dissection of a standard pelvic lymph node template. The proximal and distal extent of the lymph node packet are clipped and divided, taking great care to avoid injury to the obturator nerve and vessels, as well as the accessory obturator vein. (*Courtesy of* Li-Ming Su, MD, Gainesville, FL.)

decreased; however, there remains a strong role for surgical treatment of BPH resistant to medical therapy. Minimally invasive or endoscopic surgery for BPH predominate the landscape, but for large glands—greater than 75 g—a simple prostatectomy remains an option with long term improvement in International Prostate Symptom Score, postvoid residual urine volume, and maximal flow rate.[41] Some of the historic disadvantages with open simple prostatectomy were blood loss and incision size, which are overcome with the robotic-assisted simple prostatectomy approach.[42] The robotic-assisted version of the simple prostatectomy is typically an intra-abdominal approach in which the bladder is dropped by entering the space of Retzius; a bladder neck incision is made to reveal the Foley catheter, which is grasped with the fourth arm of the robot; the prostatic adenoma is then enucleated; and, after various hemostatic maneuvers, the posterior bladder mucosa is advanced into the posterior prostatic pseudocapsule and the cystotomy incision is closed in 2 layers with absorbable sutures. As opposed to open procedure, which typically uses a urethral catheter and a suprapubic tube, the robotic-assisted procedure typically uses a 3-way urethral catheter only. The advantage of the robotic-assisted simple prostatectomy is decreased blood loss, which leads to decreased transfusion rate and decreased length of stay.[43]

Bladder diverticulectomy

Bladder diverticula are defined as a herniation of the urinary mucosa through a weakness or absence of the detrusor muscle and can be congenital acquired or iatrogenic in nature. Classically, surgically treated diverticula, whether for reflux, obstruction, infection, or tumor, were performed with an open low midline incision; however, with continued improvements in minimally invasive techniques, robotic bladder diverticulectomy has become more common. The procedure can be performed with a transabdominal or transvesical approach. In the transabdominal approach, either selective catheterization with a council tip catheter in the diverticulum or direct illumination with a flexible cystoscope is performed to identify the diverticulum.[44] The hospital stay is 2 to 3 days, which is shorter than for open diverticulectomy.[45] Concurrent prostate procedures such as transurethral resection of the prostate, photovaporization of the prostate, or robotic simple prostatectomy can be performed concurrently.[46]

Ureteral reimplantation

Ureteral reimplant is performed for vesicoureteral reflux, ureteral obstruction, and iatrogenic transection. Obstruction can be secondary to stricture or mass lesions, strictures occurring owing to stones, infections, iatrogenic, and traumatic etiology. Ureteral reimplant can be separated into nonrefluxing and refluxing reimplants.

Nonrefluxing reimplants are performed more in the pediatric population. Transabdominal (extravesical) as well as transvesical (extraperitoneal) techniques have been described for nonrefluxing reimplantation. A 5:1 tunnel-to-ureteral diameter is preferred to minimize reflux.[47] A transvesical Cohen cross-trigonal approach can be undertaken robotically as well, distending the bladder with CO_2 to a pressure of 8 to 10 mm Hg. The ureter is mobilized by incising the mucosa circumferentially to leave a mucosal cuff, the ureter is brought into the bladder and a mucosa trough fashioned, and the mucosa is the closed over the reimplanted ureter.[48]

In adults, refluxing reimplants are usually implemented, simplifying the procedure. The transected ureter is spatulated and reimplanted without tension at the dome of the bladder with 4-0 absorbable sutures in running or interrupted fashion.[49,50]

Ureteral reimplantations sometimes require complex reconstructions for augmenting ureteral length to allow for a tension-free anastamosis. These include psoas hitches, Boari flaps and Lima advancement flaps.[51,52] Traditionally these reconstructions require a larger incision when performed open, and thus the use of the robot, in both pediatrics and adults, has made these procedures easier to perform with decreased morbidity for the patients.[52]

ROBOTIC-ASSISTED RETROPERITONEAL SURGERY
Robotic-Assisted Nephrectomy and Partial Nephrectomy

Nephrectomy was the first urologic procedure to be performed laparoscopically in 1991.[32] Less than a decade later, urologists were leading the way in robotic surgery. The laparoscopic approach to radical nephrectomy had become standard of care and the transition to robotics was not always considered necessary or convenient for radical or simple nephrectomies, with on average longer operative times[53] and similar outcomes,[54] but a higher price tag.[55]

The da Vinci robot, however, did revolutionize the current nephron-sparing era in renal surgery. It allows for significant benefits over laparoscopy, including tremor reduction, advanced visual display, and improved manual dexterity,[56] all of which play a significant role in successful retroperitoneal laparoscopic surgery. The technology has lead to improved surgical parameters, such as decreased clamp times and better resection margins.[57] Robotic-assisted laparoscopic partial nephrectomy has become the standard of care for T1 renal tumors[58] and has become so commonly performed in the United States that residents are learning to perform robotic-assisted laparoscopic partial nephrectomy with similar outcomes to those who are fellowship trained in robotics.[58]

Over the years, robotic nephron-sparing approaches have advanced significantly with better visualization, more precise movements, and technology such as intraoperative near-infrared fluorescence with indocyanine green for the localization of renal tumors. Robotic-assisted laparoscopic partial nephrectomy was one of the first single port procedures performed with the early da Vinci robotic systems more than a decade ago,[57] well before last year's latest single port version of the robot.

With regard to upper tract urinary surgery, the partial nephrectomy remains the procedure that benefits most from the use of robotics. The optimized visualization and maneuverability allow urologists to learn and perform a partial nephrectomy, traditionally one of the more difficult laparoscopic procedures to perform, much faster. With emphasis on reducing clamp time and renal ischemia, the robotic partial nephrectomy has become so effective that even large tumors (cT2) can now be undertaken as partial nephrectomies without renal hilar clamping and have similar outcomes.[57] Some investigators advocate that even pT3a tumors can safely be approached robotically in the right hands.[59] Robotic partial nephrectomy will continue to be the primary upper tract procedure that advances most and becomes standard of care as the technology advances.

Robotic-Assisted Retroperitoneal Lymph Node Dissection

Similarly to other procedures, urologists quickly adopted laparoscopic approaches to retroperitoneal lymph node dissection as early as 1992 and showed improved perioperative outcomes compared with open procedures;[56] however, this difficult procedure requires a high level of laparoscopic skill. Even with the advent of robotics in urology, robotic-assisted retroperitoneal lymph node dissection, which was first described in 2006, was not as quickly adopted as other urologic procedures.[60] Initially performed in a lateral position, a supine technique has since been developed with similar outcomes to open procedures; however, most published single-center and multicenter series remain with fewer than 50 patients[61,62] (**Fig. 4**). It is safe to assume that, given the younger patient population, the prevalence of robotic-assisted retroperitoneal lymph node dissection will only continue to grow given the advantages over the open procedures, such as improved cosmesis and convalescence, with similar outcomes.[63]

Robotic-assisted adrenalectomy

The first robot-assisted adrenalectomy was reported in 2000,[64] not long after the first robotic prostatectomy. Now there are many series that have been published, with the largest series (approximately 300 patients) showing low overall rates of conversion to open (approximately 3%) and larger tumors being approached over time.[65,66] Initially it was described with a standard transperitoneal approach (similar to

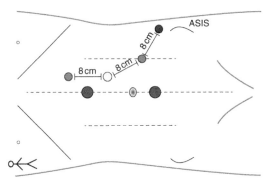

Fig. 4. Port placement for robotic-assisted retroperitoneal lymph node dissection. *Yellow* indicates camera port, *green* indicates 8-mm robotic ports, and *red* indicates 12-mm assistant ports. (*From* Allaf, ME, Kavoussi LR. Laparoscopic and robotic-assisted retroperitoneal lymphadenectomy for testicular tumors. In: Wein AJ, Kavoussi LR, Partin AW, Peters CA, eds. Campbell-Walsh Urology 11th ed. Philadelphia PA: Elsevier; 2016: 838-845; with permission.)

laparoscopic adrenalectomy) but has evolved into single-site approaches and posterior retroperitoneosopic robot-assisted approaches.[67,68] The preciseness of the robot eventually lead to the adoption of adrenal-sparing partial adrenalectomies for certain indications such as solitary metastasis[69] and hereditary adrenal masses (ie, von Hippel-Lindau, multiple endocrine neoplasia type 2) to avoid the need for steroid replacement.[70]

As with other procedures, there continues to be some debate over the benefits of robotic compared with laparoscopic approaches to adrenalectomy, with only 1 randomized control trial very early on with the original da Vinci robot.[71] Overall, similar to laparoscopic adrenalectomy, the procedure has good cosmetic and surgical outcomes in the right surgical hands with a learning curve of at least 20 cases.[72] In regards to whether there is a significant cost difference, the jury is still out with multiple studies advocating for both laparoscopic and robotic adrenalectomies in terms of cost efficiency.[68]

Pediatric robotic-assisted urologic surgery
Although the use of robotic surgery has become a part of all surgical fields, urologists once again are leading the path in terms of pediatric robotic surgery. Indications have even grown to include successful robotic-assisted retroperitoneal lymph node dissections in the adolescent population.[73] Other common robotically performed pediatric procedures include ureteral reimplantation, pyeloplasty, renal surgery and ileocystoplasty (bladder augmentation).

Future possibilities and considerations
Looking forward, the aims of robotic advancement in urologic surgery attempt to solve its current limitations: (1) cost, (2) size, (3) haptic feedback, (4) training, and (5) clinical application. A number of new systems are currently undergoing preliminary testing and development to address these issues.

Although financial limitations remain the primary reason for delayed development, new research shows that with the increased use, robotic technology may eventually become more cost effective.[74,75] New machines are also now able to provide haptic feedback information to their operators; The Senhance (TransEnterix, Morrisville, NC) and Versius Robotic System (Cambridge Medical Robotics Ltd., Cambridge, UK) systems have successfully developed this technology.[5,76]

Two types of ports exist: single-channel and multichannel (**Table 1**). The newest systems currently under development require only a single incision. Ports are inserted into the incision and allow instruments to pass through channels into the body. Single channel ports require a smaller incision to allow a single tube to enter the body. This tube houses 4 or more arms that articulate and controlled independently. Multichannel ports require a larger incision to allow multiple instruments into the body.[76] The behavior of these instruments is limited by their degrees of freedom, angles of rotation, and ability to move independently of the other instruments passed through the port.

These instrument behaviors give rise to the need for specialized training by the surgical team. Training traditional animal or cadaver models have been replaced by 3-dimensional computer-generated simulations where surgeons are able to use mock versions of the surgical systems mentioned. In addition to live training, Intuitive Surgical has also created a full catalog of simulations called SimNow available to be used for their da Vinci system. SimNow offers practice simulations with performance tracking and feedback. Performance data can be accessed remotely online. Simulation tasks range from simple skill development, to full length procedures. This solution attempts to bring formal structure for robotic surgery, something many researchers have concluded to being a necessary requirement in the field[77–82] (**Fig. 5**). Virtual

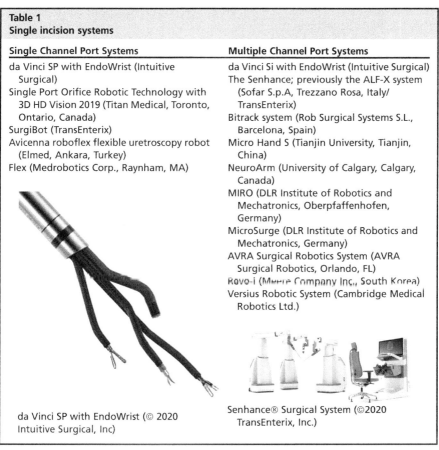

Table 1
Single incision systems

Single Channel Port Systems	Multiple Channel Port Systems
da Vinci SP with EndoWrist (Intuitive Surgical)	da Vinci Si with EndoWrist (Intuitive Surgical)
Single Port Orifice Robotic Technology with 3D HD Vision 2019 (Titan Medical, Toronto, Ontario, Canada)	The Senhance; previously the ALF-X system (Sofar S.p.A, Trezzano Rosa, Italy/TransEnterix)
SurgiBot (TransEnterix)	Bitrack system (Rob Surgical Systems S.L., Barcelona, Spain)
Avicenna roboflex flexible uretroscopy robot (Elmed, Ankara, Turkey)	Micro Hand S (Tianjin University, Tianjin, China)
Flex (Medrobotics Corp., Raynham, MA)	NeuroArm (University of Calgary, Calgary, Canada)
	MIRO (DLR Institute of Robotics and Mechatronics, Oberpfaffenhofen, Germany)
	MicroSurge (DLR Institute of Robotics and Mechatronics, Germany)
	AVRA Surgical Robotics System (AVRA Surgical Robotics, Orlando, FL)
	Rovo-i (Meere Company Inc., South Korea)
	Versius Robotic System (Cambridge Medical Robotics Ltd.)
da Vinci SP with EndoWrist (© 2020 Intuitive Surgical, Inc)	Senhance® Surgical System (©2020 TransEnterix, Inc.)

Data from Smith AD, Preminger GM, Kavoussi LR, et al. Smith's Textbook of Endourology. 4th ed. Oxford, UK: Wiley Blackwell; 2019.

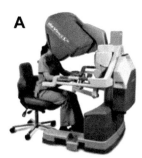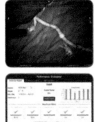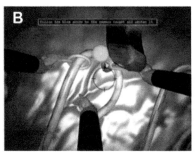

Fig. 5. da Vinci Skills Simulator (*A*) showing the ring pass (*B*) exercise for clutching and third arm manipulation. (© 2020 Intuitive Surgical, Inc.)

reality (VR) training makes use of simulation without the requirement of an entire training module (ie, the da Vinci skills simulator will not be required).[83] VR training is an efficient way to control training costs and been shown to decrease intraoperative errors, improve surgical consistency, and decrease operating time - having already been validated for transference of virtual-to-surgical skill.[84–86] VR/simulation development is even leading to patient-specific VR/simulations that surgeons can practice on before the actual procedure.[14]

Another area in need of further development is electronics and troubleshooting. Although equipment malfunction with the da Vinci systems have been shown to be rare,[87] technical training is also required to quickly identify and mediate electronic and mechanical errors.[4]

Visualization

Intraoperative visualization is also advancing. The many uses of near-infrared fluorescence imaging continue to evolve.[10] This technology has been used extensively in cases of renal cell carcinoma, where the receptors for indocyanine green dye required to visualize the fluorescence is absent, distinguishing between neoplasm and healthy tissue during the procedure.[76,88,89] This technology has also been applied to sentinel node identification.[90] PET scans with indocyanine green–labeled markers are being explored for the purposes of cancer staging.[76] Another area being explored is the use of transrectal ultrasound examination during robotic prostatectomy.[91] Augmented reality is being used to map organs and triangulate targets of surgery with greater accuracy.[92–97] These developments are limited by the speed of image processing intraoperatively, however the future is promising.[76,92,97]

Autonomous Robotics

There is some controversy in the literature regarding the use of the term robotics to describe these systems, because it falsely implies that the machines are capable of functioning autonomously. In the future, this debate may be put to rest as researchers have recently shown the feasibility of autonomous machines in animal models.[76,98] Although this approach may not be realized clinically for many years, it is an exciting step toward the advancement of urologic surgery into the future.

SUMMARY

Urology continues to lead the world of robotic surgery applications and research. In a recently published bibliometric analysis, Jackson and Patel[99] discuss the enormous growth of urologic research being conducted over the past decade. They report an increase of 845.75% during this time; and attribute this growth to the popularity of urologic robotic research being conducted.[99] These impressive figures indicate the massive interest in technological advancement and remind us that research brings to life what our imagination creates.

DISCLOSURE

D. Mikhail, J. Sarcona, M. Mekhail, and L. Richstone declare that they have no conflict of interest to be disclosed.

REFERENCES

1. Thomas R. Editorial: the evolving world of urological laparoscopy. J Urol 1995; 154(2):487–8.
2. Pasticier G, Rietbergen J, Guillonneau B, et al. Robotically assisted laparoscopic radical prostatectomy: feasibility study in men. Eur Urol 2001;40(1):70–4.
3. Otero J, Paparel P, Atreya D, et al. History, evolution and application of robotic surgery in urology. Arch Esp Urol 2007;60(4):335–41.
4. Eichel L, McDougall EM, Clayman RV. Fundamentals of laparoscopic and robotic urologic surgery. In: Wein AJ, Kavoussi LR, Novick AC, et al, editors. Campbell-Walsh Urology. Tenth Edition; 2012. p. 204–53.
5. Spinelli A, David G, Gidaro S, et al. First experience in colorectal surgery with a new robotic platform with haptic feedback. Colorectal Dis 2018;20(3):228–35.
6. Marescaux J, Leroy J, Gagner M, et al. Transatlantic robot-assisted telesurgery. Nature 2001;413(6854):35096636.
7. Challacombe BJ, Khan M, Murphy D, et al. The history of robotics in urology. World J Urol 2006;24(2):120–7.
8. Hoznek A, Zaki SK, Samadi DB, et al. Robotic assisted kidney transplantation: an initial experience. J Urol 2002;167(4):1604–6.
9. Siegel R, Ma J, Zou Z, et al. Cancer statistics, 2014. Ca Cancer J Clin 2014; 64(1):9–29.
10. Lee DJ, Mallin K, Graves AJ, et al. Recent changes in prostate cancer screening practices and epidemiology. J Urol 2017;198(6):1230–40.
11. Bill-Axelson A, Holmberg L, Ruutu M, et al. Radical prostatectomy versus watchful waiting in early prostate cancer. N Engl J Med 2005;352(19):1977–84.
12. Wilt TJ, Brawer MK, Jones KM, et al. Radical prostatectomy versus observation for localized prostate cancer. N Engl J Med 2012;367(3):203–13.
13. Wilt TJ, Jones KM, Barry MJ, et al. Follow-up of prostatectomy versus observation for early prostate cancer. N Engl J Med 2017;377(2):132–42.
14. Hamdy FC, Donovan JL, Lane J, et al. 10-year outcomes after monitoring, surgery, or radiotherapy for localized prostate cancer. N Engl J Med 2016; 375(15):1415–24.
15. Hu JC, O'Malley P, Chughtai B, et al. Comparative effectiveness of cancer control and survival after robot-assisted versus open radical prostatectomy. J Urol 2017; 197(1):115–21.
16. Novara G, Ficarra V, Mocellin S, et al. Systematic review and meta-analysis of studies reporting oncologic outcome after robot-assisted radical prostatectomy. Eur Urol 2012;62(3):382–404.
17. Gandaglia G, Sammon JD, Chang SL, et al. Comparative effectiveness of robot-assisted and open radical prostatectomy in the postdissemination era. J Clin Oncol 2014;32(14):1419–26.

18. Hu JC, Gu X, Lipsitz SR, et al. Comparative effectiveness of minimally invasive vs open radical prostatectomy. Jama 2009;302(14):1557–64.
19. Akakura K, Suzuki H, Ichikawa T, et al. A randomized trial comparing radical prostatectomy plus endocrine therapy versus external beam radiotherapy plus endocrine therapy for locally advanced prostate cancer: results at median follow-up of 102 months. Jpn J Clin Oncol 2006;36(12):789–93.
20. Rabbani F, Stapleton A, Kattan M, et al. Factors predicting recovery of erections after radical prostatectomy. The Journal of Urology 2000;164(6):1929–34.
21. Sooriakumaran P, Pini G, Nyberg T, et al. Erectile function and oncologic outcomes following open retropubic and robot-assisted radical prostatectomy: results from the LAParoscopic prostatectomy robot open trial. Eur Urol 2018; 73(4):618–27.
22. Ficarra V, Gan M, Borghesi M, et al. Posterior muscolofascial reconstruction incorporated into urethrovescical anastomosis during robot-assisted radical prostatectomy. J Endourol 2012;26(12):1542–5.
23. Hoogenes J, Bos D, Wang Y, et al. 674 Impact of posterior urethrovesical reconstruction on early return to continence after robot-assisted radical prostatectomy (RARP): results of prospective, single-blind, parallel-group, randomized controlled trial. Eur Urol Suppl 2018;17(2):e977.
24. Asimakopoulos AD, Topazio L, Angelis M, et al. Retzius-sparing versus standard robot-assisted radical prostatectomy: a prospective randomized comparison on immediate continence rates. Surg Endosc 2019;33(7):2187–96.
25. Shabsigh A, Korets R, Vora KC, et al. Defining early morbidity of radical cystectomy for patients with bladder cancer using a standardized reporting methodology. Eur Urol 2009;55(1):164–76.
26. Menon M, Hemal AK, Tewari A, et al. Nerve sparing robot assisted radical cystoprostatectomy and urinary diversion. BJU Int 2003;92(3):232–6.
27. Parekh DJ, Reis IM, Castle EP, et al. Robot-assisted radical cystectomy versus open radical cystectomy in patients with bladder cancer (RAZOR): an open-label, randomised, phase 3, non-inferiority trial. Lancet 2018;391(10139): 2525–36.
28. Rai B, Bondad J, Vasdev N, et al. Robotic versus open radical cystectomy for bladder cancer in adults. Cochrane Database Syst Rev 2019;(4):CD011903.
29. Ahmed K, Khan SA, Hayn MH, et al. Analysis of intracorporeal compared with extracorporeal urinary diversion after robot-assisted radical cystectomy: results from the international robotic cystectomy consortium. Eur Urol 2014;65(2):340–7.
30. Davis JW, Gaston K, Anderson R, et al. Robot assisted extended pelvic lymphadenectomy at radical cystectomy: lymph node yield compared with second look open dissection. J Urology 2011;185:79–84.
31. Catto JW, Khetrapal P, Ambler G, et al. Multidomain quantitative recovery following radical cystectomy for patients within the robot-assisted radical cystectomy with intracorporeal urinary diversion versus open radical cystectomy randomised controlled trial: the first 30 patients. Eur Urol 2018;74:531–4.
32. Kaouk J, Garisto J, Eltemamy M, et al. Step by step technique for single port robot assisted radical cystectomy and pelvic lymph nodes dissection using the da Vinci SPTM surgical system. BJU Int 2019. https://doi.org/10.1111/bju.14744.
33. Daneshmand S, Quek ML, Stein JP, et al. Prognosis of patients with lymph node positive prostate cancer following radical prostatectomy: long-term results. J Urol 2004;172(6):2252–5.
34. Berglund RK, Sadetsky N, DuChane J, et al. Limited pelvic lymph node dissection at the time of radical prostatectomy does not affect 5-year failure rates for

low, intermediate and high risk prostate cancer: results from CaPSURETM. J Urol 2007;177(2):526–30.

35. Cagiannos I, Karakiewicz P, Eastham J, et al. A preoperative nomogram identifying decreased risk of positive pelvic lymph nodes in patients with prostate cancer. J Urol 2003;170(5):1798–803.

36. Briganti A, Larcher A, Abdollah F, et al. Updated nomogram predicting lymph node invasion in patients with prostate cancer undergoing extended pelvic lymph node dissection: the essential importance of percentage of positive cores. Eur Urol 2012;61(3):480–7.

37. Sanda MG, Cadeddu JA, Kirkby E, et al. Clinically Localized Prostate Cancer: AUA/ASTRO/SUO Guideline, PART I. J Urology 2017;199:683–90.

38. Herr HW. Extent of surgery and pathology evaluation has an impact on bladder cancer outcomes after radical cystectomy. Urology 2003;61:105–8.

39. Maher C, Feiner B, Baessler K, et al. Surgical management of pelvic organ prolapse in women. Cochrane Database Syst Rev 2013;(4):CD004014.

40. Nygaard I. Approval process for devices and mesh for surgical treatment of pelvic organ prolapse and urinary incontinence. Clin Obstet Gynecol 2013;56(2): 229–31.

41. Varkarakis I, Kyriakakis Z, Delis A, et al. Long-term results of open transvesical prostatectomy from a contemporary series of patients. Urology 2004;64(2): 306–10.

42. Clavijo R, Carmona O, Andrade R, et al. Robot-assisted intrafascial simple prostatectomy: novel technique. J Endourol 2013;27(3):328–32.

43. Matei DV, Brescia A, Mazzoleni F, et al. Robot assisted simple prostatectomy (RASP): does it make sense? BJU Int 2012;110(11c):E972–9.

44. Khonsari S, Lee DI, Basillote JB, et al. Intraoperative catheter management during laparoscopic excision of a giant bladder Diverticulum. J Laparoendosc Adv Surg Tech A 2004;14(1):47–50.

45. Eyraud R, Laydner H, Autorino R, et al. Robot-assisted laparoscopic bladder diverticulectomy. Curr Urol Rep 2013;14(1):46–51.

46. Kural A, Atug F, Akpinar H, et al. Robot-assisted laparoscopic bladder diverticulectomy combined with photoselective vaporization of prostate: a case report and review of literature. J Endourol 2009;23(8):1281–5.

47. Smith RP, Oliver JL, Peters CA. Pediatric robotic extravesical ureteral reimplantation: comparison with open surgery. J Urol 2011;185(5):1876–81.

48. Peters CA, Woo R. Intravesical robotically assisted bilateral ureteral reimplantation. J Endourol 2005;19(6):618–22.

49. Fugita O, Kavoussi L. Laparoscopic ureteral reimplantation for ureteral lesion secondary to transvaginal ultrasonography for oocyte retrieval. Urology 2001; 58(2):281.

50. Yohannes P, Chiou RK, Pelinkovic D. Rapid communication: pure robot-assisted laparoscopic ureteral reimplantation for ureteral stricture disease: case report. J Endourol 2003;17(10):891–3.

51. Schimpf MO, Wagner JR. Case report robot-assisted laparoscopic Boari flap ureteral reimplantation. J Endourol 2008;22(12):2691–4.

52. Lima GC, Rais-Bahrami S, Link RE, et al. Laparoscopic ureteral reimplantation: a simplified dome advancement technique. Urology 2005;66(6):1307–9.

53. Hemal AK, Kumar A. A prospective comparison of laparoscopic and robotic radical nephrectomy for T1-2N0M0 renal cell carcinoma. World J Urol 2009; 27(1):89–94.

54. Asimakopoulos AD, Miano R, Annino F, et al. Robotic radical nephrectomy for renal cell carcinoma: a systematic review. BMC Urol 2014;14(1):75.

55. Boger M, Lucas SM, Popp SC, et al. Comparison of robot-assisted nephrectomy with laparoscopic and hand-assisted laparoscopic nephrectomy. JSLS 2010; 14(3):374–80.

56. Schwartz MJ, Kavoussi LR. Controversial technology: the Chunnel and the laparoscopic retroperitoneal lymph node dissection (RPLND). BJU Int 2010;106(7): 950–9.

57. Bertolo R, Simone G, Garisto J, et al. Off-clamp vs on-clamp robotic partial nephrectomy: perioperative, functional and oncological outcomes from a propensity-score matching between two high-volume centers. Eur J Surg Oncol 2019;45(7):1232–7.

58. Campbell S, Uzzo RG, Allaf ME, et al. Renal mass and localized renal cancer: AUA guideline. J Urol 2017;198. https://doi.org/10.1016/j.juro.2017.04.100.

59. Andrade HS, Zargar H, Akca O, et al. Is robotic partial nephrectomy safe for T3a renal cell carcinoma? Experience of a high-volume center. J Endourol 2017;31(2):153–7.

60. Davol P, Sumfest J, Rukstalis D. Robotic-assisted laparoscopic retroperitoneal lymph node dissection. Urology 2006;67(1):199.e7-8.

61. Stepanian S, Patel M, Porter J. Robot-assisted laparoscopic retroperitoneal lymph node dissection for testicular cancer: evolution of the technique. Eur Urol 2016;70(4):661–7.

62. Pearce SM, Golan S, Gorin MA, et al. Safety and early oncologic effectiveness of primary robotic retroperitoneal lymph node dissection for nonseminomatous germ cell testicular cancer. Eur Urol 2017;71(3):476–82.

63. Ludwig WW, Gorin MA, Pierorazio PM, et al. Frontiers in robot-assisted retroperitoneal oncological surgery. Nat Rev Urol 2017;14(12):731.

64. Horgan S, Vanuno D. Robots in laparoscopic surgery. J Laparoendosc Adv S 2001;11(6):415–9.

65. Brunaud L, Ayav A, Zarnegar R, et al. Prospective evaluation of 100 robotic-assisted unilateral adrenalectomies. Surgery 2008;144(6):995–1001.

66. Greilsamer T, Nomine-Criqui C, Thy M, et al. Robotic-assisted unilateral adrenalectomy: risk factors for perioperative complications in 303 consecutive patients. Surg Endosc 2019;33(3):802–10.

67. Park J, Kim S, Lee C-R, et al. Robot-assisted posterior retroperitoneoscopic adrenalectomy using single-port access: technical feasibility and preliminary results. Ann Surg Oncol 2013;20(8):2741–5.

68. Pahwa M. Robot-assisted adrenalectomy: current perspectives. Robot Surg 2017;4:1–6.

69. Kumar A, Hyams ES, Stifelman MD. Robot-assisted partial adrenalectomy for isolated adrenal metastasis. J Endourol 2009;23(4):651–4.

70. Boris RS, Gupta G, Linehan MW, et al. Robot-assisted laparoscopic partial adrenalectomy: initial experience. Urology 2011;77(4):775–80.

71. Morino M, Benincà G, Giraudo G, et al. Robot-assisted vs laparoscopic adrenalectomy: a prospective randomized controlled trial. Surg Endosc 2004;18(12):1742–6.

72. Brunaud L, Bresler L, Ayav A, et al. Robotic-assisted adrenalectomy: what advantages compared to lateral transperitoneal laparoscopic adrenalectomy? Am J Surg 2008;195(4):433–8.

73. Glaser AP, Bowen DK, Lindgren BW, et al. Robot-assisted retroperitoneal lymph node dissection (RA-RPLND) in the adolescent population. J Pediatr Urol 2017; 13(2):223–4.

74. Khorgami Z, Li WT, Jackson TN, et al. The cost of robotics: an analysis of the added costs of robotic-assisted versus laparoscopic surgery using the National Inpatient Sample. Surg Endosc 2019;33(7):2217–21.

75. Dandapani H, Tieu K. The contemporary role of robotics in surgery: a predictive mathematical model on the short-term effectiveness of robotic and laparoscopic surgery. Laparosc Endosc Robot Surg 2018;2:1–7.

76. Navaratnam A, Abdul-Muhsin H, Humphreys M. Updates in urologic robot assisted surgery. F1000Res 2018;7:F1000. Faculty Rev-1948.

77. Brinkman W, Schout B, Rietbergen J, et al. Training robotic surgery in urology: experience and opinions of robot urologists. Int J Med Robot 2015;11(3):308–18.

78. Janetschek G. Standardized and validated training programs for robot-assisted laparoscopy: the challenge of the future. Eur Urol 2019;75:786–7.

79. Gohil R, Khan RS, Ahmed K, et al. Urology training: past, present and future. BJU Int 2012;109(10):1444–8.

80. Stevens DJ. Urology Training: past, present and future. BJU Int 2012;109(5):E13.

81. Sarikaya S, Meneses A, Cacciamani G, et al. Future of urology training. Arch Esp Urol 2018;71(1):158–63.

82. Schlottmann F, Long JM, Brown S, et al. Low confidence levels with the robotic platform among senior surgical residents: simulation training is needed. J Robot Surg 2019;13(1):155–8.

83. Gilley DA, Sundaram CP. Impact of Virtual Reality Simulators in Training of Robotic Surgery. In: Hemal A, Menon M, editors. Robotics in Genitourinary Surgery. London: Springer; 2011.

84. Seymour NE, Gallagher AG, Roman SA, et al. Virtual reality training improves operating room performance. Ann Surg 2002;236(4):458–64.

85. Lucas SM, Zeltser IS, Bensalah K, et al. Training on a virtual reality laparoscopic simulator improves performance of an unfamiliar live laparoscopic procedure. J Urol 2008;180(6):2588–91.

86. Nagendran M, Gurusamy K, Aggarwal R, et al. Virtual reality training for surgical trainees in laparoscopic surgery. Cochrane Database Syst Rev 2013;(8):CD006575.

87. Lavery HJ, Thaly R, Albala D, et al. Robotic equipment malfunction during robotic prostatectomy a multi-institutional study. J Endourol 2008;22(9):2165–8.

88. Bates AS, Patel VR. Applications of indocyanine green in robotic urology. J Robot Surg 2016;10(4):357–9.

89. Autorino R, Zargar H, White WM, et al. Current applications of near-infrared fluorescence imaging in robotic urologic surgery: a systematic review and critical analysis of the literature. Urology 2014;84(4):751–9.

90. Manny TB, Patel M, Hemal AK. Fluorescence-enhanced robotic radical prostatectomy using real-time lymphangiography and tissue marking with percutaneous injection of unconjugated indocyanine green: the initial clinical experience in 50 patients. Eur Urol 2014;65(6):1162–8.

91. Badaan SR, Stoianovici D. Robotic Systems: Past, Present, and Future. In: Hemal A, Menon M, editors. Robotics in Genitourinary Surgery. London: Springer; 2011.

92. Hughes-Hallett A, Mayer EK, Marcus HJ, et al. Augmented reality partial nephrectomy: examining the current status and future perspectives. Urology 2014;83(2):266–73.

93. Simpfendörfer T, Baumhauer M, Müller M, et al. Augmented reality visualization during laparoscopic radical prostatectomy. J Endourol 2011;25(12):1841–5.

94. Porpiglia F, Checcucci E, Amparore D, et al. Augmented reality robot assisted radical prostatectomy using hyper accuracy three dimensional reconstruction (HA3DTM) technology: a radiological and pathological study. BJU Int 2019; 123(5):834–45.
95. Ukimura O, Gill IS. Image-fusion, augmented reality, and predictive surgical navigation. Urol Clin North Am 2009;36(2):115–23.
96. Herrell SD, Kwartowitz D, Milhoua PM, et al. Toward image guided robotic surgery: system validation. J Urol 2009;181(2):783–90.
97. Porpiglia F, Fiori C, Checcucci E, et al. Augmented reality robot-assisted radical prostatectomy: preliminary experience. Urology 2018;115:184.
98. Shademan A, Decker RS, Opfermann JD, et al. Supervised autonomous robotic soft tissue surgery. Sci Transl Med 2016;8(337):337ra64.
99. Jackson S, Patel MI. Robotic surgery research in urology: a bibliometric analysis of field and top 100 articles. J Endourol 2019;33(5):389–95.

Robotic-Assisted Laparoscopic Ventral Hernia Repair

David Earle, MD

KEYWORDS

- Hernia • Ventral • Robotic • Laparoscopic • Retrorectus • Extraperitoneal
- Preperitoneal • eTEP

KEY POINTS

- It is important to identify the patient's goals for hernia repair, then align yourself with those goals.
- Choose a technique, based on the clinical scenario, most likely to meet the patient's goals.
- The fundamental principles of ventral hernia repair should not be compromised based on the use of robotics.

INTRODUCTION

Laparoscopic ventral hernia repair was first reported by LeBlanc and Booth[1] in 1993, and even with advances in technique and equipment, the fundamentals of laparoscopic ventral hernia repair (LVHR) have not changed (**Box 1**). This approach used the intraperitoneal onlay mesh (IPOM) technique to bridge the defect, anchored by a series of full-thickness sutures and partial-thickness spiral tacks. There have been data and experience looking at a variety of fixation types (alone or in combination), and whether or not to close the defect before placing the mesh. Defect closure can be quite difficult to accomplish laparoscopically, as the angles for needle placement and knot tying on the posterior surface of the abdominal wall are challenging. This led to the use of a number of percutaneous methods for defect closure that used a variety of suture passing devices. These are still hotly debated topics, with no conclusive proof as to which technique is the best.[2] In all likelihood, there is no single best method, rather a toolbox of methods from which one can choose based on training, experience, resources, and clinical scenario.

The laparoscopic technique has been shown to have lower length of hospital stay, lower wound complications, and no increase in adverse outcomes compared with

New England Hernia Center, Tufts University School of Medicine, 20 Research Place, Suite 130, North Chelmsford, MA 01863, USA
E-mail address: DavidEarle59@gmail.com

Surg Clin N Am 100 (2020) 379–408
https://doi.org/10.1016/j.suc.2019.12.009
0039-6109/20/© 2019 Elsevier Inc. All rights reserved.

> **Box 1**
> **Fundamental principles of laparoscopic ventral hernia repair**
>
> - Avoid energy as much as possible with adhesiolysis near hollow viscera
> - Completely dissect a large area around the defect, including the entire old incision
> - Recurrence rates are lower with an increasing ratio of mesh size:defect size
> - Overlap requirements are larger for larger defects
> - Areas with less space for overlap generally need stronger fixation (Cooper's ligaments)
> - Areas with weaker fixation points available (posteriorly and diaphragm) generally need more overlap

open ventral hernia repair. Despite these patient advantages, surgeons have not overwhelmingly adopted this approach, as was done for cholecystectomy. A laparoscopic approach has been used for only approximately 20% of ventral hernia repairs for 25 consecutive years after its introduction.[3–5] This is likely because of the increased technical difficulty of the laparoscopic approach.

Using a robotic-assisted surgical device (RASD) with wristed instruments could overcome some technical challenges with LVHR, increase utilization of the laparoscopic approach, and even enable new laparoscopic techniques. Intuitive Surgical, Inc. (Sunnyvale, CA), manufacturer of the DaVinci line of RASDs, has also realized this, and has heavily invested in hernia repair and exposure to general surgeons.[6] Indeed, use of a RASD for LVHR has a low penetrance at 3.1% in New York State, but has a rising trajectory, more than doubling the number of cases from 113 in 2010 to 242 in 2013.[7] The number of standard LVHR cases also rose during that time from 4986 to 5445. New devices coming to the market forecast even more LVHR procedures in the future. Transenterix (Morrisville, NC) has already launched their Senhance RASD in the United States, but without wristed instruments, it is difficult to use for work on the anterior abdominal wall. More companies are currently developing RASDs for general surgery, including Auris Health (Redwood City, CA), CMR Surgical (Cambridge, England), Medtronic (Dublin, Ireland), and Verb Surgical (Mountain View, CA). With laparoscopy having only approximately 25% penetration for the approximately 1 million hernia operations performed annually in the United States, it is easy to see how there is plenty of room for increased adoption of the laparoscopic approach. Despite the deserved excitement regarding enabling technology, it is important to realize that the fundamentals of LVHR have not changed and should not be compromised.

One of the most commonly expressed reasons for using an RASD for an IPOM technique, for example, is to avoid the use of a tacking device (allegedly for decreased pain and cost savings), as the mesh can easily be fixed to the abdominal wall with continuous suture around its periphery using the RASD. This fixation method, however, did not have a predecessor in the prior 25 years of LVHR, and is thus unknown in terms of strength compared with existing methods of fixation.[8] Given this uncertainty, it would be prudent to study and track results of the new fixation method, and perhaps rely less on mesh fixation by increasing the mesh:defect ratio, and using known fixation methods for cases with a higher risk of recurrence. Another commonly purported advantage is the ease of defect closure. Although there is no doubt this is true, the benefit to the patient in terms of outcomes for defect closure with LVHR has not been shown.[9–11] Despite the lack of improved patient-centered outcomes, common sense dictates that defect closure for larger defects will have a more predictable impact on postoperative abdominal wall contour, and remains an important, yet unmeasured outcome for some patients. Some of the newer laparoscopic approaches that use the retrorectus and preperitoneal spaces along with myofascial flaps of the trunk rely less on fixation, and use the principle of giant prosthetic reinforcement of the visceral sac described by Rives and Stoppa in France, popularized in the United States by George Wantz in New York City.[12] Development and propagation of these laparoscopic approaches to abdominal wall reconstruction have been largely enabled by the use of an RASD, and will find their way into the armamentarium of an increasing number of hernia surgeons over time. All laparoscopic approaches, with or without an RASD, avoid the large skin excision, and thus for patients who prefer skin excision for excess skin and subcutaneous tissue, scar revision, or skin necrosis and ulceration, the open or hybrid (laparoscopic/open) approach would still be most appropriate.

This article highlights the advantages, disadvantages, and technical aspects of current approaches to LVHR using an RASD, as well as a review of the existing experience with each approach. It is beyond the scope of this article to provide a formal systematic review, or meta-analysis comparing the various techniques, details of hernia prosthetics, or the extensive body of literature with enhanced recovery after surgery programs.

PREOPERATIVE PLANNING

As each procedure has similar preoperative considerations, we include this before describing individual techniques. The first step in planning a hernia repair is to establish the goals of the patient, then align yourself with those goals. Frequently, these center around the resolution of symptoms, abdominal wall contour, and prevention of acute incarceration (ie, permanent hernia repair). The second step is to consider the clinical scenario. This includes urgency of the procedure, *past* medical/surgical history, and *future* potential for reoperation, such as pregnancy, Crohn's disease, and ostomy closure. Third, it is very important to consider the location of the defect, the size of the defect, and the size of the hernia sac. Only once these steps have been taken should the surgeon consider the best available techniques that are most appropriate, and most likely to achieve the goals. And finally, once the technique is chosen, a prosthetic most appropriate for that technique, in that clinical scenario, that is most likely to meet the goals, can be chosen (**Box 2**).

Box 2
Algorithm for robotic-assisted laparoscopic ventral hernia repair

1. *Identify patient goals*, then align yourself with those goals. Or decide those goals cannot be met (symptoms, abdominal wall contour, prevention of acute incarceration).

2. *Clinical scenario.* Urgency of operation, availability of previous records, and hospital resources (operating room time, assistants, equipment, mesh, and fixation devices).

3. *Medical/Surgical history.* Includes issues related to previous surgical site infections, mesh infections, incision locations, and increased risk of future reoperation (eg, future pregnancy, cancer interventions, Crohn disease, ostomy closure).

4. *Hernia details.* Location, defect size, sac size, associated skin changes (ulceration, necrosis, rash, and excess/stretched), and surrounding structures (implications for fixation).

5. *Choose a technique.* One most likely to realize goals, with least morbidity.

6. *Choose a prosthetic.* One that is appropriate for technique, and most likely to realize the goals of the operation, originally set forth by the patient.

Clinical Example

A 36-year-old woman with a body mass index (BMI) of 45 presents to the emergency room multiple times in the past 2 weeks for pain from a partially reducible, recurrent incisional hernia in the lower midline. She has had a hysterectomy, has no other medical problems, and is an active smoker. Physical examination reveals healed lower midline and laparoscopy incisions, no skin changes, and no abdominal wall contour abnormality. *Her primary goal is pain relief, and a lasting hernia repair.*

Her only previous hernia repair was done 6 years ago at another hospital, with no records available. Computed tomography scan reveals a polytetrafluoroethylene (PTFE) prosthetic that is flat against the abdominal wall, and fixed with multiple metal tacks. Inferiorly between the pubis and the old mesh is a defect through which fat and small bowel are herniated into a moderate-sized hernia sac. The superior portion of the mesh extends to the lateral borders of the rectus muscles, and the gap between the rectus muscles is 10 cm at its widest, but this portion is covered by the previous mesh. The portion of the current defect (not covered by mesh) is 6 cm wide × 4 cm vertical.

1. Primary goal is pain relief and durable hernia repair. Surgeon determines those goals are likely to be attainable, and aligns him/herself with those goals.
2. Clinical scenario: Urgent operation. No time for substantial weight loss or meaningful period of smoking cessation.
3. Medical/surgical history includes morbid obesity and previous hysterectomy. There is no possibility of future pregnancies, which would otherwise be a consideration for lower midline incisional hernia repair in a woman of childbearing age. Morbid obesity will likely make the operation more difficult, and may increase the risk of recurrence. Active smoking status would impair healing, and increase the chance for wound complications.
4. Hernia details. Midline defect. Gap between rectus muscles is 10 cm wide × 10 cm vertical, but is mostly covered by a previous mesh that is flat against the abdominal wall without surrounding inflammatory changes, and has adequate overlap superiorly and laterally. It appears to be made of expanded PTFE (ePTFE).
5. Choose a technique. Any open technique would have a higher risk of wound complications because of obesity and smoking. Defect closure is not necessary to restore abdominal wall contour, because this is not part of the patient's goal, in addition to not having a noticeable bulge. Any technique using defect closure will also have some dependence of healing, which is expected to be impaired by her active smoking status, as well as being technically challenging due to the previous repair. A totally preperitoneal technique would be expected to be difficult because of the previous IPOM that likely used full-thickness fixation sutures and metal tacks through the peritoneum and posterior rectus sheath. Therefore, an IPOM technique with wide pelvic preperitoneal dissection, allowing wider inferior overlap and fixation of a strong mesh to Cooper ligaments should provide a lasting hernia repair and pain relief from intermittent incarceration.
6. Choose a prosthetic. Given the technique, a prosthetic designed for intraperitoneal use, and one that is strong enough to bridge the gap would be most appropriate. The previously placed prosthetic was most likely a dual-sided ePTFE product. Lack of bunching and surrounding inflammation suggest that polymer is very biocompatible. Perhaps the most appropriate prosthetic then would be another dual-sided ePTFE product, which has the strength and biocompatibility appropriate for this specific case. Wider overlap and fixation to the pelvis and the previous mesh should provide a durable hernia repair, and most likely also relieve her symptoms, thus achieving the goals of the operation with the lowest risk of complications.

ROBOTIC-ASSISTED LAPAROSCOPIC VENTRAL HERNIA REPAIR: INTRAPERITONEAL ONLAY MESH (IPOM) TECHNIQUE

Advantages

The IPOM technique refers to the fact that all, or a portion of the prosthetic is exposed to the peritoneal cavity. This does not imply that dissection of the abdominal wall is not required to have the mesh lay flat, and on the transversalis fascia or even within the preperitoneal space. The advantage of this technique is relatively easy mesh placement, and no need to close the peritoneum, even when the preperitoneal space is dissected for mesh placement, such as creation of a large flap to expose the Cooper ligaments. Dissection of the umbilical and/or falciform ligaments may require mobilization, and are likewise not returned to their anatomic positions by the surgeon after mesh placement. Another advantage compared with extraperitoneal mesh is that there is no risk of postoperative herniation through the closed peritoneal flap or posterior rectus sheath.[13]

Disadvantages

A perceived disadvantage of IPOM relates to subsequent abdominal operation (SAO), where adhesions to the prosthetic would be expected to make the adhesiolysis more difficult, even with a prosthetic designed for intraperitoneal use. This, however, seems to be an overstated problem after LVHR. Patel and colleagues[14] reviewed SAO after 733 LVHRs and found the reoperation rate to be 17% at a mean of 2.2 years postoperatively. For the 125 who underwent an SAO, they found the overall incidence of unplanned bowel resection to be 4%, and occurred exclusively within the group of 18 patients who required operation for small bowel obstruction. Mesh infection rate after SAO was 2.4%.

Why Intraperitoneal Onlay Mesh Technique with a Robotic-Assisted Surgical Device?

The rationale for using an RASD for a laparoscopic IPOM centers around the wristed instruments, making it easier for the surgeon to laparoscopically close the defect, and fix the mesh to the abdominal wall using a variety of suturing techniques and patterns. Interestingly, all of the suturing uses partial-thickness abdominal wall sutures, with claims of less pain compared with full-thickness sutures or tacks. It is not logical that replacing one partial-thickness method of fixation (tacks) with another (sutures placed with RASD) would have an impact on pain. Indeed, a recent meta-analysis of tack versus full-thickness suture mesh fixation for LVHR revealed shorter operative times with tacks, but no difference in incidence of chronic pain, pain intensity, or hernia recurrence.[15] Regarding strength of mesh fixation with the RASD compared with full-thickness sutures and tacks, no direct comparison or long-term outcomes data exist, thus claims of improvement are premature at this time. The group led by Brent Matthews at the University of Washington in St, Louis, MO, did show that full-thickness sutures were approximately twice as strong as all available tackers at the time when they compared shear retention strength on a porcine model.[8] Palanivelu and colleagues[16] described a similar technique of defect closure with suture fixation of the mesh in 2007, and reported comparable rates of pain and hernia recurrence. They used 4 full-thickness sutures at the corners of the mesh, which were the only locations associated with significant postoperative pain, but only required oral analgesics, and all resolved by 4 weeks.

Patient Positioning

This is the same as for a non-RASD LVHR. Supine position, arms tucked at the sides. If the arms cannot be tucked on the table because of obesity, the arm boards can be placed along the side of the table. One should not place "arm holders" that project anteriorly, as they will interfere with the instrument shafts while operating on the anterior abdominal wall. Flexing the table will expand distance between costal margin and anterior superior iliac spine if more room is needed for port placement. This can also help keep the legs from colliding with the instrument placed in the lower quadrants. Another strategy is to tilt the table up on the side the ports are placed. Make sure to set the table position *before* the docking when using an RASD, as not all models allow table movement after docking. If a single side for port placement is all that is necessary, angling the feet slightly to the side opposite the ports can help avoid instrument shaft collision with the leg. This also has the advantage of requiring only a single docking of the RASD. Lower-abdominal hernias that will require exposure of Cooper ligaments should have a 3-way Foley catheter placed to aid in identification of the borders of the urinary bladder.

Positioning the Robotic-Assisted Surgical Device

The orientation of the base of the RASD adjacent to the operating table will depend on the make and model used. It will also depend on the port site locations, which for an IPOM technique, will often be all on one side, as lateral to the defect as possible. If there is a requirement for ports on the opposite side, the RASD will have to be "double-docked": undocked, moved to the other side of the table, then redocked with the same orientation. In relation to the table, the base can be positioned at the side of the table either perpendicular, parallel, or at an angle, and should be located on the side of the table opposite the ports. For lower-abdominal hernias, the device can also be positioned near the patient's perineum if the patient is placed in a lithotomy-type position. The exact position will depend on the size and setup of the operating room, patient body habitus, model of RASD, and surgeon preference.

Surgical Technique

Step 1. Three ports are placed laterally, 8 to 10 cm apart from one another depending on which RASD is being used. Longer ports will give more clearance for the instrument shafts from the edge of the table. Ports should be positioned within the abdominal wall according to manufacturer's recommendations, and in general, placed in a position ready to use (angled anteriorly), then tension transiently released on the RASD arm (or "burped") before starting to work at the console. If using a single dock, the ports must be far enough from the edge of the defect to allow room for the instruments to reach and suture the ipsilateral side of the mesh, but not so far as the tucked arm would collide with the RASD arms. Being able to adequately place and secure the mesh on the ipsilateral side is critical. If this cannot be accomplished with ports placed on one side, then a set of ports will need to be placed on the opposite side, and the RASD will have to be double-docked to properly place and fix the mesh on both sides **(Fig. 1)**.

Step 2. Abdominal wall exposure. This is the same for LVHR with any technique, and should involve safe, complete adhesiolysis, exposure of the entire old incision, takedown of the umbilical and falciform ligaments for midline defects, and exposure of the Cooper ligaments for lower midline defects.[2]

Step 3. Measuring the defect and using an appropriately sized mesh is no different from with standard LVHR,[2] and details are beyond the scope of this article. The

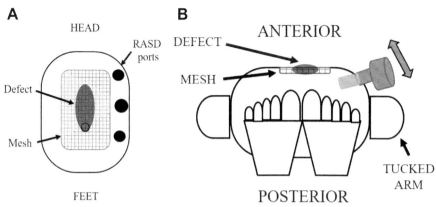

Fig. 1. Schematic (not to scale) of port placement relative to defect, mesh, and arms. (*A*) Overhead view of a typical port setup for IPOM, TAPP, and TARUP techniques. (*B*) View from feet for port setup for IPOM, TAPP, and TARUP techniques. Note the ports should be placed laterally enough to access the ipsilateral side of the mesh and/or tissue flap (depending on technique), but not so lateral as to cause collision between the RASD arms and the tucked arms. If this cannot be accomplished, additional ports will need to be placed on the opposite side, and the RASD "double-docked."

fundamental principles and potential pitfalls include accurate measurement of the defect, and use of an appropriate-sized mesh for the defect. For repairs in which the defect is not closed, and the mesh will bridge the defect, many surgeons focus on centimeters of overlap, or the distance between the defect edge, and edge of the mesh. Because the abdomen is cylindrical, a linear relationship is not the best way to think about mesh size. Rather, a 3-dimensional perspective is most appropriate, such as mesh:defect ratio. Although there is no precise ratio shown to be advantageous, and no practical way to measure the ratio intraoperatively, we know from the preponderance of data that larger defects have higher recurrence rates, and should require a larger ratio. Mesh fixation strength is also dependent on this ratio. Using extreme examples, a 2 × 2-cm midline defect at the umbilicus in a thin patient that is covered by a 20 × 30-cm prosthetic of sufficient strength will have a small amount of force exerted on the mesh covering the defect, and therefore not require comparatively strong fixation. Alternatively, 10 × 15-cm midline defect from a lower midline defect on an obese patient that is covered by a 20 × 30-cm prosthetic of sufficient strength will have a much larger force exerted on the mesh, and thus require stronger fixation, a larger mesh, or both.

> - Defect should be accurately measured, and dictated in the operative report.
>
> - Measurements on the skin will overestimate defect size compared with measurements taken on the abdominal wall itself. This mismatch is gradually increased with increasing size of the hernia sac and increasing obesity.

Step 4. Mesh fixation. Intracorporeal, partial-thickness abdominal wall suture fixation of the prosthetic is a new concept born with a robotic approach and has many variations. These include choices regarding suture size and type, as well as the suturing pattern (**Box 3**). Interrupted sutures can be placed alone, or in conjunction with continuous sutures. Sutures may be placed along the edge, to bony structures, to

> **Box 3**
> **Considerations for suture fixation of mesh**
>
> - Suture type: permanent, long/short-acting absorbable.
> - Suture size: note that barbed suture is the same strength as one size smaller because of the barbs.
> - Suture design: monofilament, braided, barbed.
> - Suture pattern: (1) continuous versus interrupted; (2) mesh-tissue bites (along mesh edge) versus mesh-tissue-mesh bites (away from mesh edge); (3) around periphery, with or without central fixation.
> - Suture depth: this will be variable among surgeons, and will depend on needle size and angle of approach.

the diaphragm, and/or in a quilting pattern (**Fig. 2**). There is no consensus regarding mesh suturing other than not fixing the mesh solely to the peritoneum, and this is different compared with full-thickness sutures placed through separate stab incisions.

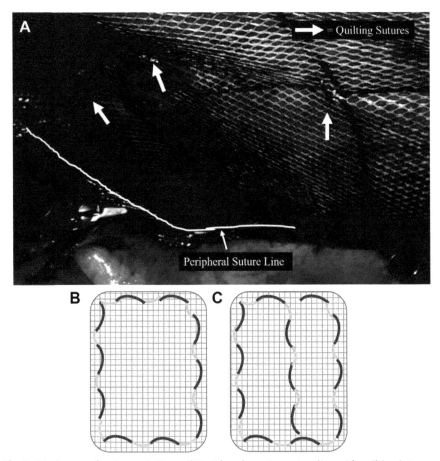

Fig. 2. Mesh suture fixation variations. A) Peripheral running suture line with quilting interrupted sutures (*Courtesy of* Karl LeBlanc, MD, Baton Rouge, LA). B) Running suture around the periphery only C) Running suture around the periphery and along the center of the mesh.

Use of additional fixation with a mechanical device with a variety of permanent and absorbable constructs also may be used depending on the clinical situation and surgeon preference. These can be used alone, or in conjunction with sutures. There are no data supporting one method of mesh fixation is clinically better than another.[2]

Given the lack of a standard approach, and no long-term data, one should generally take measures to reduce the tension on the fixation points, such as increasing the mesh:-defect ratio compared with what would be used for full-thickness sutures and tacks.

Immediate Postoperative Care, Rehabilitation, and Recovery

Postoperative care is no different from a standard LVHR. Patients can be discharged from the hospital when able to ambulate, void, and tolerate per os intake sufficiently to avoid dehydration. There is generally no formal restriction of activity or diet, allowing patients to guide their activity level based on pain and discomfort. If the defect is closed, some surgeons will recommend light activity until the scar strength of the defect closure is approximately 90% completed, typically 6 to 8 weeks postoperative. This of course depends on how well the tissue holds the sutures, the size of the defect, and direction of closure. Transversely closed defects in the midline will have much less postoperative tension compared with midline defects, given that simultaneous contraction of the oblique muscles during coughing, flexing the trunk with a fixed pelvis, and straining for bowel movements all conspire to pull the midline apart vertically. Patients are typically able to bathe normally within a day or two.

Clinical Results in the Literature

A decade after LeBlanc and Booth's LVHR IPOM technique[1] was reported, the first 2 cases of LVHR using an RASD in humans were reported by Ballantyne and colleagues[17] in Hackensack, New Jersey. Over the next 12 years, only 3 small, single-surgeon/center series were reported.[18-20] All of these reports placed the mesh in the IPOM location and used suture mesh fixation, albeit with different types of sutures and patterns. The first 2 reports were small series of 11 and 13 patients, and looked at small to medium-sized defects (2–10 cm). Tayar and colleagues[18] from Créteil Cedex, France, reported their experience with 11 patients. Their mean operative time was 180 minutes, but mean anesthesia time was 270 minutes, suggesting setup of the RASD averaged 90 minutes per case. Median length of stay (LOS) was 3 days, and recurrence rate with a median follow-up of 25 months was zero. In addition, they reported one missed enterotomy, and attributed this complication to lack of haptic feedback from the RASD. Allison and colleagues[19] in Houston, Texas, reported on defect sizes ranging in area from 6 to 11/ cm² that were all closed with absorbable suture, with an average operating time of 131 minutes, and mean LOS of 2.4 days. Notably, 2 patients had prolonged LOS (6 and 10 days) because of need for inpatient pain control. No patient, however, had long-term pain, with a median follow-up of 23 months. They had one recurrence of a lumbar hernia in that group. The largest of these reports is from Gonzalez and colleagues[20] from Miami, Florida, had 67 patients in each of 2 comparison groups, 1 with defect closure (PCD) using the RASD, and one without defect closure (NPCD) and no RASD. This study revealed a longer operating time for the RASD/defect closure group by 20 minutes, and no other statistically significant differences, including complications (3% PCD vs 10.4% NPCD; $P = .08$), LOS (2.5 PCD vs 3.7 days NPCD; $P = .46$), and recurrence rate (1.5% PCD vs 7.5% NPCD; $P = .10$) with a median follow-up of 17 to 21 months. The study, however, used 2 different types of mesh, one of which had a very low strength, was used to bridge defects, and was ultimately recalled from the marketplace because of higher recurrence rates.

In 2015, Kudsi and colleagues[21] from Boston, Massachusetts, described their personal series of 106 consecutive patients who all underwent LVHR with a RASD. Mean defect size was 4.3 cm (range 2–25 cm), and defects were "selectively" closed in 98 cases using a size 0 barbed suture. The mean operative time was 85.7 minutes (35–335 minutes), and mean LOS was 0.2 days (0–5). With a median follow-up of 6 months (1–24), the complication rate was 6%, and recurrence rate was 1.8%.

In 2016, Chen and colleagues[22] from New York City compared LVHR IPOM between LVHR with standard laparoscopic equipment and LVHR with a RASD. Both groups had small defects (2–3 cm), and used permanent mesh that bridged the defect. The standard LVHR group used full-thickness, transfascial sutures and tacks for mesh fixation. The RASD group used partial-thickness abdominal wall sutures for mesh fixation. Of the 72 patients studied (33 standard, 39 with RASD), they found the RASD group had a longer operative time by an average of 91 minutes, and no difference in LOS (all outpatient), or number of patients requiring admission for pain control, suggesting the new mesh fixation method is not less painful compared with the standard method described. Also in 2016, Gonzalez and colleagues[23] reported their multicenter experience with 368 patients. It was not mentioned if these patients represented all ventral hernia repairs performed during that timeframe, thus there could be selection bias. No defect size was mentioned; however, the defect was closed in 69% of the patients. In addition, there were a variety of prosthetics used, with the permanent synthetic category being used 99% of the time. There were also a variety of mesh fixation techniques, with some sort of suture fixation alone being used in 58% of cases. Mean operative time was 102 minutes, and mean LOS was 1 day. Thirty-day complication rate was 8.4%, and 1.9% required reoperation within 30 days for infected mesh (n = 2), enterotomy (2), abscess (1), small bowel obstruction (1), and recurrent hernia (1).

In 2017, Prabhu and colleagues[24] analyzed prospectively collected data from the Americas Hernia Society Quality Collaborative database for LVHR performed with standard laparoscopic equipment (454 cases) and LVHR performed with a RASD (177 cases). The groups were matched using a propensity score analysis to ensure equivalency of the groups. Although some minor differences existed between the groups, most of the mesh in the standard LVHR group was fixed with full-thickness sutures and tacks (74%), whereas most of the mesh in the RASD group was fixed with sutures alone (86%). The suturing pattern and depth of sutures placed with the RASD were not recorded. Operative time greater than 2 hours was more common in the RASD group (47% vs 31%; P<.05), as was fascial closure (93% vs 56%; P<.05). There was a statistically significant difference in mean LOS for the groups as a whole (Standard = 1 day, RASD = 0 days); however, when analyzing surgeons that performed both techniques within their practice, there was no difference in LOS, which was 1 day for each group. This suggests that factors other than the technique may be responsible for hospital LOS. Regarding surgical site occurrences, there were more seromas in the standard LVHR group compared with the RASD group (10% vs 3%; P = .006), but no difference in the rate of surgical site occurrence requiring procedural intervention (1% vs 0%; P = 1.0), making this a less clinically relevant finding. Although "any complication" was more likely in the standard group (Standard 19% vs RASD 8%; P<.001), there were no statistically significant differences between the groups with regard to postoperative deep venous thromboembolism, pulmonary embolism, myocardial infarction, cardiac arrest, ileus, intraoperative complications, or readmissions. Also in 2017, Oviedo and colleagues[25] from Tallahassee, Florida, reported LVHR with RASD with (n = 33) and without (n = 14) bilateral endoscopic component separation (external oblique release). All patients had primary defect closure and IPOM mesh placement. They found no significant difference in operative time, blood loss, LOS, or complications.

They did note the noncomponent separation group had a higher recurrence rate (23% vs 0%; $P<.02$) with a median follow-up of 28 and 19 months, respectively.

In 2018, Walker and colleagues[26] from Houston, Texas, published a retrospective review comparing standard LVHR with RASD LVHR. They looked at 215 patients (73 standard, 142 RASD) and found the RASD group had a mean BMI 6 points lower than the standard group, yet longer mean operative times by 18 minutes. There was no difference in mean LOS, but a significant increase in surgical site infection for the standard group (6.8% vs 0%; $P<.01$). Although there was a higher rate of defect closure in the RASD group (71% vs 55%), there was no difference in recurrence rate. The recurrence rate was 6.8% (mean follow-up 23.6 weeks) for the standard group, and 7.7% (mean follow-up 12.3 weeks) for the RASD group. After propensity score matching, they found the standard group had higher rates of surgical site occurrence (19% vs 4%; $P<.001$) and recurrence (4.2% vs 2.1%; $P<.01$) with a median follow-up of 5 to 6 weeks. That same group has recently completed a randomized trial comparing standard with RASD LVHR with the IPOM technique (Shinil K. Shah, DO, FACS. Associate Professor, Department of Surgery, Medical Director of Research, Division of Minimally Invasive and Elective General Surgery. McGovern Medical School at UT Health, personal communication, 2019). They recruited 124 patients, and found longer operative times in the RASD group, with no difference in LOS, postoperative emergency room visits, morbidity, or mortality. Finally, in 2019, Zayan and colleagues[27] from Ohio State University reported a retrospective review comparing standard (n = 33) with RASD (n = 14) LVHR. The type of mesh and location of mesh placement were not described; 87% of the standard group and 100% of the RASD group had defect closure, but the techniques were not described. Mesh fixation for the standard group was an absorbable tacking device alone in 97% of cases, and for the RASD group was a self-fixating mesh (44%) or sutures (56%). They found the RASD group had a longer average operative time by a mean of 63 minutes (2:29 vs 1:26; $P = .009$) and a shorter LOS (1 vs 2 days; $P = .001$). With a mean follow-up of 14 to 15 months, there were no statistically significant differences in 1 year Carolinas Comfort Scale scores and recurrence.

ROBOTIC-ASSISTED LAPAROSCOPIC VENTRAL HERNIA REPAIR: TRANSABDOMINAL PREPERITONEAL (TAPP) TECHNIQUE
Advantages

This technique refers to preperitoneal placement of the mesh, posterior to the posterior rectus sheath, and anterior to the peritoneum and/or transversalis fascia. The preperitoneal placement of mesh has the advantage of the ability to use a less expensive, nonbarrier mesh. There is also a perception that even mesh designed for intraperitoneal use is problematic. The perceived problems with intraperitoneal mesh designed for intraperitoneal use are theoretic. Patel and colleagues[14] from Greenville, North Carolina, showed low complication rates for subsequent reoperation after LVHR using an IPOM technique. Another theoretic advantage is the need for less mesh fixation, particularly along the edges of the mesh, which is often used to prevent herniation of viscera between the abdominal wall and the mesh. Mesh fixation for strength is another matter altogether, and has to do with defect size, defect closure, and use of myofascial flaps of the trunk. Finally, some have commented that the mesh position against the abdominal wall, rather than the peritoneum allows the mesh to contact more abdominal wall. However, a proper IPOM dissection should expose the abdominal wall and preperitoneal space when necessary (eg, taking down falciform and umbilical ligaments, exposing the Cooper ligaments), and thus will also position the mesh immediately adjacent to the abdominal wall in many circumstances.

Disadvantage

The primary disadvantage for the transabdominal preperitoneal (TAPP) technique is the need to close the peritoneum, which is often thin, and may not hold sutures well. This takes extra time, and may need to be converted to an IPOM if peritoneal closure is not possible. Finally, this technique is only feasible for relatively small defects, typically less than 5cm in diameter.

Patient and Robotic-Assisted Surgical Device Positioning

This is the same as for the IPOM technique, described in detail previously.

Surgical Technique

Step 1. Port placement is the same as for the IPOM technique, described in detail previously (see **Fig. 1**).

Step 2. Abdominal wall exposure. This is the same for LVHR with any technique, and should involve safe, complete adhesiolysis, and exposure of the entire old incision.[2] The difference with a TAPP approach is that the peritoneum is incised lateral to defect at a distance large enough to be able to accommodate an appropriate-sized mesh. Therefore, the maximum mesh size must be determined before incising the peritoneum. For midline defects, the peritoneum is incised on the same side as the ports in a craniocaudad direction, and the peritoneal flap dissected toward the midline. When the hernia defect is encountered, the sac and hernia contents are dissected away from their attachments anteriorly, and usually remain intact as the flap is developed to the contralateral side (**Fig. 3**). If the sac must be divided, the rent in the peritoneum can be closed later. Any additional holes in the peritoneal flap can be closed

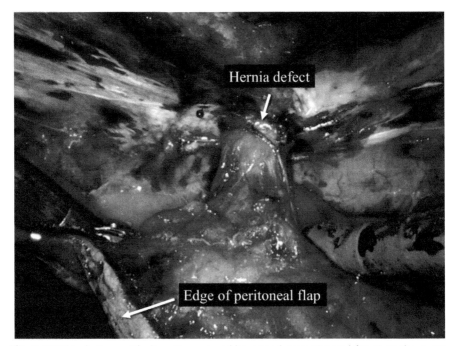

Fig. 3. TAPP technique with dissection around herniated preperitoneal fat. Note the posterior rectus sheath, which remains intact. (*Courtesy of* Conrad Ballecer, MD, Phoenix, AZ.)

later as well. The development and dissection within the preperitoneal plane may enable the surgeon to limit some adhesiolysis between the peritoneum and bowel, and will mobilize the falciform and umbilical ligaments.

Step 3. Measuring the defect and using an appropriately sized mesh is no different than standard LVHR[2], and is described in Step 3 of the preceding IPOM section in further detail. Although there is no standard, a bare polypropylene mesh is used by most surgeons. If there are rents in the peritoneum that cannot be closed, some will use a mesh designed for intraperitoneal use, or interpose omentum between the bowel and abdominal wall to avoid the possibility of adhesions between the mesh and the bowel.

Step 4. Mesh fixation. The TAPP approach creates a pocket within the extraperitoneal space, thus making formal mesh fixation less relevant, especially when the defect is closed and/or there is a large mesh:defect ratio. There is no standard, or even a generally accepted method for mesh fixation with this approach. Options for mesh fixation include none, adhesives, intermittent or running sutures (permanent or absorbable; partial or full-thickness), and mechanical tacks/fasteners (permanent or absorbable) (**Fig. 4**).

Step 5. Closure of the peritoneal flap. This is typically accomplished with a running, absorbable suture in the same direction as the initial incision to create the flap along the ipsilateral side of the ports. If a barbed suture is used, use of the loop at the end of the strand is used to pass the needle through, and anchor the beginning of the suture line, and no knot is necessary to anchor the end of the suture line. It would be prudent

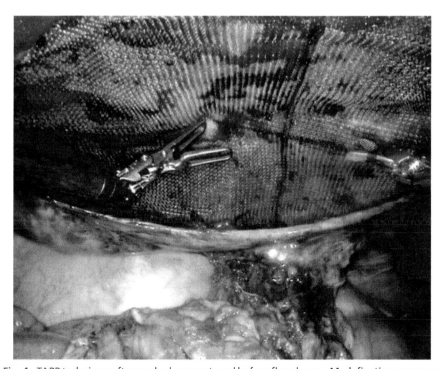

Fig. 4. TAPP technique after mesh placement, and before flap closure. Mesh fixation can range from none, to adhesives, mechanically placed fasteners, and/or sutures. If the flap closure is done using barbed suture, take care to cut the tail very short, as protrusion in to the peritoneal cavity can cause bowel obstruction. (*Courtesy of* Conrad Ballecer, MD, Phoenix, AZ)

to cut the suture flush with the peritoneum at the end to prevent a long tail of barbed suture from projecting into the peritoneal cavity, as this can cause bowel obstruction, but is uncommon.[28] Alternatively, one can simply hold the peritoneal flap over the mesh, then desufflate the abdomen by placing a suction device above the flap to avoid trapping gas in this location. It is important to turn off the insufflator for this maneuver. Jorge Daes has demonstrated that re-insufflation after 10 minutes reveals the peritoneal flap completely stuck to the prosthetic, with no gap at the edge of the flap (Jorge Daes, MD, FACS. Department of Minimally Invasive Surgery, Clinica Portoazul, Barranquilla, Colombia, personal communication, 2019).

Immediate Postoperative Care, Rehabilitation, and Recovery

This is the same as for the IPOM technique, described in detail previously.

Etiology of Adhesions to Mesh and Clinical Results in the Literature

The purpose for placing extraperitoneal mesh is to avoid adhesions between the mesh and the viscera. It is quite clear that these adhesions can be completely absent, or present at variable density, with the extreme of eventually eroding into hollow viscera, such as the bowel or urinary bladder. Even though the frequency of extreme adhesions is low, the consequences can be high, and thus a determination of etiology, and strategies for prevention are worth investigating. Let's explore some logical reasoning regarding etiology of adhesions between mesh and viscera. We presume that adhesions will not form between mesh and viscera if there is an intervening layer of autogenous tissue, such as the peritoneum or posterior rectus sheath; however, we know that adhesions between viscera and peritoneum, and between loops of bowel can occur in the absence of mesh. This is most likely due to tissue injury in response to a traumatic or nontraumatic inflammatory event. When we do observe adhesions between mesh and viscera, the adhesions are almost always *not uniform* across the mesh, even though the polymer is uniform throughout the mesh. For a single patient, the foreign body response would also be expected to be uniform across the mesh, but it is not. Therefore, the logical explanation of why mesh adheres to viscera is due to a mechanical force that causes tissue trauma. Some of this trauma will have occurred during the operation, and this may at least partially explain why there are fewer adhesions after a laparoscopic approach compared with laparotomy: less tissue trauma. But some tissue trauma may occur after the operation, because of folding or buckling of the mesh. The areas in which the mesh is not flat may actually cause trauma to the viscera, and subsequent adhesions. And because this buckling is not uniform throughout the mesh, the adhesions are also not uniform. An adhesion barrier or microporous polymer may limit adhesion formation to mesh, but will do little to avoid mechanical trauma to the viscera from areas that are folded or buckled. Therefore it is less likely the polymer that the mesh is constructed from is responsible for the adhesions, and more likely due to mechanical properties. The architecture of the mesh, pore size, and shape and/or knitting pattern would also be expected to play a role in the mechanical interaction between the mesh and the viscera. This gives rise to a very logical explanation for placing mesh in the extraperitoneal space, because mesh folding or buckling of the mesh would be expected to cause less tissue trauma postoperatively because the peritoneum or posterior rectus sheath would become a barrier to smooth out the folded or buckled areas of mesh where they would otherwise be in direct contact with the viscera. This in turn would be expected to cause less mechanical visceral trauma, and hence a lower risk of developing adhesions between the mesh and viscera. Indeed, any folding or buckling would be in direct contact with the abdominal wall, and thus be expected to cause more adhesions between the mesh and abdominal wall, which would serve to promote abdominal wall fixation to the mesh. Further, the mesh would be expected to have less folding or buckling in this space, because intra-abdominal pressure would serve to compress the mesh between the layers, and thus have a tendency to flatten it out.

There have been only been a few studies looking at postoperative adhesions between viscera and mesh after LVHR with an IPOM technique in humans. One notable study by Koehler and colleagues[29] looked at patients who underwent LVHR with the IPOM technique between 1993 and 2001. They reviewed 65 cases of SAO during that time, and rated the adhesions to the previous mesh based on review of the operative report. Most SAOs were for a new diagnosis (38/65), and the remainder were for recurrent hernia (17/65) or complications of the initial LVHR performed in the early postoperative period (10/65). Mean time to SAO was 420 days (2–1739 days). Adhesions to the mesh were absent or flimsy in 91% of patients; vascular, dense, or both in 9%; and "cohesive" in none.

Chelala and colleagues[30] looked at 125 reoperations after LVHR with the IPOM technique in 1326 patients operated on between 2000 and 2014. They found no patient to have dense adhesions between the mesh and the viscera, and only 12.7% classified as "easily cleavable or mild serosal intestinal adhesions." The vast majority (87.3%) of patients were almost evenly split between no adhesions and "loose adhesions of the omentum."

In 2010, Wassenaar and Colleagues[31] from the Netherlands reviewed 695 LVHR cases done between 2011 and 2009, and found approximately 10% required SAO. They divided those 72 cases into 2 groups: early SAO, which occurred within a few days because of a complication or suspected complication from LVHR, and late SAO, which occurred at least 1 month postoperative. All cases used an IPOM technique with ePTFE dual-sided mesh fixed with a double-crown permanent spiral tack technique, or a combination of tacks and sutures. In the early SAO group, 6 of 7 had peritonitis due to enterotomy or infection, and the mesh was removed. One patient had a suspicion of enterotomy, and diagnostic laparoscopy confirmed no injury, and the mesh was left in situ. In the late SAO group, 65 patients were reoperated on a median of 14 months after initial LVHR, 83% with a laparoscopic approach only, and 17% with laparotomy. The most common reason for SAO was hernia related (64%), with recurrent hernia responsible for 22% (14/65), chronic pain for 18% (12/65), new abdominal wall hernias for 13% (8/65), and port site hernias in 11% (7/65). Bowel obstruction related to adhesions accounted for only 2 cases of SAO.

Type of prosthetic may have a role in adhesion formation, possibly due to postoperative tissue trauma, as mentioned previously. An interesting report from Alkhoury and colleagues[32] from New Haven, Connecticut, in 2011 reviewed their experience with LVHR IPOM technique using plain polypropylene mesh anchored with a double crown of titanium spiral tacks. This was a single-surgeon series of 141 patients with a mean follow-up of 40 months in 123 patients (87%). During the follow-up period, 3 patients developed small bowel obstruction that all resolved without operative intervention, and 6 patients developed recurrent hernias. Four patients underwent repair of their recurrence, all with a laparoscopic approach. Two patients had moderate adhesions that were taken down using sharp and electrocautery dissection, and 2 were converted to an open approach due to extensive adhesions.

Snyder and colleagues[33] reviewed data from their National Surgical Quality Improvement Program database for ventral hernia repair at 16 Veterans Affairs Medical Centers in the United States. They evaluated 1444 cases, and found that 366 (25.3%) patients required SAO at a median follow-up period of 79.7 months, which occurred at a median of 18.9 months after hernia repair. They stratified the cases by 7 different hernia repair techniques, and found that LVHR IPOM had the lowest incidence of SAO at 20.6%, equivalent to onlay mesh. They also found that LVHR IPOM was associated with extensive/difficult adhesions for 38% of SAOs (range for different techniques was 25%–50%); however, it was the only technique not associated with enterotomy or unplanned bowel resection. Finally, the operative time for SAO did not differ between LVHR IPOM and the suture (nonmesh), underlay ePTFE, and onlay polypropylene groups.

ROBOTIC-ASSISTED LAPAROSCOPIC VENTRAL HERNIA REPAIR: ENHANCED VIEW TOTALLY EXTRAPERITONEAL (eTEP) TECHNIQUE
Advantages

A main advantage of the enhanced view totally extraperitoneal (eTEP) technique is initiating the operation within the abdominal wall space where the mesh will ultimately be placed. It largely stays out of the peritoneal cavity, thus limits the need for extensive adhesiolysis, and only requires adhesiolysis of the midline. Entrance into the peritoneal cavity is commonly done at the level of the hernia sac, and is used for inspection and adhesiolysis only when necessary to avoid bowel injury. In addition, the approach can use mobilization of the posterior rectus sheath alone, or in combination with transversus abdominus release (TAR).

Disadvantages

By dissecting outside of the hernia sac, direct or delayed thermal injury of bowel is a possibility. This can be avoided by entering the peritoneal cavity through the falciform ligament superior to any old incision or hernia sac, or via a separate port before this portion of the dissection has been completed to inspect for and even perform the adhesiolysis. Hernia defects that extend close to the pubis and the xiphoid process would require "double docking" of the RASD, which increases the need to go back and forth from the console to add ports, and adds time to the operation. There is also a possibility of contained hematoma within the retrorectus space, and the possibility of disruption of the posterior rectus sheath closure causing early postoperative bowel obstruction.

Patient and Robotic-Assisted Surgical Device Positioning

Table flexed (trunk in lordosis), arms tucked (**Fig. 5**). The RASD boom can be placed parallel, perpendicular, or at an angle depending on the specific model.

Surgical Technique

Step 1. Access to the retrorectus space. We describe this technique for midline hernias only. There is no single port setup for every hernia repair using this technique, but the concept is that the ports will be as far from the hernia defect as possible, without placing them too close to the costal margin, pelvis, or laterally to avoid RASD arm collision with the patient's chest, thighs, or arms. There are generally 3 port setups used: (1) "top-down" (superiorly placed ports working toward an operative field inferiorly), single dock, (2) "bottom-up" (inferiorly placed ports working toward an operative field superiorly), single dock, and (3) lateral, single-dock. Choice between superior or inferior port placement will depend on hernia defect location along the midline, defect size, and body habitus. When using a "top-down" or "bottom-up" approach, there are typically 4 ports used, 1 for initial entry, and subsequent use by a bedside assistant, and 3 ports for the RASD camera and instruments (**Fig. 6**). Regardless of exact location, initial access is performed through the rectus muscle at a location above the arcuate line. It is typically accomplished toward the lateral aspect of the rectus

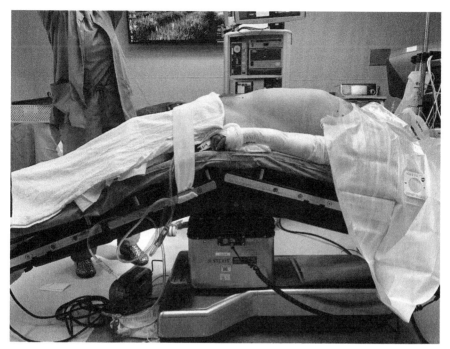

Fig. 5. Patient position for eTEP approach from with "top-down" or "bottom-up" approaches. Flexing the trunk minimizes the risk of collision between the RASD and the thighs or face, depending on the port placement.

muscle near the costal margin or near the umbilicus on either the right or left side depending on the surgeon's preference and anatomy. The first port can be done with an open technique, or an optical entry port depending on surgeon preference. The scope can be used to bluntly dissect the retrorectus space until another port can be safely placed, then an instrument through the second port can facilitate dissection until there is enough space to safely place the remaining ports.

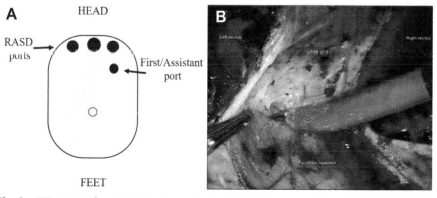

Fig. 6. eTEP approach – "Top-Down", single-dock. (A) Port setup of dissection after the cross-over. Scope port is in the subxiphoid location with a field of view towards the feet; (B) Representative view of the dissection after the crossover, before the hernia defect is encountered. (*Courtesy of* Igor Belyansky, MD, Annapolis, MD).

Another option is a lateral port placement, using only 3 ports. The first port entry is typically done near the costal margin and through the rectus muscle relatively close, and medial to the linea semilunaris. The scope is used to bluntly dissect the retrorectus space until the other 2 ports can be safely placed under direct vision (**Fig. 7**).

Regardless of which port setup is used, the surgeon has the option to also place intraperitoneal ports for assessment and/or lysis of adhesions at any time during the operation. Alternatively, the surgeon can carefully open the hernia sac and inspect the contents and/or perform lysis of adhesions.

Step 2. Development of the retrorectus space. Much of this will be done to gain enough space to place the additional ports. The space is developed primarily with blunt dissection and sparing use of an energy source. When beginning superiorly, after the initial port is placed in the space, the scope itself is used to develop the space enough to allow placement of a second port just superior to the initial port. These 2 ports are then used to bluntly dissect the space as far as possible inferiorly, and all the way to the xiphoid process superiorly. Once the space has been adequately developed, the medial posterior rectus sheath on the ipsilateral side is detached just before it fuses with the linea alba to expose the falciform ligament. The falciform ligament is bluntly pushed away from the linea alba, and the contralateral posterior rectus sheath is identified and divided in a similar fashion. This will expose the contralateral rectus muscle and retrorectus space, which is developed enough superiorly to allow the placement of 2 additional ports under direct vision, one in the midline subxiphoid location, and one along the opposite costal margin. Care should be taken to place the

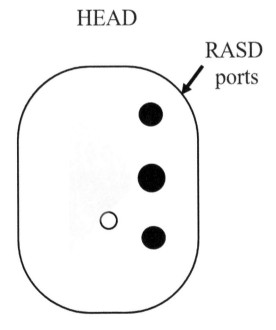

Fig. 7. Port set-up for a lateral eTEP approach. This is also a "single-dock" approach, and the ports are all placed medial to the linea semilunaris, in contrast to the TARUP, which places ports lateral to the linea semilunaris, similar to the IPOM and TAPP approaches.

ports far enough apart to avoid collision of the RASD arms after docking. Once all the ports are placed, the RASD can be docked, and the operation can continue with the surgeon at the console.

When beginning inferiorly, the first port is placed above the arcuate line, through the rectus muscle just medial to the linea semilunaris, and the scope is used to dissect inferiorly into the space of Retzius to expose the ipsilateral epigastric vessels and the Cooper ligament. A second port can then be placed just lateral to the epigastric vessels to facilitate dissection of the space of Retzius so the remaining 2 ports can be safely placed. Unlike the "top-down" setup, no crossover is necessary before placing all of the ports because the space of Retzius has no posterior rectus sheath. The ports should be placed far enough apart to avoid collision of the RASD arms, and superiorly enough to avoid collision with the pelvis and thighs. Once all the ports are placed, the RASD can be docked. Similarly, a unilateral dissection is completed as far superiorly as possible. What differs, is the opposite side also can be dissected superiorly before dividing the medial borders of the posterior rectus sheath just before they fuse with the linea alba. Once both sides have been dissected as far as feasible, the medial borders of the posterior rectus sheath are divided, with the use of an energy source as needed (**Fig. 8**).

Step 3. The crossover. This simply refers to the division of the medial aspect of the posterior rectus sheath bilaterally, just before it fuses with the linea alba. When beginning superiorly, this is partially accomplished before docking the RASD, as the surgeon is moving from one side to the other to create enough space to place all the ports. When beginning inferiorly, because all the ports are placed in the space of Retzius, the RASD can be docked before most of the retrorectus dissection and the crossover are accomplished.

Step 4. Management of the hernia defect. During the dissection of the retrorectus space and division of the posterior rectus sheaths, one will encounter the hernia defect and its contents. Small hernia sacs (<5 cm width) or herniated preperitoneal fat, particularly with primary hernias, can simply be reduced and left intact as the dissection of the midline continues. Larger defects or incisional hernias will have a higher probability of containing bowel, with or without adhesions. If the surgeon has not already performed an intraperitoneal inspection and/or adhesiolysis, the surgeon should have a low threshold to open the hernia sac (typically without the use of an energy source) to inspect for adherent bowel. Reduction of hernia contents can then be accomplished

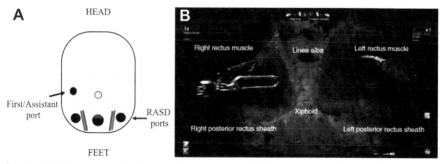

Fig. 8. eTEP approach – "Bottom-Up", single-dock. (*A*) Port setup. Note that all three ports can be placed before the cross-over, because there is no posterior sheath behind the rectus muscles below the arcuate line. Scope port is in the suprapubic location with a field of view towards the head; (*B*) Representative view of the dissection looking towards the head. (*Courtesy of* Igor Belyansky, MD, Annapolis, MD.)

under direct vision, taking into account the fundamental principles of adhesiolysis (eg, avoid energy source near bowel, avoid excessive traction, inspect for enterotomy carefully). The hernia sac can then be closed separately, or together with the posterior rectus sheath closure at the surgeon's discretion. If the posterior rectus sheath will be left open, the sac should generally be closed.

Step 5. Management of the midline. There are 3 aspects to this step of the operation: the hernia defect, the linea alba away from the hernia defect, and the posterior rectus sheath. If the hernia defect is going to be closed, vertical or horizontal closure can be accomplished according to the specific anatomy of the patient, favoring a direction that is under the least amount of tension intraoperatively. Suture type and technique are at the discretion of the surgeon, but size 0 barbed suture using the short-stitch technique are routinely practiced by the author. This also applies to the management of the linea alba away from the hernia defect, typically only important when plicating a diastasis. There is no consensus or data to dictate whether or not to plicate a rectus diastasis above and below a hernia defect, but the principles of closure are the same as for the hernia defect, with the exception that a plication is always performed vertically. The posterior sheath can be closed with the same principles, or if there is too much tension for closure, simply left open, provided the hernia sac has been closed. Closing the posterior rectus sheath under tension exposes the patient to the risk of disruption of the closure in the early postoperative period, with bowel herniation and obstruction becoming a possibility. If the hernia sac cannot be closed, and there would be excessive tension on the posterior sheath closure, a TAR can be performed unilaterally or bilaterally to facilitate this. The amount of dissection and mobilization are at the discretion of the surgeon. Once the TAR has been completed, the posterior rectus sheath should come together without any tension.

Step 6. Placement of mesh/drain. Once the dissection is complete, the defect closed, and further closure of the posterior sheath and/or linea alba plication is complete, there will be a confluent retrorectus space that is separated from an intact linea alba, and separated from the peritoneal cavity. There is no need for a mesh designed for intraperitoneal use in this situation, and the mesh should be strong enough to be able to bridge a gap, should the defect closure and/or plication fail in the future. The mesh can be trimmed to fit the size of the space, and should extend to the lateral borders of the posterior rectus sheath (semilunar line), unless these were divided as part of a TAR, in which case the mesh can extend beyond the semilunar lines. The mesh should extend in the craniocaudad direction for distance enough to allow for mesh coverage of the defect in the event the defect closure fails, and allow for mesh contracture. Mesh fixation will depend on patient anatomy. Options include partial fixation, such as to the Cooper ligaments, or fixation with sutures or devices placed with a mechanical device or created by the surgeon. These can be placed in a quilting-type manner, or any manner at the surgeon's discretion. The mesh should fit the space appropriately so that excessive buckling and folding are avoided. There may be some unevenness of the mesh, which will promptly flatten when the gas is released, and intra-abdominal pressure increases after the patient is extubated. If the defect has been closed, there is theoretically no need for any formal mesh fixation, as the prosthetic should incorporate into the abdominal wall over time, and cannot migrate out of the contained retrorectus space. Mesh fixation, type, and amount will be determined by the surgeon based on the patient's goals, clinical scenario, anatomy, and intraoperative tissue characteristics.

There are no data or enough experience to guide the surgeon on whether or not to place a drain in the retrorectus space. The rationale for drain placement is to prevent accumulation of fluid and blood that could prevent the muscles from adhering to the mesh/posterior rectus sheath. It is also unclear that any significant bleeding within this space would not accumulate, as blood tends to clot quickly, and the drain diameter is too small to allow drainage of clot. If a drain is placed, it should probably be removed after a shorter period of time compared with drains left in the subcutaneous space that does not contain a synthetic prosthetic device. Theoretically, shorter drain times would be expected to reduce infection rates related to the drain itself. It is the author's practice to place a single, 19-French fluted drain, and remove it when the drainage is ≤30 mL/d or at approximately 7 days regardless of the amount of output. By 7 days, there should be no active bleeding, the mesh should be anchored to the muscle well enough that any fluid accumulation will not separate it, and serosanguinous fluid should reabsorb.

Immediate Postoperative Care, Rehabilitation, and Recovery

Postoperative care is the same for any ventral hernia repair or midline laparotomy closure that involves reapproximation of the midline. In general, activity is restricted in some fashion for 6 to 8 weeks, with the caveat that the patient should ambulate and perform most activities of daily living. If a drain was placed in the retrorectus space, over the mesh, this should probably be left in for a relatively shorter period of time compared with a drain left in a space without a mesh. If posterior rectus sheath closure was performed without a TAR, and the patient develops a small bowel obstruction, the surgeon should have a relatively low threshold to return to the operating room for a diagnostic laparoscopy to search for the existence of a posterior sheath disruption with bowel herniation under the mesh, and above the posterior rectus sheath. If a TAR was done, the dramatic decrease in tension of the posterior sheath closure makes this much less likely.

Clinical Results in the Literature

The concept of performing laparoscopic hernia repair in the retrorectus space primarily came from a report in 2002 by Miserez and Penninckx in Belgium.[34] They reported on 15 patients, mostly with midline defects, but also included a lumbar and parastomal defect. They used standard laparoscopic instruments, and did not reapproximate the posterior rectus sheath after the crossover, or close the hernia defect. Mean defect width was 3 cm, and plain polypropylene or ePTFE mesh was used depending on potential exposure to bowel. All mesh was anchored anteriorly with metal spiral tacks, and closed suction drains were used selectively. Operative time was not reported. Median LOS was 5 days, with 2 prolonged stays due to ileus and stroke. Three patients required antibiotics for documented or presumed infection, and no mesh had to be removed. With a median follow-up of 126 ± 37 days, there was 1 recurrence. A decade later, Dr Jorge Daes from Barranquilla, Colombia,[35] used the retrorectus space to develop a larger space of Retzius for a TEP approach to more difficult inguinal hernia repairs. Belyansky and colleagues,[36] learning from the experience of Daes,[35] then applied the same approach for midline ventral hernia repair with standard laparoscopic equipment, and subsequently with a RASD, with what turns out to be very similar to what Miserez and Penninckx[34] described in 2002. The multi-institutional report of Belyansky and colleagues[36] reviewed their experience with standard laparoscopic instrumentation in 79 patients with a mean BMI of 31, one-third of whom had a previous ventral hernia repair. A total of 41 patients underwent TAR. Mean defect width was 6.2 cm without TAR and 11.1 cm with TAR, mean operative time was 219 minutes overall, and mean LOS was 1.0 days without TAR and 2.7 days with TAR. There was 1 case converted to an open procedure for excision of a bone fragment, and the overall complication rate was 3.8%, primarily due to seroma and wound dehiscence. There were no readmissions within 30 days, and 1 recurrence with a mean follow-up of 322 ± 122 days. The subsequent single-institution report of Belyansky and colleagues[37] that used a RASD described 37 patients, 8 of whom underwent a TAR performed by 2 surgeons. In addition to midline defects, they included 1 parastomal and 3 flank defects. Mean defect size (greatest dimension) was 7.4 cm (5.9 cm without, and 11.3 cm with TAR), mean operative time was significantly longer for patients undergoing TAR (141 vs 240 minutes), and varied substantially between surgeons. There were no conversions to an open approach. Complication rate was 7.4% overall, due solely to seromas and oral intolerance. Mean LOS was significantly longer for patients undergoing TAR (0.3 vs 2.1 days). Follow-up was less than 2 months, so recurrence rates were not reported. Penchev and colleagues[38] performed a retrospective comparison of eTEP and IPOM techniques using standard laparoscopic instrumentation, with 27 patients in each group. Both groups were similar in terms of medical history and BMI (mean 25 and 27), as well as hernia defect area (71 and 76 cm^2). Mean operative time was significantly longer for the eTEP approach (186 ± 62 vs 90 ± 31 minutes). There was no significant difference in LOS (mean 2.9 vs 3.4 days) or complications (n = 6 vs 4; primarily seroma) between the groups. There were no conversions to another technique. Postoperative pain gradually decreased at a similar rate in both groups to a level lower than preoperatively, and was lower in the eTEP group at each time point, but the difference seemed to be minimal at 30 days. There was no statistical analysis of the pain scores. Follow-up was only 30 days, and there was 1 readmission and 1 recurrence, both in the IPOM group, and not statistically different from the eTEP group.

ROBOTIC-ASSISTED LAPAROSCOPIC VENTRAL HERNIA REPAIR: TRANSABDOMINAL RETRORECTUS UMBILICAL PROSTHETIC (TARUP) TECHNIQUE

Advantages

Theoretic advantages of the transabdominal retrorectus umbilical prosthetic (TARUP) technique are the mechanical advantage of a mesh placed posterior to the repair. In addition, keeping the mesh in an extraperitoneal location is more likely to cause fewer adhesions between bowel and viscera, but the true clinical impact of this is unknown. The use of a single set of laterally based ports requires docking of the RASD only once, thus avoiding the need to "double dock" the RASD.

Disadvantages

When comparing this to an open approach with a ventral hernia patch designed for small defects, this approach is significantly longer, but the clinical implications are unknown. The approach also presents some significant pitfalls, particularly the risk of dividing the linea semilunaris while accessing the ipsilateral posterior rectus sheath. Posterior rectus sheath hematoma and umbilical skin necrosis are possible disadvantages, but can be seen with other techniques. This technique is limited to relatively small midline hernias, and thus has the disadvantage that it is not useful for larger defects, particularly those that would require a mesh to be placed beyond the lateral borders of the rectus muscle.

Patient and Robotic-Assisted Surgical Device Positioning

Supine, arms tucked. No flexion required. Boom of the RASD placed on the opposite side of the ports.

Surgical Procedure

Step 1. Placement of the ports is no different from a standard IPOM approach. Typically, the first port is placed along the anterior axillary line near the costal margin, usually on the left, but occasionally on the left depending on the clinical circumstances. The secondary ports are placed under direct vision, taking care to be as far lateral of the ipsilateral semilunar line as possible, but not lateral enough to cause a collision between the RASD arms and the tucked arm. For this reason, an arm-holding device that projects anteriorly and is rigid should be avoided (see **Fig. 1**).

Step 2. Dissection of any incarcerated visceral contents and adhesion can be performed as necessary with all standard precautions.

Step 3. Open the ipsilateral posterior rectus sheath. This should be done well within the body of the rectus muscles to avoid injury to the neurovascular bundles and linea semilunaris. This is typically performed with a monopolar scissor, but a monopolar hook, or ultrasonic device also could be used. The opening should be performed in the craniocaudal direction, and long enough to have adequate visualization of the operative field, and dissect an adequate space for mesh placement.

Step 4. Dissection of the ipsilateral retrorectus space. This is largely accomplished with blunt dissection and sparing use of an energy source for hemostasis.

Step 5. The crossover. This is accomplished by first dividing the posterior rectus sheath before it fuses with the linea alba, and gaining access to the preperitoneal space above the falciform and/or umbilical ligaments. The contralateral rectus sheath is the divided just beyond the fusion with the linea alba. It is important not to divide the linea alba here, as it will lead to a subcutaneous plane, and not the contralateral retrorectus space. Once the contralateral posterior rectus sheath is divided, the retrorectus space is then developed up to the linea semilunaris.

Step 6. Defect closure. This can be done at the discretion of the surgeon, and is performed the same as any other defect closure previously described.

Step 7. Mesh placement. Mesh is then placed flat, against the rectus muscles. An appropriately sized mesh should be placed that accounts for mesh contraction, and defect bridging in the event the defect is not closed, or if defect closure fails.

Step 8. Closure of the ipsilateral posterior rectus sheath. This can be accomplished by any method, but is typically performed with a long-acting absorbable, barbed suture in a running fashion. When using a barbed suture, care should be taken to avoid leaving a tail of this protruding into the peritoneal cavity, as that would probably increase the incidence of bowel adhesion.

Immediate Postoperative Care, Rehabilitation, and Recovery

This technique depends less on healing the defect closure, thus restriction of activities would be expected to be less important. Monitoring for complications of umbilical skin necrosis and posterior rectus sheath space hematoma are performed as appropriate.

Clinical Results in the Literature

Muysoms and colleagues[39] reported their multi-institutional experience with TARUP in 41 patients with a mean BMI of 30. All cases were for small (2 × 2 cm) primary or trocar incisional hernias at the umbilicus, and all operations used an RASD. There were 3 ports used, and each case placed all suture material and a 15 × 15-cm self-gripping mesh in the peritoneal cavity before docking the RASD. All defects were closed anteriorly, and the posterior rectus sheath was not closed where it was divided during the crossover, but all peritoneal defects were closed. Mesh was placed with the grips facing anteriorly. Mean operative time was 73 minutes, and decreased with experience to a mean of 61 minutes for the last 13 cases. There were no conversions to another technique, and the LOS was outpatient for 68%, 1 night for 29%, and 2 night for 3%. There were 2 complications requiring intervention. One return to the operating room for laparoscopic evacuation of a retro-muscular hematoma, and one for drainage and antibiotics of a peri-umbilical wound infection 1 month postoperative. No mesh required removal. They did not report on recurrence rate.

ROBOTIC-ASSISTED LAPAROSCOPIC VENTRAL HERNIA REPAIR: SUBCUTANEOUS ONLAY LAPAROSCOPIC APPROACH (SCOLA) TECHNIQUE

Subcutaneous onlay laparoscopic approach (SCOLA) is an emerging technique described primarily with standard laparoscopic instrumentation, and very limited experience with an RASD. This approach should afford all the advantages of a laparoscopic approach compared with an open approach in terms of reduction of postoperative pain, recovery time, and wound complications. Compared with a posterior approach (intra-abdominal or eTEP), the SCOLA technique may be easier for some surgeons because the suture line is placed on the posterior aspect of the the operative field (the "floor"), rather than the anterior aspect (the "ceiling"). The articulation of the RASD instruments, however, can overcome this issue to some extent. The advantage of an anterior approach is the avoidance of the peritoneal cavity, and thus a potential for lower risk of injury to intra-abdominal organs. The one exception is when dissecting herniated contents, particularly if they are hidden beneath a hernia sac. It may be best in this situation to keep the sac intact, then reduce this in its entirety. If there is concern about herniated viscera, one can always open the sac and directly inspect the contents, taking care to avoid inadvertent visceral injury while opening the sac. This is much less likely for small midline hernias; however, cannot be underestimated because of the serious nature of missed or delayed visceral injury.

Advantages

Using a laparoscopic technique (with or without an RASD) compared with an open onlay technique would be expected to have all the benefits of laparoscopic surgery, including less pain, shorter recovery, and fewer wound complications. In addition, by staying completely extraperitoneal, there would be a lower chance for inadvertent bowel injury. The one exception would be the case in which there were adhesions to a hernia sac, and an energy source was used too close to the bowel, which was hidden within the sac, or injured while dissecting and/or opening the sac.

Disadvantages

Theoretically, there is a mechanical disadvantage with the mesh anterior to the repair compared with posterior. There is also a risk of retraction/fibrosis of the elevated subcutaneous tissue, which does not exist with techniques that do not use subcutaneous flaps. There is also a theoretically increased risk of skin necrosis due to devascularization, if the flap dissection divides all the peri-umbilical perforators, although this has not been reported to date.

Patient and Robotic-Assisted Surgical Device Positioning

Supine, slight hip extension, legs abducted. Abduction can be performed with a split-leg table, or stirrups. If using stirrups, it is important to keep the thighs level or slightly posterior to the trunk (via hip extension), and not anterior to the trunk. Legs do not need to be abducted for use with an RASD. Flexing the bed is helpful when using the RASD to avoid collision between the RASD arms and the patient's thighs and pelvis. The boom of the RASD is placed along the side of the bed, parallel, perpendicular, or at an angle, depending on the model.

Surgical Technique

Step 1. A 1-cm to 2-cm transverse incision in the suprapubic region. The subcutaneous tissue is lifted off the aponeurosis with a combination of monopolar energy and blunt dissection for an area large enough to place a laparoscopic port. A standard port can be placed, but will require suture fixation. Alternatively, a blunt port with a collar for suture fixation, or a balloon-tipped port can be used. Two ports are then placed laterally on either side of the camera port at a distance large enough to avoid collision of the arms. The device is then docked according to surgeon preference (**Fig. 9**A).

Step 2. The dissection of the subcutaneous fascia off the aponeurosis is then carried all the way to the xiphoid process, also using an energy source and blunt dissection. This is a very straightforward dissection, except at the umbilical stalk and areas of herniation. The umbilical stalk is simply divided at the level of the abdominal wall. Hernia defects require reduction and or resection of the preperitoneal fat, or hernia sac. It is ok to open the hernia sac to inspect for adhesions, and the resulting pneumoperitoneum should not compromise the working space. The defect should be fully dissected free of herniated contents. The width of the dissection will depend on the width of the diastasis, size of the hernia defect(s), and planned size of the mesh. Typically, this width would be 12 to 15 cm, or 6 to 7 cm on each side. Any perforators encountered are controlled with sutures or an energy source as appropriate.

Step 3. Closure of the diastasis and hernia defect. There is no standard for suture type or technique. If not using an onlay mesh, most surgeons would recommend a permanent suture of sufficient strength for reapproximation of the diastasis. If using an onlay mesh, suture type may be less important in terms of long-acting absorbable versus permanent. Use of the short-stitch technique, described by Millbourn and colleagues[40] in 2009, will distribute tension over a greater surface area of the closure, and theoretically will increase the chance of staying together. Use of barbed suture is generally thought to be technically easier because it maintains tension while creating the suture line, and theoretically may even increase the surface area over which the tension is distributed, potentially lowering the risk of the suture pulling through the tissue. The suture line will encompass any and all hernia defects as well (**Fig. 9**B).

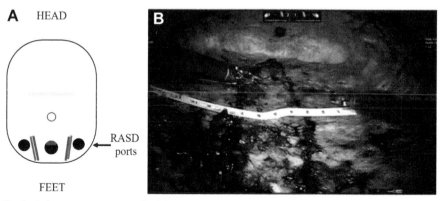

Fig. 9. Subcutaneous approach. (*A*) Port setup. Note that all three ports can be placed in the beginning, similar to the eTEP approach, but the plane of dissection is subcutaneous, not the space of Retzius. The scope port is in the suprapubic location with a field of view towards the head; (*B*) Photo showing dissection before plication and mesh placement. The medial borders of the rectus muscles have been traced with a surgical marker to easily identify needle placement during plication and closure of the hernia defect. (*Courtesy of* F. Malcher, MD, Bronx, NY.)

Step 4. Mesh placement. Placement of a mesh over the suture line is accomplished in whatever manner the surgeon is accustomed to for laparoscopic hernia repair. The important point of mesh placement is that the mesh lays flat against the abdominal wall. Fixation of the mesh can be performed with mechanically placed fasteners, sutures, or adhesives. The mesh also could be left in place without fixation. Lack of data and experience with this technique in general prohibit recommendation of one fixation method over another, and surgeons should use their best judgment.

Step 5. Reapproximation of subcutaneous tissue and umbilical stalk can be accomplished with a series of interrupted absorbable sutures. If a mesh is placed, the sutures should encompass the subcutaneous tissue, mesh, and a superficial bite of aponeurosis. A closed suction drain may be placed at the surgeon's discretion.

Immediate Postoperative Care, Rehabilitation, and Recovery

Use of an abdominal binder is at the surgeon's discretion. Activity restriction is also at the surgeon's discretion, but because a successful plication and repair is at least partially dependent on healing of the suture line, heavy activity may be restricted for 6-8 weeks, at which time the strength of the suture line should be approximately 90% of its final strength. The remainder of the postoperative care is a matter of local preferences and routine.

Clinical Results in the Literature

Bellido Luque and colleagues[41] in Spain reviewed their experience in 2014 with 21 patients with a mean BMI of 27. They described the technique with standard laparoscopic instrumentation used via 3 ports in the suprapubic region. After their dissection, which included disconnecting the umbilical stalk, hernias were repaired with a preperitoneal ventral hernia patch with the straps anchored to the defect edges with absorbable suture. Mean hernia defect size was 3.4 cm diameter, and were all in the midline. The diastasis was closed with permanent barbed suture. Mean values were 99 minutes for operative time, 1.5 days for LOS, and 4.2 days for drain removal. Seromas occurred in 23% of patients, but only 1 required percutaneous drainage. Subcutaneous emphysema occurred in 2 patients, and resolved spontaneously without clinical consequences. There was no skin necrosis or wound infection. Mean follow-up of all patients was 20 months. There was no hernia recurrence. The diastasis was measured by ultrasound preoperatively and postoperatively, and decreased from 24 to 39 mm to 2.9 to 3.7 mm at 24 months.

Muas and colleagues[42] in Argentina described a similar technique for 2 cases of diastasis associated with small midline hernias of 1 to 2 cm. Both cases plicated the diastasis and repaired the hernia defect with a permanent, running barbed suture line, and placement of a plain polypropylene mesh on the anterior surface of the abdominal wall, and fixed with interrupted absorbable sutures. One patient also had a unilateral external oblique release. Mean operative time was 107 minutes, and drains were removed at 48 hours. No intraoperative or postoperative complications were noted, but there was no long-term follow-up.

Dr Faria-Correa in Singapore[43] used a long history of endoscopic-assisted abdominoplasty and applied this to 5 cases using a RASD with a similar technique: 3 ports in the suprapubic region. No data were presented regarding operative time, LOS, or follow-up, as the article focused on technique. It was noted that there were no complications.

Cuenca and colleagues[44] reported a single case in 2017 using a nearly identical technique for repair of a 2-cm epigastric and 1-cm midline hernias associated with a diastasis. They used standard laparoscopic instrumentation; however, they closed the hernia defect as part of the plication with barbed suture, and placed an onlay of 20 × 15-cm plain polypropylene mesh, anchored with interrupted absorbable suture. There were no complications, but LOS, operative time, and follow-up were not provided.

Köckerling and colleagues[45] from Germany reported a slightly different technique in 2019 with an endoscopic-assisted approach. Between June 2015 and February 2016, they operated on 40 patients with umbilical and epigastric hernias with associated diastasis using a curved incision around the umbilicus with a short extension superiorly in the midline. Once the subcutaneous dissection is complete, the anterior rectus sheath is incised longitudinally on both sides 2 to 3 cm lateral to the linea alba. The medial cut edges are then sewn together to create a new, narrow linea alba and close the hernia defect(s). A coated polypropylene mesh is then sewn in place to the lateral cut edge of the anterior rectus sheath to essentially replace the anterior rectus sheath flaps that have been sewn together in the midline. Mean values for BMI were 32.6 and operative time 120 minutes. No LOS was reported, and there were 3 complications: 2 delayed umbilical wound healing and 1 seroma, none of which required intervention.

Most recently, the same approach was used in Brazil, where a minority of the procedures (4 of 48 cases) were performed using an RASD. Claus and colleagues[46] performed 48 cases for repair of small midline hernias (mean defect size 2.3 cm), and used a variety of prosthetics in 94% of cases. They did not specify the number of patients followed, but noted a 27% incidence of seroma formation, approximately half of which required 1 or more percutaneous drainage procedures, and 1 required subsequent open excision combined with panniculectomy. One patient also developed retraction and fibrosis of the subcutaneous tissue, presumably under the skin flaps. After a mean follow-up period of only 8 months, the investigators noted 1 recurrent hernia. The remainder of the patients (94%) reported being satisfied with their results.

The surgeons who performed operations with both standard and RASD instrumentation noted the RASD platform afforded improved ergonomics and stability of the scope.

SUMMARY

LVHR with an RASD has many options for specific techniques. The articulating nature of the instruments significantly improves the surgeon's ability to suture in a variety of positions compared with standard, nonarticulating laparoscopic instrumentation. In addition, control of the scope gives a much more stable image of the operative field compared with manual control by an assistant, further improving the ability of the surgeon to use this technique in a reproducible fashion. These benefits have given rise to a host of laparoscopic repair techniques previously performed only in an open fashion (retrorectus repair with mesh placement with or without TAR, and onlay repair with mesh), laparoscopically without an RASD (IPOM), or not at all (TAPP for ventral hernia).

Importantly, rather than provide a technique using laparoscopy with an RASD for each patient, the surgeon should apply the technique that best fits the clinical scenario, and is most likely to meet the goals of the patient in terms of restoration of abdominal wall contour, scar revision, symptom resolution, and permanence of repair. We must focus on avoiding projection of what is important for each case, and ask our patients what is most important to them. Then we should critically listen to their concerns to establish realistic goals, and align those goals with our available techniques and prosthetics, for a given clinical scenario.

All of these techniques are evolving, as have all techniques over time. We must not lose sight, however, of some basic surgical tenants, such as delicate tissue handling, avoidance of inadvertent use of potentially damaging energy adjacent to bowel, operating with a clear view of the operative field, distribution of tension along a suture line, meticulous hemostasis, and obliteration of dead space. So, rather than perform every hernia repair with an RASD, or never use an RASD for hernia repair, match the patient to the best technique for the patients as an individual. Ideally, we should collect our short-term and long-term outcomes data for these techniques, and use this feedback to continuously innovate and improve.

DISCLOSURE

Anchora Medical, Auris Health Inc., Bard/Davol, CMR Surgical, Medtronic, and Verb Surgical: consulting fee/consulting. Gordian Surgical: honoraria/proctoring/consulting fee/consulting. New View Surgical and Via Surgical: stock/scientific advisory board/ownership stake/advisory board. Surgiquest: honoraria/stock/scientific advisory board. Standard Bariatrics Consulting Fee/Regulatory consulting.

REFERENCES

1. LeBlanc KA, Booth WV. Laparoscopic repair of incisional abdominal hernias using expanded polytetrafluoroethylene: preliminary findings. Surg Laparosc Endosc 1993;3(1):39–41.
2. Earle D, Roth SJ, Saber A, et al, SAGES Guidelines Committee. SAGES guidelines for laparoscopic ventral hernia repair. Surg Endosc 2016;30(8):3163–83.
3. Earle D. Open versus laparoscopic incisional/ventral hernia repair in the Medicare population. Oral presentation. American Hernia Society annual meeting. Orlando, FL, March 13-16, 2013.
4. Earle D. Hospital based outcomes of open versus laparoscopic ventral hernia repair. Oral presentation. American Hernia Society annual meeting. Orlando, FL, March 13-16, 2013.
5. Poulose B, Shelton J, Phillips S, et al. Epidemiology and cost of ventral hernia repair: making the case for hernia research. Hernia 2012;16:179–83.
6. Lois A, Ehlers A, Minneman J, et al. Disclosure at #SAGES2018: an analysis of physician-industry relationships of invited speakers at the 2018 SAGES national meeting. Surg Endosc 2019. https://doi.org/10.1007/s00464-019-07037-w.
7. Altieri M, Yang J, Xu J, et al. Outcomes after robotic ventral hernia repair: a study of 21,565 patients in the state of New York. Am Surg 2018;84(6):902–8.
8. Melman L, Jenkins E, Deeken C, et al. Evaluation of acute fixation strength for mechanical tacking devices and fibrin sealant versus polypropylene suture for laparoscopic ventral hernia repair. Surg Innov 2010;17(4):285–90.
9. Papageorge CM, Funk LM, Poulose BK, et al. Primary fascial closure during laparoscopic ventral hernia repair does not reduce 30-day wound complications. Surg Endosc 2017;31(11):4551–7.
10. Wennergren JE, Askenasy EP, Greenberg JA, et al. Laparoscopic ventral hernia repair with primary fascial closure versus bridged repair: a risk-adjusted comparative study. Surg Endosc 2016;30(8):3231–8.
11. Tandon A, Pathak S, Lyons NJ, et al. Meta-analysis of closure of the fascial defect during laparoscopic incisional and ventral hernia repair. Br J Surg 2016;103(12):1598–607.
12. Wantz GE. Giant prosthetic reinforcement of the visceral sac. Surg Gynecol Obstet 1989;169(5):408–17.
13. Warren JA, Cobb WS, Ewing JA, et al. Standard laparoscopic versus robotic retromuscular ventral hernia repair. Surg Endosc 2017;31(1):324–32.

14. Patel PP, Love MW, Ewing JA, et al. Risks of subsequent abdominal operations after laparoscopic ventral hernia repair. Surg Endosc 2017;31(2):823–8.

15. Ahmed MA, Tawfic QA, Schlachta CM, et al. Pain and surgical outcomes reporting after laparoscopic ventral hernia repair in relation to mesh fixation technique: a systematic review and meta-analysis of randomized clinical trials. J Laparoendosc Adv Surg Tech A 2018;28(11):1298–315.

16. Palanivelu C, Jani KV, Senthilnathan P, et al. Laparoscopic sutured closure with mesh reinforcement of incisional hernias. Hernia 2007;11(3):223–8.

17. Ballantyne GH, Hourmont K, Wasielewski A. Telerobotic laparoscopic repair of incisional ventral hernias using intraperitoneal prosthetic mesh. JSLS 2003; 7(1):7–14.

18. Tayar C, Karoui M, Cherqui D, et al. Robot-assisted laparoscopic mesh repair of incisional hernias with exclusive intracorporeal suturing: a pilot study. Surg Endosc 2007;21(10):1786–9.

19. Allison N, Tieu K, Snyder B, et al. Technical feasibility of robot-assisted ventral hernia repair. World J Surg 2012;36(2):447–52.

20. Gonzalez AM, Romero RJ, Seetharamaiah R, et al. Laparoscopic ventral hernia repair with primary closure versus no primary closure of the defect: potential benefits of the robotic technology. Int J Med Robot 2015;11(2):120–5.

21. Kudsi OY, Paluvoi N, Bhurtel P, et al. Robotic repair of ventral hernias: preliminary findings of a case series of 106 consecutive cases. Am J Robot Surg 2015; 2(1):22–6.

22. Chen YJ, Huynh D, Nguyen S, et al. Outcomes of robot-assisted versus laparoscopic repair of small-sized ventral hernias. Surg Endosc 2017;31(3):1275–9.

23. Gonzalez A, Escobar E, Romero R, et al. Robotic-assisted ventral hernia repair: a multicenter evaluation of clinical outcomes. Surg Endosc 2017;31(3):1342–9.

24. Prabhu AS, Dickens EO, Copper CM, et al. Laparoscopic vs robotic intraperitoneal mesh repair for incisional hernia: an Americas Hernia Society Quality Collaborative Analysis. J Am Coll Surg 2017;225(2):285–93.

25. Oviedo RJ, Robertson JC, Desai AS. Robotic ventral hernia repair and endoscopic component separation: outcomes. JSLS 2017;21(3) [pii:e2017.00055].

26. Walker PA, May AC, Mo J, et al. Multicenter review of robotic versus laparoscopic ventral hernia repair: is there a role for robotics? Surg Endosc 2018;32(4):1901–5.

27. Zayan NE, Meara MP, Schwartz JS, et al. A direct comparison of robotic and laparoscopic hernia repair: patient-reported outcomes and cost analysis. Hernia 2019;23(6):1115–21.

28. Clapp B, Klingsporn W, Lodeiro C, et al. Small bowel obstructions following the use of barbed suture: a review of the literature and analysis of the MAUDE database. Surg Endosc 2019. https://doi.org/10.1007/s00464-019-06890-z.

29. Koehler RH, Begos D, Berger D, et al. Minimal adhesions to ePTFE mesh after laparoscopic ventral incisional hernia repair: reoperative findings in 65 cases. JSLS 2003;7(4):335–40.

30. Chelala E, Baraké H, Estievenart J, et al. Long-term outcomes of 1326 laparoscopic incisional and ventral hernia repair with the routine suturing concept: a single institution experience. Hernia 2016;20(1):101–10.

31. Wassenaar EB, Schoenmaeckers EJ, Raymakers JT, et al. Subsequent abdominal surgery after laparoscopic ventral and incisional hernia repair with an expanded polytetrafluoroethylene mesh: a single institution experience with 72 reoperations. Hernia 2010;14(2):137–42.

32. Alkhoury F, Helton S, Ippolito RJ. Cost and clinical outcomes of laparoscopic ventral hernia repair using intraperitoneal nonheavyweight polypropylene mesh. Surg Laparosc Endosc Percutan Tech 2011;21(2):82–5.

33. Snyder CW, Graham LA, Gray SH, et al. Effect of mesh type and position on subsequent abdominal operations after incisional hernia repair. J Am Coll Surg 2011; 212(4):496–502 [discussion: 502–4].

34. Miserez M, Penninckx F. Endoscopic totally preperitoneal ventral hernia repair. Surg Endosc 2002;16(8):1207–13.

35. Daes J. The enhanced view-totally extraperitoneal technique for repair of inguinal hernia. Surg Endosc 2012;26(4):1187–9.

36. Belyansky I, Daes J, Radu VG, et al. A novel approach using the enhanced-view totally extraperitoneal (eTEP) technique for laparoscopic retromuscular hernia repair. Surg Endosc 2018;32(3):1525–32.

37. Belyansky I, Reza Zahiri H, Sanford Z, et al. Early operative outcomes of endoscopic (eTEP access) robotic-assisted retromuscular abdominal wall hernia repair. Hernia 2018;22(5):837–47.

38. Penchev D, Kotashev G, Mutafchiyski V. Endoscopic enhanced-view totally extraperitoneal retromuscular approach for ventral hernia repair. Surg Endosc 2019;33(11):3749–56.

39. Muysoms F, Van Cleven S, Pletinckx P, et al. Robotic transabdominal retromuscular umbilical prosthetic hernia repair (TARUP): observational study on the operative time during the learning curve. Hernia 2018;22(6):1101–11.

40. Millbourn D, Cengiz Y, Israelsson LA. Effect of stitch length on wound complications after closure of midline incisions: a randomized controlled trial. Arch Surg 2009;144(11):1056–9.

41. Bellido Luque J, Bellido Luque A, Valdivia J, et al. Totally endoscopic surgery on diastasis recti associated with midline hernias. The advantages of a minimally invasive approach. Prospective cohort study. Hernia 2015;19(3):493–501.

42. Muas DMJ, Verasayb GF, Garcíac WM. Endoscopic prefascial repair of the recti diastasis: description of new technique. Rev Hispanoam Hernia 2017;5(2):47–51.

43. Faria Correa MA. Minimally invasive robotic abdominoplasty. Adv Plast Reconstr Surg 2017;1(2):82–90.

44. Cuenca O, Rodríguez A, Segovia A. Reparacion endoscopica de diastasis de recto y defectos de la linea alba media. Cir Parag 2017;41(2):37–40.

45. Köckerling F, Botsinis MD, Rohde C, et al. Endoscopic-assisted linea alba reconstruction plus mesh augmentation for treatment of umbilical and/or epigastric hernias and rectus abdominis diastasis - early results. Front Surg 2016;3:27.

46. Claus CMP, Malcher F, Cavazzola LT, et al. Subcutaneous onlay laparoscopic approach (SCOLA) for ventral hernia and rectus abdominus diastasis repair: technical description and initial results. Arq Bras Cir Dig 2018;31(4):e1399.

Robotic Inguinal Hernia Repair

Dina Podolsky, MD, Yuri Novitsky, MD*

KEYWORDS

- Inguinal hernia • Robotic • Robotic surgery • TAPP

KEY POINTS

- Robotic inguinal hernia repair is the natural progression of this process, using the same operative principles but with critical advances that change both the patient and the surgeon experience.
- For the surgeon, robotic surgery allows for a 3-dimensional view of the operating field while providing an articulating wrist, greatly improving the ergonomics experience.
- As with laparoscopy, both a robotic totally extraperitoneal approach (rTEP) and a robotic transabdominal preperitoneal repair (rTAPP) are feasible.
- Because of technical factors, the rTAPP is done with considerably more frequency than rTEP; it is also the author's preferred method of repair.

INTRODUCTION

Ger and colleagues[1,2] first introduced laparoscopic inguinal hernia repair in 1990, as a minimally invasive approach to the classic preperitoneal repair. Robotic inguinal hernia repair is the natural progression of this process, using the same operative principles but with critical advances that change both the patient and the surgeon experience. For the surgeon, robotic surgery allows for a 3-dimensional view of the operating field while providing an articulating wrist, greatly improving the ergonomics experience from the traditional "straight sticks" used in laparoscopic surgery. For the patient, robotic inguinal hernia repairs offer the benefit of a minimally invasive approach without the need for any penetrating fixation (tacks), as well as allowing for benefits of a minimally invasive surgery approach in very challenging scenarios.

As with laparoscopy, both a robotic totally extraperitoneal approach (rTEP) and a robotic transabdominal preperitoneal repair (rTAPP) are feasible. However, because of technical factors, the rTAPP is done with considerably more frequency than

Columbia University Medical Center, Comprehensive Hernia Center, Department of Surgery, 161 Fort Washington Avenue, New York, NY 10032, USA
* Corresponding author.
E-mail address: ynovit@gmail.com

Surg Clin N Am 100 (2020) 409–415
https://doi.org/10.1016/j.suc.2019.12.010
0039-6109/20/© 2019 Elsevier Inc. All rights reserved.

rTEP; it is also the author's preferred method of repair. Therefore, this article focuses primarily on rTAPP robotic inguinal hernia repair.

PREOPERATIVE PLANNING
Diagnosis

A physical examination is usually the only preoperative test needed to confirm the presence of an inguinal hernia. When in doubt, a dynamic groin ultrasound might be the next best test to rule in an inguinal hernia. For patients who have previous repairs, it is important to obtain operative reports to understand which mesh and approach was used. Although a mesh patch will not be encountered in the preperitoneal space, a "plug" might be.

Mesh Choice

In the author's practice, mesh utilization remains an important part of most inguinal hernia repairs. The author's practice routinely uses a macroporous polypropylene midweight mesh, sized at least 12 × 15 cm. For large direct defects, greater than 2 to 3 cm, they use a heavyweight polypropylene mesh to ensure proper reinforcement.

Indications

The primary indication for an rTAPP procedure is the presence of a symptomatic inguinal or femoral hernia. Secondary indications include the presence of an inguinoscrotal, incarcerated, and/or sliding hernia. These hernias will benefit from the fine dissection offered by robotic surgery. Last, a recurrent hernia that has previously been repaired via an anterior approach should be approached from the posterior direction. A robotic approach is particularly useful for patients with a history of open prostatectomy, pelvic/lower abdominal procedures, select failed posterior repairs, and hernias in obese patients.

Contraindications

The only absolute contraindication to an rTAPP repair is an inability to tolerate either general anesthesia or pneumoperitoneum. However, there are relative contraindications to the procedure. A "hostile" abdomen, previous extensive pelvic surgery, and/or the presence of either a right- or a left-sided ostomy will complicate the procedure. Although not an absolute contraindication, a previously placed preperitoneal mesh will increase the difficulty of the procedure and should only be approached by an experienced hernia surgeon.

PREPARATIONS AND PATIENT POSITION

Patients void before entering the operating room. Routine placement of a Foley catheter is avoided, except for patients in whom difficult dissection is anticipated. Standard preoperative antibiotics, usually a first general cephalosporin, are given within 30 minutes of incision. The patient is placed on the operating room table in the supine position. Both arms are tucked at the sides.

SURGICAL APPROACH

The Xi da Vinci robotic boom is positioned to the right of the operating room table. The instruments required for this operation are three 8-mm robotic ports, a bipolar fenestrated grasper, a Monopolar scissors, and a Mega Suture Cut Needle Driver. In addition, a Force Bipolar could be used in cases of large hernia sac to facilitate effective retraction. Furthermore, in those cases with a large chronically incarcerated inguino-scrotal hernia, a fourth port is placed for better retraction.

SURGICAL PROCEDURE
Step 1: Access to the Peritoneal Cavity

Access to the peritoneal cavity is usually obtained via a standard cut-down technique at the umbilicus. A 10-mm incision is made at the umbilicus, and the umbilical stalk is grasped and traced down to the linea alba. The fascia is then incised under direct visualization, and an 8-mm trocar is inserted into the abdominal cavity. For patients with previous periumbilical scars, the author uses an optical trocar peritoneal cavity entry in either upper quadrant.

The abdomen is insufflated, and a camera is used to make a general sweep of the peritoneal cavity and groin. Two more ports are placed bilaterally at the level of the umbilicus, roughly 6 to 8 cm apart from one another. Before docking the robot, the patient is placed in the Trendelenburg position.

Step 2: Docking the Robot

At this point, the robot is docked; a monopolar scissor is placed in the right port, and a fenestrated bipolar grasper is placed in the left port. A 30° camera is placed in the center port. Attention is drawn to the groin. Any easily lysed adhesions and/or incarcerated viscera are reduced. However, if a sliding hernia is present, it is best to leave it attached to the peritoneum and reduce both the viscera and the peritoneum "en bloc."

Step 3: Peritoneal Flap Creation

Next is the creation of the peritoneal flap. The flap should be created 4 to 5 cm cephalad to the internal ring in a medial to lateral direction. As landmarks, the author uses the median umbilical ligament medially and the anterior superior iliac spine (ASIS) laterally. It is important to not drift caudally when creating your peritoneal flap to avoid any injury to the nerves, which run inferior medial to the ASIS.

Step 4: Preperitoneal Dissection

Once the peritoneum is incised, an avascular plane between the peritoneum and transversalis fascia is created. The transversalis fascia should stay ventral, or "on the ceiling," to protect the epigastric vessels and nerves. Medially, this dissection is carried out to the space of Retzius by bluntly pushing the bladder down, exposing the Cooper ligament. Of note, large direct hernias may obscure the Cooper ligament; in these cases, it is better to reduce the hernia first. Laterally, the dissection is carried out to the psoas muscle. Once the medial and lateral preperitoneal dissection is completed, the next step is reduction of the hernia sac.

Step 5: Reduction of Hernia Sac

For indirect defects, the hernia sac is traditionally found in the anterolateral position relative to the cord structures. A combination of blunt dissection and electrocautery is used to separate the sac from both the vas deferens medially and the testicular vessels laterally. For chronic, thickened sacs, it might be difficult to identify the edge of the indirect hernia sac. In these cases, it is easiest to first identify the testicular vessels more laterally and cephalad and trace them down toward the internal ring. For chronically incarcerated sacs that cannot be reduced, the sac can be ligated at the internal ring, making sure to protect the vas deferens, which tends to be closely adherent to the tip of the hernia sac.

Direct defects are simpler to reduce. The direct hernia is grasped and reduced; a pseudosac, which is an invagination of the transversalis fascia, is identified. The pseudosac is typically left in place as the direct defect is reduced. Reduction of a direct defect will help to expose the Cooper ligament. It is advisable to reduce the sac only with blunt rather than sharp dissection or electrocautery, because sometimes the bladder may herniate through a direct defect. Once reduced, the hernia sac is parietalized at least 5 cm in the cephalad direction, making sure to create a large enough inferior pocket for a mesh to lie flat. Last, some investigators advocate suturing a large direct hernia sac to the ileopubic track or anterior abdominal wall to reduce the rate of seroma. The author has found no reliable supporting data on this technique, and thus, the author's practice does not routinely perform this. They also strongly advocate against closing defects to avoid nerve injuries.

After the direct and indirect spaces have been addressed, it is prudent to rule out a femoral hernia. The femoral canal lies just lateral to the lacunar ligament. Reduction of a femoral hernia must be done with great care, because the iliac vein will be immediately lateral to the hernia.

At the conclusion of the dissection, the author aims to obtain a so-called critical view of the myopectineal orifice (**Fig. 1**). The Cooper ligament and pubic symphysis are visualized medially. The vas (in men) and testicular vessels are parietalized and clearly seen. The distal 4 to 5 cm of the psoas muscle is seen to ensure an adequate inferior pocket. Hemostasis is ensured.

Step 6: Mesh Placement

The mesh should be sized at least 15 × 12 cm and should cover the entire myopectineal orifice, including the direct, indirect, and femoral spaces (**Fig. 2**). The medial aspect of the mesh is secured to the Cooper ligament with an absorbable 2-0 Vicryl suture. Great care is taken to not place any fixation in the areas where the neurovascular structures lie.

Step 7: Flap Closure

The peritoneal flap is then reapproximated using a running 3-0 absorbable V-Loc suture. No tissue bites should be taken below the level of the ASIS to avoid injury to the ilioinguinal or ileohypogastric nerves. Once the peritoneal flap is reattached, the ports are removed and the abdomen is desufflated.

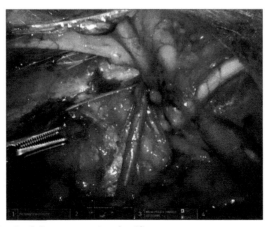

Fig. 1. "Critical view" of the myopectineal orifice.

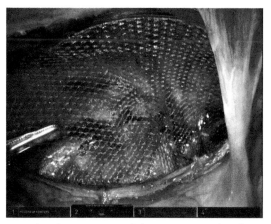

Fig. 2. Mesh placement showing coverage of the myopectineal orifice.

POSTOPERATIVE CARE, REHABILITATION, AND RECOVERY

Robotic inguinal hernia repairs are typically performed on an outpatient basis. In anticipation of swelling, the author recommends icepacks to the groin for the first 48 hours.

There are no limitations on physical activity; patients should not "do anything through pain," but they are encouraged to return to physical activity whenever they see fit. Most patients recover within 2 weeks. Few, if any, narcotic pain pills are required for this surgery. The main complications following a robotic inguinal hernia repair are seroma and hematoma formation, and to a lesser frequency, chronic groin pain. These complications can usually be managed via symptomatic relief with warm compresses, external compression, and nonsteroidal anti-inflammatory drugs. Studies show that approximately 8% will need percutaneous drainage. Surgical site infections are low, frequently quoted as less than 1%. Finally, the risk of recurrence exists for all types of hernia repairs. The risk of recurrence following an rTAPP repair is somewhere between 2% and 4%. The most common mechanism of recurrence is similar to the traditional laparoscopy inferiorly, either if the bottom of the mesh is lifted during peritoneal flap closure or if the peritoneum is not properly reduced during dissection.

CLINICAL RESULTS IN THE LITERATURE

An increasing amount of literature has been published on robotic inguinal hernia repair over the past decade. Most studies are single-institution retrospective reviews. Overall, the data have shown robotic inguinal hernia repairs to be a safe and effective alternative to laparoscopy in the treatment of unilateral and bilateral inguinal hernias.

In a meta-analysis of published data on rTAPP by Aiolfi and colleagues,[3] the intraoperative complication and conversion rate were found to be 0.03% and 0.14%. Postoperative complications included urinary retention (4.1%), seroma/hematoma (3.5%), and an overall complication rate of 7.5%. Recurrence rates are low and also comparable to laparoscopic inguinal hernia repair; although follow-up is short in the published robotic literature (<365 days), recurrence rates are less than 1%.[3–12] There are currently no published data on robotic inguinal hernia repair and the prevalence of chronic pain.

In a national database review, Pokala and colleagues[13] found that overall complications of robotic inguinal hernia repairs were significantly lower than both open and laparoscopic (0.67% robotic vs 4.44% laparoscopic vs 3.85% open, $P<.05$). Robotic inguinal hernia repairs were associated with lower postoperative infections, 30-day readmissions, and length of stay when compared with open repairs.[13] Of note, robotic repairs had a significantly higher direct cost ($9431) when compared with both laparoscopic ($6502) and open ($8837).[13]

Robotic inguinal hernia repairs also trend higher in operative times than both open and laparoscopic repairs, most likely attributable to surgeon learning curve and the need for instrument exchange. The exact number of cases needed for proficiency for rTAPP is yet to be determined, and there is a range in the literature. In a 2018, Muysoms and colleagues[14,15] found the operative time for rTAPP to drastically reduce over a learning curve of 50 cases, whereas Tam and colleagues[16] found their single-institution learning curve to be closer to 11 to 12 cases.

REFERENCES

1. Ger R, Monroe K, Duvivier R, et al. Management of indirect inguinal hernias by laparoscopic closure of the neck of the sac. Am J Surg 1990;159:370–3.
2. Bittner R, Schwarz J. Primary unilateral not complicated inguinal hernia: our choice of TAPP, why, results and review of literature. Hernia 2019;23(3):417–28.
3. Aiolfi A, Cavalli M, Micheletto G, et al. Primary inguinal hernia: systematic review and Bayesian network meta-analysis comparing open, laparoscopic transabdominal preperitoneal, totally extraperitoneal, and robotic preperitoneal repair. Hernia 2019;23(3):473–84.
4. Aiolfi A, Cavalli M, Micheletto G, et al. Robotic inguinal hernia repair: is technology taking over? Systematic review and meta-analysis. Hernia 2019;23(3):509–19.
5. Wu JJ, Way JA, Eslick GD, et al. Transabdominal pre-peritoneal versus open repair for primary unilateral inguinal hernia: a meta-analysis. World J Surg 2018;5:1304–11.
6. Waite KE, Herman MA, Doyle PJ. Comparison of robotic versus laparoscopic transabdominal preperitoneal (TAPP) inguinal hernia repair. J Robot Surg 2016;10:239–44.
7. Butters M, Redecke J, Köninger J. Long-term results of a randomized clinical trial of Shouldice, Lichtenstein and transabdominal preperitoneal hernia repairs. Br J Surg 2007;94:562–5.
8. Pokorny H, Klingler A, Schmid T, et al. Recurrence and complications after laparoscopic versus open inguinal hernia repair: results of a prospective randomized multicenter trial. Hernia 2008;12:385–9.
9. Eklund AS, Montgomery AK, Rasmussen IC, et al. Low recurrence rate after laparoscopic (TEP) and open (Lichtenstein) inguinal hernia repair: a randomized, multicenter trial with 5-year follow-up. Ann Surg 2009;249:33–8.
10. Gong K, Zhang N, Lu Y, et al. Comparison of the open tension-free mesh-plug, transabdominal preperitoneal (TAPP), and totally extraperitoneal (TEP) laparoscopic techniques for primary unilateral inguinal hernia repair: a prospective randomized controlled trial. Surg Endosc 2011;1:234–9.
11. Abbas AE, Abd Ellatif ME, Noaman N, et al. Patient-perspective quality of life after laparoscopic and open hernia repair: a controlled randomized trial. Surg Endosc 2012;26:2465–70.
12. Charles EJ, Mehaffey JH, Tache-Leon CA, et al. Inguinal hernia repair: is there a benefit to using the robot? Surg Endosc 2018;32:2131–6.

13. Pokala B, Armijo PR, Flores L, et al. Minimally invasive inguinal hernia repair is superior to open: a national database review. Hernia 2019;23(3):593–9.
14. Muysoms F, Van Cleven S, Kyle-Leinhase I, et al. Robotic-assisted laparoscopic groin hernia repair: observational case-control study on the operative time during the learning curve. Surg Endosc 2018;32:4850–9.
15. Colvin HS, Rao A, Cavalli M, et al. Glue versus suture fixation of mesh during open repair of inguinal hernias: a systematic review and meta-analysis. World J Surg 2013;37:2282–92.
16. Tam V, Rogers DE, Al-Abbas A, et al. Robotic inguinal hernia repair: a large health system's experience with the first 300 cases and review of the literature. J Surg Res 2019;235:98–104.

Robotic Primary and Revisional Bariatric Surgery

Pouya Iranmanesh, MD[a], Kulvinder S. Bajwa, MD[a], Melissa M. Felinski, DO[a], Shinil K. Shah, DO[a,b,]*, Erik B. Wilson, MD[a]

KEYWORDS

- Robotic surgery • Bariatric surgery • Revisional surgery • Roux-en-Y gastric bypass
- Sleeve gastrectomy • Adjustable gastric band

KEY POINTS

- Potential advantages of robotics in bariatric surgery include instrumentation, easier suturing allowing for handsewn anastomoses, multiquadrant access, and improved ergonomics for the surgeon.
- The most commonly performed robotic bariatric procedures include sleeve gastrectomy, Roux-en-Y gastric bypass, and biliopancreatic diversion with duodenal switch.
- Robotic bariatric surgery is at least as safe as laparoscopic bariatric surgery, with some smaller studies suggesting potential advantages.
- Large, high-quality, randomized studies are missing in the field of robotic bariatric surgery.

INTRODUCTION

According to the World Health Organization, the prevalence of obesity, defined as a body mass index of greater than 30 kg/m^2, has tripled across the world since 1975.[1] It has reached pandemic levels and currently affects 650 million individuals, representing 13% of the world's adult population.[1] Statistics are even more alarming in western countries (93.3 million obese adults [39.8%] in the United States).[2] Bariatric surgery is a well-established treatment option for patients with morbid obesity and obesity-related comorbidities.[3–7]

The first historical procedures performed for the treatment of obesity such as the jejunoileal bypass described by Kromen and Linner at the University of Minnesota in 1954[8] and, several years later, the jejunocolic bypass described by Payne and colleagues,[9] resulted in major morbidity, not only because of the lack of knowledge about

[a] Division of Minimally Invasive and Elective General Surgery, Department of Surgery, McGovern Medical School, University of Texas Health Science Center at Houston, Houston, TX, USA; [b] Michael E Debakey Institute for Comparative Cardiovascular Science and Biomedical Devices, Texas A&M University, College Station, TX, USA
* Corresponding author. Department of Surgery, McGovern Medical School, UT Health, 6431 Fannin Street, MSB 4.156, Houston, TX 77030.
E-mail address: shinil.k.shah@uth.tmc.edu

Surg Clin N Am 100 (2020) 417–430
https://doi.org/10.1016/j.suc.2019.12.011
0039-6109/20/© 2019 Elsevier Inc. All rights reserved.
surgical.theclinics.com

the complex metabolic interactions linked to obesity, but also owing to the invasiveness of laparotomies in patients with excess weight. A better understanding of the metabolic processes in obesity and lessons learned from complications such as malnutrition, vitamin deficiencies, bacterial overgrowth, and severe diarrhea prompted surgeons to refine their surgical techniques and find new, more effective procedures to decrease perioperative morbidity. The advent of laparoscopy was a major surgical revolution and it was naturally adopted in the field of bariatric surgery as a solution to decrease morbidity and overcome the challenges of open surgery in patients with obesity.[10]

Publication of the first case of laparoscopic adjustable gastric band (AGB) placement in 1993 by Broadbent and colleagues[11] and the first laparoscopic gastric bypass in 1994 by Wittgrove and colleagues[12] launched the era of minimally invasive bariatric surgery. In 1998, Guy-Bernard Cadière and his team performed the first robotic-assisted bariatric surgery.[13] They were followed in 2001 by Horgan and Vanuno,[14] who showed the feasibility of robotically-assisted laparoscopic sleeve gastrectomy (SG) and Roux-en-Y gastric bypass (RYGB). Currently, the most commonly performed procedures include SG, RYGB, and biliopancreatic diversion with duodenal switch (BPD-DS), the vast majority of which are performed using minimally invasive approaches.[15] Other procedures such as AGB placement or vertical banded gastroplasty have fallen out of favor and are infrequently performed nowadays.[15] In this article, we discuss the specificities of robotic-assisted bariatric surgery and their outcomes. Even though robotic surgical systems work according to a master–slave principle and are not able to perform automated tasks, we use the term "robotic" instead of "robotic-assisted" throughout this article for sake of simplification.

TECHNICAL ADVANTAGES OF ROBOTICS FOR BARIATRIC SURGERY

General purported advantages of robotic surgical systems over traditional laparoscopy include 3-dimensional high-definition visualization, tremor filtration, and direct camera control by the surgeon and wristed instruments, which make relatively complex laparoscopic tasks such as suturing easier.[16–18] In the field of bariatric surgery, these characteristics translate, for example, into the ability to perform fully handsewn anastomoses versus the more commonly performed stapled anastomoses with the laparoscopic approach.[19]

Robotic systems may also provide ergonomic advantages. Patients with obesity often have large amounts of abdominal wall fatty tissue, often resulting in leverage forces on trocars and instruments. Robotic arms help to compensate the weight of the abdominal wall, sparing the surgeon tedious physical efforts to overcome these counterproductive forces, and avoiding instruments bending or breaking.

Multiquadrant access is another benefit of recent robotic platforms.[20] During bariatric surgery (eg, RYGB and BPD-DS), the surgeon often has to work in different abdominal quadrants to measure small bowel and perform anastomoses, and unexpected findings will sometimes require working in unplanned abdominal areas. A common example is the discovery of pelvic adhesions preventing bowel mobilization during RYGB or BPD-DS. With a traditional laparoscopic approach, it may be challenging to perform a lysis of adhesions with the upper abdominal trocar setup, unless additional ports are introduced. In more complex situations, the surgeon sometimes decides to perform another bariatric procedure not involving the small bowel such as an SG or even abort the surgery.[21] Recent robotic platforms overcome this difficulty to a certain extent by allowing multiquadrant access without the need to move or redock the robotic system. This advance could potentially help the surgeon to successfully perform the initially planned procedure in these situations.

Until recently, stapling tasks had to be performed by a bedside assistant during robotic surgery. The advent of robotic staplers has enabled surgeons to avoid this limitation by positioning and firing staplers themselves. Combined with the surgeon's ability to control the camera and 3 different robotic arms at the surgeon console, robotic stapling can potentially obviate the need for a surgically trained bedside assistant during bariatric procedures. This feature may be useful in situations in which surgeons do not have bedside assistance readily available.

OPERATING ROOM SETUP AND TROCAR PLACEMENT

The principles behind operating room setup and trocar placements are similar between laparoscopic and robotic bariatric surgery. Our team leaves both of the patient's arms untucked. The bedside assistant and the scrub nurse or surgical technologist stand on the patient's right. Even though different positions for the robotic cart have been described, we usually place it on the patient's left side to provide easy access to the head for the anesthesia team and ample space on the patient's right side for the bedside assistant.

We use a similar trocar setup for most of our bariatric and foregut procedures (**Fig. 1**). We enter the abdomen in the right upper quadrant with a 5-mm trocar using an optical viewing technique. This trocar will later be changed for a robotic trocar. After a pneumoperitoneum of 15 mm Hg CO_2 has been created, a first robotic trocar is placed periumbilically (or supraumbilically for patients with higher body mass index) for the camera. We generally place the camera trocar just to the left of midline to improve visualization (especially in the case of a large falciform ligament) as well as

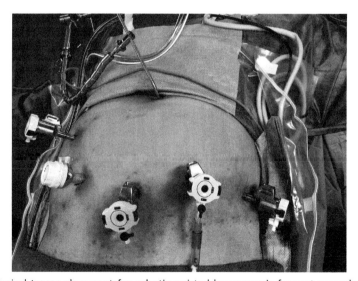

Fig. 1. Typical trocar placement for robotic-assisted laparoscopic foregut procedures. A 5-mm trocar is initially placed in the right upper quadrant (RUQ) to establish peritoneal access. The camera port is generally placed superior and to the left of the umbilicus. Two left-sided robotic trocars are placed for instrumentation, and the 5-mm RUQ trocar is exchanged for a robotic trocar. When bedside stapling is used, the accessory port can be placed in the right mid abdomen. A subxiphoid port is placed to accommodate an external liver retractor.

to decrease the incisional hernia risk. A robotic trocar is subsequently placed along the left anterior axillary line, at the level of the camera port. An additional robotic trocar is placed midway between the camera trocar and the lateral left upper quadrant trocar (if hiatal dissection is planned, this trocar can be placed more cephalad to ensure better access). Depending on the robotic platform, the camera trocar will either be an 8-mm robotic trocar or a standard 12-mm camera trocar, and the other robotic trocars will be 8 mm or 5 mm. Finally, a 12-mm or 15-mm (if planning to use a larger stapler or to facilitate specimen extraction during a SG) standard trocar is placed midway between the lateral right upper quadrant and the camera trocars for the bedside assistant and for stapling (if a robotic stapler is not being used). If the surgeon desires, an external liver retractor can be placed through a small subxiphoid incision. Internal liver retractors (such as the FreeHold Trio Retractor, Freehold Surgical, New Hope, PA) can also be used as per surgeon preference. The robotic system is then generally docked from the patient's left side (**Fig. 2**).

ROBOTIC BARIATRIC PROCEDURES
Adjustable Gastric Band

The largest study comparing robotic versus laparoscopic AGB placement found no significant difference in intraoperative times or outcomes, except for patients with a body mass index of greater than 50 kg/m^2, for which operative times were shorter in the robotic group.[22] Even though gastric band placements are rarely performed nowadays,[15] a significant number of patients with previously placed AGB are converted to other bariatric procedures because of weight loss failure or band-related complications such as slippage, erosion, or leakage.[23] The robotic system may have some advantages in this indication, as will be discussed in the Robotic Reoperative Bariatric Surgery section. Aside from possible assistance with suturing for gastrogastric plication, robotic systems generally do not provide an obvious advantage during AGB placement. Given the significant decrease in placement of AGB, there is little literature over the past several years on this topic.

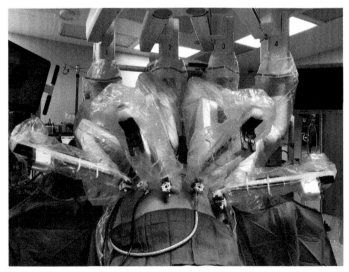

Fig. 2. Robotic patient side cart. The robotic patient side cart is generally placed on the left side of the patient to allow for easy access for anesthesia as well as the bedside assistant.

Robotic Roux-en-Y Gastric Bypass

The potential benefits of robotic surgery are more apparent in a procedure such as the RYGB, which involves multiple suturing tasks, including the possibility to use a hand-sewn technique for both gastrojejunal and jejunojejunal anastomoses.[24] Our team performs a double-layer, handsewn gastrojejunal anastomosis with a 2-0 absorbable suture. We use a standard or robotic stapler to create the jejunojejunal anastomosis and enterotomies are closed with a handsewn technique as well. Our detailed, fully robotic RYGB technique has previously been published elsewhere.[25]

Most comparative data between laparoscopic and robotic RYGB come from observational and/or database studies and not from high-quality randomized controlled trials. The majority of these series report longer overall operating room times and costs[26] when using the robotic platform, with increasing surgeon and operating room staff experience being a factor to partially overcome this time difference.[27–29] There are studies that demonstrate potential advantages of the robotic approach. One of the largest published series, including 1100 robotic RYGB, showed a gastrojejunal leak rate of 0.09% (1 leak), which is much lower than the published laparoscopic RYGB leak rates of 1% to 5%.[30] A lower anastomotic leak rate with robotic RYGB was also demonstrated in a series published by Snyder and colleagues[31] (0% vs 1.7%, robotic vs laparoscopic; $P = .04$). A series of 777 RYGBs (388 robotic compared with 389 laparoscopic procedures) demonstrated lower leak rates, early reoperations, hospital length of stay, complications, and conversion rates with the robotic technique. There were longer operative times with the robotic approach.[32] A lower stricture rate with robotic RYGB was demonstrated by Rogula and colleagues,[33] but only when compared with laparoscopic RYBG performed with a 21-mm circular stapler. This finding suggests that this may have been related to anastomotic technique, and not necessarily to the robotic technique.

Although there are studies that demonstrate potential advantages to the robotic RYGB technique, the vast majority of studies note no significant clinical outcome difference between the 2 approaches. There are a number of systematic reviews and meta-analyses that have been performed. They have to be interpreted carefully, because the majority of included studies are small, often single center, and are retrospective/nonrandomized. One of the most recent systematic reviews on robotic versus laparoscopic RYGB demonstrated that the robotic approach was associated with increased operative time without any other differences.[34] Two prior published meta-analyses demonstrated decreased stricture rates with robotic RYGB[35,36]; however, this finding was not demonstrated in the most review systematic review.

Recent interest has focused on large database studies to account for some of the limitations of prior studies. A propensity matched analysis of the Bariatric Outcomes Longitudinal Database (BOLD) evaluating robotic (2415 patients) versus laparoscopic (135,040 patients) RYGB (2007–2012) demonstrated longer operative times, as well as higher rates of reoperation (30 and 90 days), strictures, anastomotic leak, ulcers, nausea/emesis, and overall complications with the robotic approach.[37] A number of studies have been published recently from analyses of the Metabolic and Bariatric Accreditation and Quality Improvement Program (MBSAQIP) database. The studies sometimes demonstrate differing results based on study design and statistical methods used for analysis. Studies evaluating robotic as compared with laparoscopic RYGB has demonstrated increased operative times[29,38–40] and readmission rates with robotics[29,39] and decreased blood transfusions with robotics.[29,41] Some of the comparative studies have demonstrated increased reoperation rates with robotics but a decreased number of patients with a hospital length of stay of greater than 2 days with the robotic approach.[29]

Most of these studies use propensity matching techniques to adjust for confounders. In the study performed by Sebastian and colleagues,[41] a secondary propensity matching analysis was performed also accounting for operative time and conversion rates. This analysis then demonstrated additional advantages for the robotic approach, including deceased hospital length of stay, anastomotic leaks, renal complications, and venous thromboembolism related complications. A criticism of this approach (adjusting for operative time/conversion rates) may lead to comparing more difficult laparoscopic operations to more straightforward robotic operations or vice versa, which leads to some caution with the interpretation of these data. Acevedo and colleagues[40] also performed a case-control matching analysis, with a secondary analysis accounting for operative time and conversion rates. Before controlling for these 2 variables, they demonstrated higher 30-day readmission rates and lower rates of mortality, bleeding and transfusion rates, and wound infections with the robotic approach. After controlling for operative time and conversion rates in a manner similar to Sebastian and colleagues,[41] they demonstrated increased 30-day readmission rates and lower wound infection rates with the robotic approach.

The preponderance of the data suggests that robotic and laparoscopic approaches to RYGB are equivalent, with the robotic approach taking longer and costing more. High-quality randomized trials comparing the outcomes of robotic and laparoscopic RYGB among expert surgeons would be valuable to truly assess outcomes differences.

Robotic Longitudinal Sleeve Gastrectomy

SG has become the most commonly performed bariatric procedure in the United States since 2015.[42] Even though SG is a relatively straightforward laparoscopic procedure, using the robotic platform has potential advantages, especially when associated suturing tasks are required. These include, for instance, staple line oversewing and staple line omentopexy, which are routinely done by some teams, or concomitant hiatal hernia repair. A robotic SG technique without staples has also been described, where the stomach is divided between clamps and subsequently sutured with absorbable material.[43] Robotic SG can also be used as a relatively easy training procedure to familiarize the surgeon and associated team with the robotic system and prepare them for more complex robotic surgeries. Our team uses the same trocar placement as in the RYGB, with a 15-mm assistant trocar to accommodate larger staple loads and to help retrieve the gastric specimen. The omentum and short gastric vessels along the greater curvature are divided first using an advanced hemostatic device. After dissection of the angle of His and the left crus, gastric stapling with or without buttressing material is performed by the bedside assistant or, if the robotic stapler is used, by the surgeon over a 36F or 40F bougie. Our technique does not include staple line oversewing or omentopexy.

The data on robotic versus laparoscopic SG parallels some of the same challenges as the data on RYGB. There are few high-quality data evaluating potential outcome advantages of robotic SG and most studies are small. Vilallonga and colleagues[44] compared 100 laparoscopic and 100 robotic SG, noting increased operating times in the robotic group, whereas Romero and colleagues[45] found a shorter length of stay in the robotic group when comparing 134 robotic SG with a literature review of 3148 SG. No significant differences in outcomes were found in these studies. Most studies demonstrate increased costs for robotic SG, although there are some that demonstrate equivalent costs between the robotic and laparoscopic approaches.[46]

There are few published systematic reviews or meta-analyses on robotic versus laparoscopic SG. They demonstrate increased costs and hospital length of stay without differences in other outcomes.[47,48] Similarly, analyses of the MBSAQIP database (2015 and/or 2016) demonstrate uniformly longer operative time with the robotic approach to SG.[29,41,49,50] No mortality difference has been observed between the 2 approaches in these studies.[50] Decreased stricture and postoperative bleeding rates were noted with robotic SG as compared with laparoscopic SG in an analysis by Sebastian and colleagues.[41] However, there is no consistent theme of outcome advantages with robotic SG. Several studies have demonstrated worst outcomes with robotics including higher rates of organ space infection.[49] Papasavas and colleagues[29] demonstrated that robotic SG was associated with higher 30 day reintervention rates and percentage of patients with a hospital length of stay of more than 2 days. Fazl Alizadeh and colleagues[50] reported higher morbidity, leak (1.5% vs 0.5%, robotic vs laparoscopic SG; $P<.01$), and surgical site infection rates with robotic SG. It is important to note that the vast majority of studies on robotic SG do not demonstrate clinical inferiority or superiority.

Robotic Biliopancreatic Diversion with Duodenal Switch

This procedure traditionally includes 2 anastomoses (duodenoileal and ileoileal). More recently, a single duodenoileal anastomosis technique has also been described with promising results.[51] The robotic platform allows the surgeon to perform these anastomoses with a handsewn technique. Our team uses the same overall trocar placement scheme as described elsewhere in this article, with the difference that all trocars will be placed a few centimeters more caudal to optimize access to the duodenal area and the terminal ileum, especially in patients with previous SG (2-stage BPD-DS) where no dissection in the hiatal region is required. We perform a fully handsewn, double-layered, end-to-side duodenoileal anastomosis with a 2-0 absorbable suture. If performing a traditional BPD-DS (2 anastomoses), we usually perform a stapled side-to-side ileoileal anastomosis, with handsewn closure of enterotomy defect. The length of the common channel is 100 to 150 cm in a double anastomoses BPD-DS and 250 to 300 cm in a single anastomosis BPD-DS. Even though there is no randomized, controlled trial comparing laparoscopic and robotic BPD-DS, a single-center study including 179 consecutive patients who underwent robotic BPD-DS showed longer operative times, similar weight loss results, and decreased leak rates as compared with the laparoscopic approach.[52] Other published series of robotic BPD-DS demonstrate acceptable outcomes; Sudan and Podolsky[53] reported no leaks or mortality in a series of 59 procedures.

Robotic Reoperative Bariatric Surgery

The overall incidence of reoperative procedures after bariatric surgery is estimated to go from 5% to 54%.[54] Reoperative bariatric surgery mainly includes 3 types of procedures[54]:

- Revisions, where the anatomy of the initial procedure is preserved. These procedures are often performed to manage complications of an effective procedure, such as redo of a gastrojejunal anastomosis because of intractable marginal ulcer or stricture.
- Conversions, where anatomy of a different bariatric procedure is created. Insufficient weight loss, weight regain, or recurrence of obesity-related comorbidities are the most frequent reasons leading to this type of surgery (eg, conversion from a AGB or vertical banded gastroplasty to an RYGB). A different example is

conversion from an SG to an RYGB for the management of severe postoperative gastroesophageal reflux disease.

- Reversals, where the original anatomy is restored. Reversals are usually a last resort treatment option in patients with catastrophic nutritional deficiencies or excessive weight loss.

Even if every bariatric procedure can fail or result in complications requiring reoperation, the number of reoperative bariatric procedures in the past decade has mainly been driven by high complication rates or treatment failure of past weight loss procedures, which have largely been abandoned, such as adjustable or fixed gastric bands and gastroplasty-type procedures.[54] This pattern might continue in the future, because recent studies have suggested higher incidence of Barrett's esophagus than previously thought after SG,[55] which is currently the most commonly performed bariatric procedure in the United States and other countries.[15,42] Hence, combined with the overall increase of bariatric procedures performed worldwide, the number of reoperative procedures will most likely continue to increase in the coming years.

In addition to the usual difficulties of surgery in patients with obesity, such as abdominal wall thickness, visceral fat, and hepatomegaly, reoperative surgery adds the challenge of working in a hostile environment with varying degree of adhesions, modified tissue planes, and decreased vascularization. These challenges can potentially explain the higher complications rates seen after laparoscopic reoperative bariatric surgery, with leak rates ranging from 6% to 22%.[56–58] Besides the ability to perform handsewn anastomoses, articulated instruments and 3-dimensional high-definition visualization could potentially result in a more precise dissection and better handling of tissues, which might result in better postoperative outcomes. Although no large, randomized trials are available, several studies have suggested potential advantages of the robotic approach, with lower leak rates, lower laparotomy conversion rates, and shorter lengths of hospital stay[59] compared with laparoscopic surgery.[60,61] These data suggest that robotic surgery may provide the highest benefit for reoperative bariatric surgery, resulting in complications rates similar to primary weight loss procedures.

An analysis of the MBSAQIP database does offer some insight in revisional robotic bariatric surgery. Acevedo and colleagues[62] performed a case-matched study and demonstrated longer operative time, increased hospital length of stay, and increased rate of unplanned intensive care unit admissions with robotic revisional bariatric surgery. When specifically comparing matched cohorts for RYGB and SG, robotics was associated with longer operative time in both groups. Laparoscopy was associated with increased transfusion rates (RYGB) and decreased postoperative sepsis (SG). The other published analysis of the MBSAQIP database specifically evaluating laparoscopic versus robotic revisional bariatric surgery demonstrated increased operative time and length of stay for robotic-assisted revisional surgery.[63] An important limitation of these studies as the types of revision are not specified (eg, revisions from prior AGB, fixed gastric bands, SG, vertical banded gastroplasty, RYGB).[62] It is difficult to decipher the effects of patient selection (ie, more or less difficult cases performed with laparoscopic or robotic techniques).

Robotic Surgery Training and Learning Curve

Advanced technologic devices such as robotic platforms require surgeon and operating room staff training. In addition to improving patients outcomes, appropriate training of the whole operating room team allows for time efficiency in robotic set-up and docking.[27] Even though no formal robotic surgery training is required at the time being by national surgery boards across the world, a growing number of institutions use various training curriculums or credentialing systems to grant robotic surgery privileges. These include dry laboratories, live animal or cadaveric laboratories, as well as proctoring from experienced robotic surgeons for live human procedures. Because robotic platforms are by nature computer interfaces between the patient and the surgeon, their possibilities can be enhanced by virtual reality. A promising example are the robotic simulators, which offer a full range of exercises, going from basic knowledge of the robotic platform to performing entire surgical procedures such as cholecystectomies. In this context, it is probably only a matter of time until the possibility to perform a simulated robotic RYGB or SG becomes real. In addition, several studies suggest a shorter learning curve for robotic bariatric procedures compared with the laparoscopic approach. Buchs and colleagues[64] found the RYGB learning curve to be around 20 to 25 cases, compared with 100 cases for laparoscopic RYGB, whereas Vilallonga and colleagues[65] considered 10 cases as the learning curve for robotic SG.

Cost Considerations

Controlling costs is undoubtedly a major concern for health care systems, especially in developed countries where new, costly technologies are marketed and where expectations of the general population are constantly increasing. The costs of a robotic system can be divided into 3 categories: initial purchase, maintenance, and disposable parts. Even though these costs can initially seem prohibitive, Hagen and colleagues[24] have shown that establishing a business plan, optimizing robotic operative times, and, most important, decreasing severe complications of bariatric surgery such as gastrointestinal leak rates can at least partially compensate these costs. Surgeon experience and the learning curve play a critical role as well, because shorter operating times decrease overall costs and can result in higher income by allowing more surgeries to be performed in a defined time slot. The advent of new robotic platforms, currently being developed by a number of companies across the world, hopefully will stimulate market competition and decrease overall costs.

SUMMARY

Even though robotic surgery offers potential technological advantages such as wristed instrumentation, 3-dimensional high-definition visualization, tremor filtration, and ergonomic positioning, its widespread adoption has been limited by high costs, longer operative times, and controversy in the literature about its potential to improve patients outcomes compared with traditional laparoscopy. In general, robotics has been shown to be safe and generally equivalent to the laparoscopic approach with the exception of costs and operative time, as mentioned.

In the field of bariatric surgery, the robotic approach is associated with often conflicting data. Although certain studies suggest it may help to decrease anastomotic stricture and leak rates, this finding has not been uniformly demonstrated in large database studies. There are even conflicting outcomes when different investigators analyze the same database. Although this is secondary generally to choices of analysis techniques, there are several points to consider when evaluating papers based on analysis of these large databases (BOLD and MBSAQIP).

The article published from the BOLD database evaluated patients who underwent operations from 2007 to 2012. Articles published from the MBSAQIP database regarding robotic versus laparoscopic RYGB and SG evaluated data from 2015 and 2016. Although evaluating these data is important, it may not reflect the current state of outcomes with robotics. There is an element to measuring the national learning curve of robotic surgery in these studies. These databases include data from high- and low-volume robotic centers and surgeons. As with most operations, there may be better outcomes with higher volume centers, and the database studies are generally not able to tease out these differences. Database studies do not account for nuances of patient selection, that is, choosing more or less complicated operations for robotic and/or laparoscopic approaches depending on surgeon preferences, comfort levels and technical skills. Cohort matching and propensity analyses attempt to do this; however, there are certainly criticisms to this approach. There have been changes to robotic platforms and technology. Additionally, robotic techniques may differ (totally robotic vs using robotic assistance for portions of the operation and performing some portions with traditional laparoscopic methods).

Although robotic surgery continues to increase in popularity, large single-center or multicenter experiences and analysis of national databases will continue to help clarify the role of robotics in primary and revisional bariatric surgery as well as lay the framework for high-quality, randomized studies.

DISCLOSURE

E.B. Wilson has received teaching honoraria from Intuitive Surgical. S.K. Shah has received research grant support from Intuitive Surgical.

REFERENCES

1. World Health Organization. Obesity and overweight. 2018. Available at: https://www.who.int/news-room/fact-sheets/detail/obesity-and-overweight. Accessed October 26, 2019.
2. Hales CM, Carroll MD, Fryar CD, et al. Prevalence of obesity among adults and youth: United States, 2015-2016. NCHS Data Brief 2017;(288):1–8.
3. Poirier P, Cornier MA, Mazzone T, et al. Bariatric surgery and cardiovascular risk factors: a scientific statement from the American Heart Association. Circulation 2011;123(15):1683–701.
4. Garvey WT, Mechanick JI, Brett EM, et al. American Association of Clinical Endocrinologists and American College of Endocrinology Comprehensive Clinical Practice Guidelines for Medical Care of Patients with Obesity. Endocr Pract 2016;22(Suppl 3):1–203.
5. Mechanick JI, Youdim A, Jones DB, et al. Clinical practice guidelines for the perioperative nutritional, metabolic, and nonsurgical support of the bariatric surgery patient–2013 update: cosponsored by American Association of Clinical Endocrinologists, The Obesity Society, and American Society for Metabolic & Bariatric Surgery. Obesity (Silver Spring) 2013;21(Suppl 1):S1–27.
6. Dixon JB, Zimmet P, Alberti KG, et al. Bariatric surgery: an IDF statement for obese Type 2 diabetes. Arq Bras Endocrinol Metabol 2011;7(4):433–47.
7. Weiner RA. Indications and principles of metabolic surgery. Chirurg 2010;81(4):379–94 [quiz: 395] [in German].
8. Kremen AJ, Linner JH, Nelson CH. An experimental evaluation of the nutritional importance of proximal and distal small intestine. Ann Surg 1954;140(3):439–48.
9. Payne JH, Dewind LT, Commons RR. Metabolic observations in patients with jejunocolic shunts. Am J Surg 1963;106:273–89.
10. Reoch J, Mottillo S, Shimony A, et al. Safety of laparoscopic vs open bariatric surgery: a systematic review and meta-analysis. Arch Surg 2011;146(11):1314–22.
11. Broadbent R, Tracey M, Harrington P. Laparoscopic gastric banding: a preliminary report. Obes Surg 1993;3(1):63–7.

12. Wittgrove AC, Clark GW, Tremblay LJ. Laparoscopic gastric bypass, Roux-en-Y: preliminary report of five cases. Obes Surg 1994;4(4):353–7.

13. Cadiere GB, Himpens J, Vertruyen M, et al. The world's first obesity surgery performed by a surgeon at a distance. Obes Surg 1999;9(2):206–9.

14. Horgan S, Vanuno D. Robots in laparoscopic surgery. J Laparoendosc Adv Surg Tech A 2001;11(6):415–9.

15. Angrisani L, Santonicola A, Iovino P, et al. IFSO Worldwide Survey 2016: primary, endoluminal, and revisional procedures. Obes Surg 2018;28(12):3783–94.

16. Corcione F, Esposito C, Cuccurullo D, et al. Advantages and limits of robot-assisted laparoscopic surgery: preliminary experience. Surg Endosc 2005; 19(1):117–9.

17. Van Koughnett JA, Jayaraman S, Eagleson R, et al. Are there advantages to robotic-assisted surgery over laparoscopy from the surgeon's perspective? J Robot Surg 2009;3(2):79–82.

18. Ho C, Tsakonas E, Tran K, et al. Robot-assisted surgery compared with open surgery and laparoscopic surgery. CADTH Technol Overv 2012;2(2):e2203.

19. Jiang HP, Lin LL, Jiang X, et al. Meta-analysis of hand-sewn versus mechanical gastrojejunal anastomosis during laparoscopic Roux-en-Y gastric bypass for morbid obesity. Int J Surg 2016;32:150–7.

20. Protyniak B, Jorden J, Farmer R. Multiquadrant robotic colorectal surgery: the da Vinci Xi vs Si comparison. J Robot Surg 2018;12(1):67–74.

21. Joo P, Guilbert L, Sepulveda EM, et al. Unexpected intraoperative findings, situations, and complications in bariatric surgery. Obes Surg 2019;29(4):1281–6.

22. Edelson PK, Dumon KR, Sonnad SS, et al. Robotic vs. conventional laparoscopic gastric banding: a comparison of 407 cases. Surg Endosc 2011;25(5):1402–8.

23. Koh CY, Inaba CS, Sujatha-Bhaskar S, et al. Laparoscopic adjustable gastric band explantation and implantation at academic centers. J Am Coll Surg 2017; 225(4):532–7.

24. Hagen ME, Pugin F, Chassot G, et al. Reducing cost of surgery by avoiding complications: the model of robotic Roux-en-Y gastric bypass. Obes Surg 2012;22(1): 52–61.

25. Shah SK, Walker PA, Snyder BE, et al. Essentials and future directions of robotic bariatric surgery. In: Kroh M, Chalikonda S, editors. Essentials of robotic surgery. Cham, Switzerland: Springer International Publishing; 2015. p. 73–80.

26. Bailey JG, Hayden JA, Davis PJ, et al. Robotic versus laparoscopic Roux-en-Y gastric bypass (RYGB) in obese adults ages 18 to 65 years: a systematic review and economic analysis. Surg Endosc 2014;28(2):414–26.

27. Iranmanesh P, Morel P, Wagner OJ, et al. Set-up and docking of the da Vinci surgical system: prospective analysis of initial experience. Int J Med Robot 2010; 6(1):57–60.

28. Bustos R, Mangano A, Gheza F, et al. Robotic-assisted Roux-en-Y gastric bypass: learning curve assessment using cumulative sum and literature review. Bariatr Surg Pract Patient Care 2019;14(3):95–101.

29. Papasavas P, Seip RL, Stone A, et al. Robot-assisted sleeve gastrectomy and Roux-en-y gastric bypass: results from the metabolic and bariatric surgery accreditation and quality improvement program data registry. Surg Obes Relat Dis 2019;15(8):1281–90.

30. Tieu K, Allison N, Snyder B, et al. Robotic-assisted Roux-en-Y gastric bypass: update from 2 high-volume centers. Surg Obes Relat Dis 2013;9(2):284–8.

31. Snyder BE, Wilson T, Scarborough T, et al. Lowering gastrointestinal leak rates: a comparative analysis of robotic and laparoscopic gastric bypass. J Robot Surg 2008;2(3):159–63.

32. Buchs NC, Morel P, Azagury DE, et al. Laparoscopic versus robotic Roux-en-Y gastric bypass: lessons and long-term follow-up learned from a large prospective monocentric study. Obes Surg 2014;24(12):2031–9.

33. Rogula T, Koprivanac M, Janik MR, et al. Does robotic Roux-en-Y gastric bypass provide outcome advantages over standard laparoscopic approaches? Obes Surg 2018;28(9):2589–96.

34. Wang L, Yao L, Yan P, et al. Robotic versus laparoscopic Roux-en-Y gastric bypass for morbid obesity: a systematic review and meta-analysis. Obes Surg 2018;28(11):3691–700.

35. Economopoulos KP, Theocharidis V, McKenzie TJ, et al. Robotic vs. laparoscopic Roux-En-Y gastric bypass: a systematic review and meta-analysis. Obes Surg 2015;25(11):2180–9.

36. Markar SR, Karthikesalingam AP, Venkat-Ramen V, et al. Robotic vs. laparoscopic Roux-en-Y gastric bypass in morbidly obese patients: systematic review and pooled analysis. Int J Med Robot 2011;7(4):393–400.

37. Celio AC, Kasten KR, Schwoerer A, et al. Perioperative safety of laparoscopic versus robotic gastric bypass: a propensity matched analysis of early experience. Surg Obes Relat Dis 2017;13(11):1847–52.

38. Lundberg PW, Wolfe S, Seaone J, et al. Robotic gastric bypass is getting better: first results from the Metabolic and Bariatric Surgery Accreditation and Quality Improvement Program. Surg Obes Relat Dis 2018;14(9):1240–5.

39. Sharma G, Strong AT, Tu C, et al. Robotic platform for gastric bypass is associated with more resource utilization: an analysis of MBSAQIP dataset. Surg Obes Relat Dis 2018;14(3):304–10.

40. Acevedo E Jr, Mazzei M, Zhao H, et al. Outcomes in conventional laparoscopic versus robotic-assisted primary bariatric surgery: a retrospective, case-controlled study of the MBSAQIP database. Surg Endosc 2019. [Epub ahead of print].

41. Sebastian R, Howell MH, Chang KH, et al. Robot-assisted versus laparoscopic Roux-en-Y gastric bypass and sleeve gastrectomy: a propensity score-matched comparative analysis using the 2015-2016 MBSAQIP database. Surg Endosc 2019;33(5):1600–12.

42. Surgery ASfMaB. Estimate of bariatric surgery numbers, 2011-2017. 2018. Available at: https://asmbs.org/resources/estimate-of-bariatric-surgery-numbers. Accessed October 26, 2019.

43. Rezvani M, Sucandy I, Antanavicius G. Totally robotic stapleless vertical sleeve gastrectomy. Surg Obes Relat Dis 2013;9(5):e79–81.

44. Vilallonga R, Fort JM, Caubet E, et al. Robotic sleeve gastrectomy versus laparoscopic sleeve gastrectomy: a comparative study with 200 patients. Obes Surg 2013;23(10):1501–7.

45. Romero RJ, Kosanovic R, Rabaza JR, et al. Robotic sleeve gastrectomy: experience of 134 cases and comparison with a systematic review of the laparoscopic approach. Obes Surg 2013;23(11):1743–52.

46. El Chaar M, Gacke J, Ringold S, et al. Cost analysis of robotic sleeve gastrectomy (R-SG) compared with laparoscopic sleeve gastrectomy (L-SG) in a single academic center: debunking a myth! Surg Obes Relat Dis 2019;15(5):675–9.

47. Magouliotis DE, Tasiopoulou VS, Sioka E, et al. Robotic versus laparoscopic sleeve gastrectomy for morbid obesity: a systematic review and meta-analysis. Obes Surg 2017;27(1):245–53.
48. Tasiopoulou VS, Svokos AA, Svokos KA, et al. Robotic versus laparoscopic sleeve gastrectomy: a review of the current evidence. Minerva Chir 2018;73(1): 55–63.
49. Lundberg PW, Stoltzfus J, El Chaar M. 30-day outcomes of robot-assisted versus conventional laparoscopic sleeve gastrectomy: first analysis based on MBSAQIP. Surg Obes Relat Dis 2019;15(1):1–7.
50. Fazl Alizadeh R, Li S, Inaba CS, et al. Robotic versus laparoscopic sleeve gastrectomy: a MBSAQIP analysis. Surg Endosc 2019;33(3):917–22.
51. Sanchez-Pernaute A, Rubio MA, Perez Aguirre E, et al. Single-anastomosis duodenoileal bypass with sleeve gastrectomy: metabolic improvement and weight loss in first 100 patients. Surg Obes Relat Dis 2013;9(5):731–5.
52. Antanavicius G, Rezvani M, Sucandy I. One-stage robotically assisted laparoscopic biliopancreatic diversion with duodenal switch: analysis of 179 patients. Surg Obes Relat Dis 2015;11(2):367–71.
53. Sudan R, Podolsky E. Totally robot-assisted biliary pancreatic diversion with duodenal switch: single dock technique and technical outcomes. Surg Endosc 2015;29(1):55–60.
54. Lo Menzo ES, Szomstein S, Rosenthal RJ. Reoperative bariatric surgery. In: Nguyen NT, BRP, Morton JM, et al, editors. The ASMBS textbook of bariatric surgery, vol. 1. New York: Springer; 2015. p. 269–82.
55. Sebastianelli L, Benois M, Vanbiervliet G, et al. Systematic endoscopy 5 years after sleeve gastrectomy results in a high rate of Barrett's esophagus: results of a multicenter study. Obes Surg 2019;29(5):1462–9.
56. Abdelgawad M, De Angelis F, Iossa A, et al. Management of complications and outcomes after revisional bariatric surgery: 3-year experience at a bariatric center of excellence. Obes Surg 2016;26(9):2144–9.
57. Shimizu H, Annaberdyev S, Motamarry I, et al. Revisional bariatric surgery for unsuccessful weight loss and complications. Obes Surg 2013;23(11):1766–73.
58. Brethauer SA, Kothari S, Sudan R, et al. Systematic review on reoperative bariatric surgery: American Society for metabolic and bariatric surgery revision task force. Surg Obes Relat Dis 2014;10(5):952–72.
59. Gray KD, Moore MD, Elmously A, et al. Perioperative outcomes of laparoscopic and robotic revisional bariatric surgery in a complex patient population. Obes Surg 2018;28(7):1852–9.
60. Snyder B, Wilson T, Woodruff V, et al. Robotically assisted revision of bariatric surgeries is safe and effective to achieve further weight loss. World J Surg 2013; 37(11):2569–73.
61. Buchs NC, Pugin F, Azagury DE, et al. Robotic revisional bariatric surgery: a comparative study with laparoscopic and open surgery. Int J Med Robot 2014; 10(2):213–7.
62. Acevedo E, Mazzei M, Zhao H, et al. Outcomes in conventional laparoscopic versus robotic-assisted revisional bariatric surgery: a retrospective, case-controlled study of the MBSAQIP database. Surg Endosc 2019. [Epub ahead of print].
63. Clapp B, Liggett E, Jones R, et al. Comparison of robotic revisional weight loss surgery and laparoscopic revisional weight loss surgery using the MBSAQIP database. Surg Obes Relat Dis 2019;15(6):909–19.

64. Buchs NC, Pugin F, Bucher P, et al. Learning curve for robot-assisted Roux-en-Y gastric bypass. Surg Endosc 2012;26(4):1116–21.

65. Vilallonga R, Fort JM, Gonzalez O, et al. The initial learning curve for robot-assisted sleeve gastrectomy: a surgeon's experience while introducing the robotic technology in a bariatric surgery department. Minim Invasive Surg 2012; 2012:347131.

Pediatric Robotic Surgery

Naomi-Liza Denning, MD[a,b,1], Michelle P. Kallis, MD[a,b,1],
Jose M. Prince, MD[a,b,*]

KEYWORDS

- Robotic surgery • Pediatric urology • Robotic urologic surgery • Pediatric surgery
- Robotic gastrointestinal surgery • Children • Pediatric • Minimally invasive surgery

KEY POINTS

- Pediatric robotic-assisted surgery is increasing in prevalence.
- Patient size is a consideration in selection for robotic-assisted surgery, but small size, less than 10 kg, is not necessarily a contraindication, depending on the specific patient and procedure.
- Operative success rates and complications of pediatric robotic-assisted surgery seem to be similar to those seen with laparoscopic surgery.
- Short learning curves for robotic-assisted surgery allows for quick implementation of this technology into a surgeon's practice.

HISTORY

The first described use of robotic surgery in a child occurred in 2001, nearly 10 years after its use was first described in adults, with a case report describing the use of this technology in the creation of a Nissen fundoplication.[1–5] Since these initial reports, robotic surgery has seen widespread application within the adult population, especially in urologic and gynecologic procedures.[3,4] As is often the case for new devices, technology, and therapeutic options in surgery, the application of robotic surgery for children has occurred more slowly than in adults. This caution is due in large part to technical limitations with developing appropriately sized instrument for the pediatric patient; however, recent years have seen broader implementation.[4,6]

As a new field, pediatric robotic surgery has had more than 200 articles published since its advent in 2001.[4] The majority of this work has focused on the development of robotic pediatric urology with a case volume increasing an average of 236.6%

The author M.P. Kallis holds stock in Intuitive Surgical and Transenterix.

[a] Department of Surgery, Donald and Zucker School of Medicine at Hofstra/Northwell, 300 Community Drive, Manhasset, NY 11030, USA; [b] Cohen Children's Medical Center at Northwell Health, 269-01 76th Avenue, CH 158, New Hyde Park, New York, NY 11040, USA
[1] Denning and Kallis co-first authors
* Corresponding author. Division of Pediatric Surgery at Cohen Children's Medical Center, 1111 Marcus Ave, New Hyde Park, NY 11042.
E-mail address: jprince@northwell.edu

per year.[7] As a result, the most common procedures described using robotics are pyeloplasty and ureteral implantation, followed by fundoplication in the pediatric general surgery literature.[4,7] By 2012, 2393 robotic procedures in 1840 pediatric patients were reported in the literature, and of these 36.8% are gastrointestinal procedures.[8] Over time, more complex and a wider variety of cases are being described using a robotic approach, including thoracic cases, Kasai portoenterostomies, and excision of choledochal cysts.[8]

Although the surgical robotics marketplace is growing, currently the only robotics system that is approved for pediatric use is the da Vinci Surgical System (Intuitive Surgical, Sunnyvale, CA).[6] The da Vinci system was the first robotic surgery system to be approved by the US Food and Drug Administration for intra-abdominal surgery and is the predominant robotic surgery platform used in the United States.[5,6,9,10] However, the only available instrument sizes on the da Vinci system are 5 mm and 8 mm, thus limiting the ability of this system to be used in neonates and small children.[6] More recently, the Senhance robotics system (Transenterix, Morrisville, NC) has begun to offer 3 -mm instrument sizes, which could make robotic surgery more technically feasible for even the smallest pediatric patient[6] (**Fig. 1**).

TECHNICAL BENEFITS, LIMITATIONS, AND COSTS
Benefits

Broadly, the advantages of robotic surgery include many of the same technical improvements and benefits to patient recovery as laparoscopic surgery and other minimally invasive techniques that came before it, including minimizing operative trauma, decreasing postoperative pain, limiting the need for postoperative opioid use, reducing hospital stays, a quicker return to work or school, and improving cosmetic outcomes.[10,11] Supporters of robotic surgery argue that it supersedes the capabilities of traditional laparoscopy by the very nature of its design. As opposed to the traditional

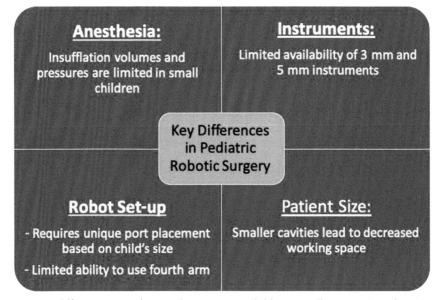

Fig. 1. Key differences in pediatric robotic surgery. Children's small size require adaptations in robotic set up, instrument use, operative technique, and anesthetic considerations.

laparoscopic instruments that are long, rigid, and thus incapable of bending, robotic instruments were designed specifically to mimic the movements of the human wrist.[9,10] Further eliminating instrumental constraint is the new EndoWrist technology implemented in the da Vinci Surgical System by Intuitive Surgical. These instruments created with a snake-wrist design allow for 7° of freedom, compared with the 4° of freedom of traditional laparoscopic instruments.[10] Such improved dexterity may be particularly advantageous for pediatric surgery where the smaller body habitus of newborns, infants, and young children can make certain anatomic areas more difficult to access.[3] Moreover, robotic systems are equipped with motion scaling, which reduces the scale of the surgeons movements 5:1, supporting precise movements in small and narrowed spaces.[10]

The visualization of anatomy in pediatric patients can prove particularly difficult given their small size. In open surgery, visualization is augmented through the use of surgical loupes, and in traditional laparoscopy magnified endoscopes similarly enhance visualization. Although loupes and endoscopes aid surgeons in acquiring an appropriate visual field, the highly magnified 3-dimensional images provided by the robotic surgeon console allows for a degree of visualization that cannot be achieved with either open or traditional laparoscopic methods.[10] Robotic systems are capable of magnifying images between 10 and 15 times, allowing for enhanced depth perception and surgeon control.[10,12] Beyond magnification capabilities, robotic cameras provide tremor filtration and operator-controlled views, making for steadier and more precise visualization.[13] Furthermore, all robotic surgical systems consist of a surgeon console that is physically separate from the operative cart at the patient's bedside, which lends itself to the application of telesurgery and telementoring.[10,11] The ability for a senior pediatric surgeon to carry out or oversee an operation in another part of the country or world where access to advanced pediatric surgical care is limited could have immense training and humanitarian potential.

Although improved dexterity, manual control, and visualization are important for conducting any type of surgical procedure, pediatric surgical oncology cases are particularly high risk given the often poorly accessible locations of some tumors. These cases are often marred by limited visualization and significant anatomic constraints.[14] These technical challenges often preclude the use of conventional minimally invasive surgical techniques and create an opportunity to develop robotic-assisted approaches that circumvent these limitations for complex oncological procedures.[14]

Limitations

The primary disadvantage of robotic surgical technology in pediatric surgery is related to the size of the surgical robot and its associated instruments (**Table 1**).[5,9,10] As mentioned, robotic instruments approved for pediatric use are only available in 2 sizes—8 mm and 5 mm—which are both significantly larger than the 3-mm instruments that are commonly used in traditional laparoscopic procedures. Similarly, robotic endoscopes are currently only available as 12.0 mm and 8.5 mm, as a previously available 5-mm scope was discontinued owing to low use.[5] Although the 8.5-mm scope may be useable in larger children, this size would be prohibitively large for the intercostal space of a child weighing 5 kg or less.[15] Along these lines, the manufacturer of the da Vinci surgical platform recommends placement of ports 8 cm apart. This distance would be difficult to achieve in small children or neonates where anatomic space is limited.[5]

Although not currently approved for use in pediatric surgery, the Senhance robotic platform (Transenterix) has created a system compatible with 3-mm instruments. Bergholz and colleagues[6] examined the potential use of this technology in pediatric

Table 1
Comparison of North American robotic systems

Company (System Name)	Degrees of Freedom	Smallest Available Instrument Size	Haptic Feedback
Intuitive Surgical (Da Vinci Surgical System)	7	5 mm	None
TransEnterix (Senhance)	7	3 mm	Available
Medrobotics Corp (Flex)	180	3 mm	None
Titan Medical Inc (SPORT)	Multiple	25-mm single port platform	None
J&J/Alphabet (Verb Surgical)	In development	In development	In development
Medtronic (Hugo)	In development	In development	In development

Data from Refs.[5,6,10]

patients by examining the ability of surgeons to complete specific operative tasks in experimental boxes designed to mimic the small body cavities of pediatric patients. This study demonstrated that surgeons were successfully able to perform intracorporal suturing and knot tying in body cavities as small as 90 mL, and that instruments were able to be inserted directly without the need for ports, thus, decreasing the necessary distance between ports.[6] This study illustrates that, although pediatric robotic surgery is currently limited by the size of instruments available on the market, this limitation can feasibly be circumvented through the research and development of pediatric-sized instruments.

Costs

The cost analysis for the use of the robot is not strictly measured by numerical cost in dollars, but should be considered as value equating to quality (as defined by positive outcomes/cost). Naturally, there is the initial cost of purchasing and maintaining the robot itself, as well as the increased costs from the disposable robotic equipment and the longer operative times.[5] Analysis of financial data from Intuitive Surgical revealed that, in 2017, the average cost per procedure of the robot itself was $3568, with $1866 for instruments and accessories, $1038 for robot systems, and $663 for a service contract.[16] It should be noted that these estimates do not account for other expenses or savings associated with the robotic portion of a procedure, such as increased operating room or anesthesia time, staff training, cost of marketing campaigns, or improvement in patient volume and, as a result, required infrastructure improvements or decreased length of stay after minimally invasive surgery.[16] In contrast, patient satisfaction as well as emotional and professional gains may also be taken into account when determining the worth of this kind of investment.[17] Parental satisfaction after pediatric robotic-assisted surgery has been argued to be improved compared with other approaches.[12]

Several studies have examined the relationship of caseload volume to cost, primarily within the adult literature. Palmer and colleagues[18] found that 3 to 5 cases per week are necessary to demonstrate a net gain from robotic surgery. Other studies have demonstrated that increased caseload is required to maintain profits when switching from laparoscopic to robotic procedures. As a result, costs remain problematic for pediatric hospitals, particularly given the frequently lower operating budgets and the smaller volume of patients requiring or eligible for robotic procedures.[5] Many pediatric medical centers are unable to absorb the initial costs of a pediatric robotic-assisted surgery program. For example, over 15 years of pediatric urologic robotic surgery, published material stems only from 48 institutions, with the vast majority of those in the United States.[7]

TRAINING CONSIDERATIONS

Several decades ago, conventional laparoscopy was a novel and unfamiliar surgical technique that required dedicated and focused training, but today it has become the clinical standard for a multitude of procedures and has been seamlessly integrated into surgical residency training.[10] Today, it is robotic surgery that is the new surgical technique that may be unfamiliar to many surgeons and thus requires focused training. However, compared with conventional laparoscopic training, it is reported that comfort levels can be attained more quickly with robotic surgery than with the laparoscopic equivalent. Many have attributed the short learning curve for robotic procedures, in part, to the intuitive symmetric movement of the robotic system that moves in line with the surgeon's hands, as opposed to traditional laparoscopy that requires movement in reverse. The intuitive movement of robotic systems allows for ease of use even for the most naïve users.[3,9]

When examining operative time for new robotic users, novice users who have had significant prior conventional laparoscopy training tended to have decreased operative times when beginning to preform robotic surgery as opposed to novice robotic users that had minimal prior conventional laparoscopic training.[11] Additionally, as novice robotic users garnered more experience with the robotic platform, their robotic operative times decreased for both simple and more complex procedures.[11]

In 2007, Meehan and colleagues[19] examined their experience teaching robotic fundoplication to both staff surgeons and general surgery residents and, similar to other published studies, found that surgeons quickly reduced their robotic operative time with repeated experience. Looking at the learning curve of a single staff surgeon, after only 5 robotic fundoplications, operative time dropped 50%, from 3 hours to 90 minutes. This short learning curve allowed for the attending surgeon to quickly gain a level of mastery with robotic procedures sufficient to train residents in these robotic techniques. After the fifth case, subsequent procedures were conducted by the general surgery resident and the attending surgeon served as the bedside assistant.[19]

Less complex cases, such as a fundoplication, make excellent robotic training cases not only for residents, but for nursing and technical staff assisting in the operating room as well. These simpler cases are typically more common and allow residents, nursing staff, and even anesthesia personnel to repetitively complete the same tasks and commit these tasks to memory.[19] Increasing familiarity of everyone in the operating room to the nuisances of the robot and the associated room setup with simple cases translates into improved performance in more complex cases.[19] It is imperative to have a core group of specific staff familiar with robotic procedures to decrease setup and turnover times and increase case efficiency.

CURRENT APPLICATIONS, SAFETY, AND OUTCOMES

Robotic surgery has been used in almost all pediatric surgical subspecialties including otolaryngology, urology, general and thoracic surgery, and surgical oncology. Among pediatric disciplines, robotic surgery is most frequently used in urology. Although robotic surgery is increasing in use in both adult and pediatric surgery, pediatric robotic-assisted surgery is still very much in its infancy.

Urologic Applications

Urologic procedures are the most common application of pediatric robotic surgery.[2] Procedures that have been performed using robotic assistance include pyeloplasty, ureteral reimplantation, complete and partial nephrectomies, bladder augmentation, Mitrofanoff appendicovesicostomy, bladder outlet procedures, and treatment of utricular cysts, among many others.[2] A 2018 publication categorized all reported robotic-assisted urologic procedures (total of 3688) in pediatrics from 2003 to 2016. By far, the most common were pyeloplasty (n = 1923), ureteral reimplantation (n = 1120), with heminephrectomy (n = 136) and nephrectomy or nephroureterectomy (n = 117) a distant third and fourth.[7]

Pyeloplasty

Robotic-assisted pyeloplasty is the most common procedure performed robotically in pediatric patients, both within urology and overall.[20] The first pediatric laparoscopic pyeloplasty was performed in 1995; the procedure is technically difficult and has a steep learning curve. The first robotic-assisted pediatric pyeloplasty was done in 2002. Robotic-assisted surgery offers all the benefits of traditional laparoscopic surgery, but with the added benefits of 3-dimensional visualization and an articulating instrument for ease of intracorporeal suturing, allowing a shorter learning curve for this procedure compared with traditional laparoscopy.[20]

Numerous authors have reported series of robotic-assisted pyeloplasty with success rates ranging from 78% to 100%, with the majority of studies reporting success rates in excess of 90%.[20] Comparisons between robotic-assisted, laparoscopic, and open procedures have found robotic procedures typically have shorter hospital length of stay and require less pain medication; however, operative times are longer.[20,21]

Pyeloplasty in infants less than 10 kg has been performed successfully. Avery and colleagues[22] published a multi-institutional study of 60 infants less than 12 months old with a 91% success rate and an 11% complication rate, which is similar to other studies on larger children and adults. The authors recommended modifications for infants less than 10 kg, including midline port placement to avoid collision of the robotic arms and suturing of the trocars to the fascia or skin to avoid dislodgement.[22] Kafka and colleagues[23] recently evaluated the safety of robotic-assisted pyeloplasty in infants weighing less than 10 kg by prospectively comparing outcomes of patients undergoing robotic-assisted pyeloplasty with a matched cohort from their retrospectively acquired database of open procedures. They found no significant differences in outcomes or complications.

Ureteral reimplantation

Ureteral reimplantation for vesicoureteral reflux is the second most common pediatric robotic-assisted procedure.[8] Of all ureteral reimplantation procedures performed minimally invasively, 81% are done robotically.[24] Robotic-assisted ureteral reimplantation can be done by an extravesical or intravesical approach and, of these approaches, the extravesical is much more widely reported.[24,25] Despite initial challenges associated with a steep learning curve, multi-institutional studies now describe robotic-assisted ureteral reimplantation as effective and safe. Boysen and colleagues[26] reported a series of 260 patients at 9 academic centers with a radiographically confirmed reflux resolution rate of 87.9%. They reported 25 complications (9.6%), among which there were no Clavien-Dindo grade IV or V complications and 7 (2.7%) grade III complications. A prospective evaluation by the same group subsequently reported a 93.8% radiographic resolution of reflux.[27]

Conversely, a 2016 study comparing robotic versus open ureteral reimplantation in 17 centers and more than 1600 patients (of which 1494 were open procedures) demonstrated longer operating times with robotic procedures. The 90-day complication rate was higher for robotic-assisted surgery compared with open procedures (13.0% vs 4.5%) and the median hospital cost increased with robotic surgery by $1855 per procedure. However, it should be noted that 51% of the robotic cases occurred in 2012 and 2013,[28] which is a significant number of years ago given the speed with which improvements in robotic surgical skill and comfort level have improved.[25]

Partial or complete nephrectomy

In pediatric patients, complete or partial nephrectomies are more often indicated for benign disease rather than malignancy.[2] Currently, many nephrectomies performed in children are still performed using an open approach. A 2019 study of pediatric nephrectomies done for multicystic dysplastic kidney disease over a 10-year period demonstrated that, of 569 nephrectomies, 84.2% were completed using an open approach and 15.8% were done minimally invasively (10.0% laparoscopic and 5.8% robotic). However, it was noted that the frequency of minimally invasive nephrectomies increased annually, from a low of 8% in 2006% to 29% in 2015.[29]

Although the majority of pediatric minimally invasive complete or partial nephrectomies are performed using a conventional laparoscopic approach, there are several reports of robotic complete or partial nephrectomies, particularly in older children.[30,31] However, robotic-assisted nephrectomy has been described in smaller children and infants as well. A 2016 case report demonstrated a successful partial nephrectomy in an 11-month-old, 10.7-kg child.[32] A 2019 two-center review compared open, laparoscopic, robotic-assisted, or laparoendoscopic single site partial nephrectomy for benign disease in 59 pediatric patients over a 10-year period.[33] The median patient age was 16 months (interquartile range, 9.0–49.7 months) and median weight was 10.7 kg (interquartile range, 8.8–16.4 kg); there were no differences between the groups. Not surprisingly, they found open procedures were associated with a greater opioid requirement postoperatively. Operative times were shortest in the open group, and both the open and the laparoendoscopic single site groups had significantly shorter operative times than either the laparoscopic or robotic-assisted groups. There were no intraoperative complications. Six patients experienced postoperative complications, all of which were Clavien-Dindo grade II: 4 postoperative urinary tract infections, 1 patient with fever, and 1 respiratory distress requiring pharmacologic treatment.[33]

Preliminarily, given the limited data that exist in the pediatric literature, outcomes seem to be similar between open and robotic-assisted complete or partial nephrectomies. Most complications are not specific to the robotic-assisted approach, but rather are intrinsic to the procedure itself. Malik and colleagues[34] compared their robotic-assisted partial nephrectomy complications to published open or laparoscopic partial nephrectomy complication rates over a 6-year period and found similar lengths of stay and complication rates as reported laparoscopic approaches. Bansal and colleagues[35] reported an 8.3% complication rate (all Clavien-Dindo grade I) in a recent study of 24 pediatric patients undergoing robotic-assisted nephroureterectomy. Mason and colleagues[36] described a series of 21 pediatric patients undergoing robotic-assisted partial nephrectomies for duplicated collecting systems and reported 2 postoperative complications, a urinary tract infection and an incarcerated port site hernia requiring reoperation.

Dangle and colleagues[37] recently reported one of the largest descriptions of 90-day perioperative complication rates after pediatric urologic robotic-assisted surgery in a multi-institutional study. Of 880 procedures, high-grade complications were rare. There were 41 patients (4.8%) who had a grade IIIa or IIIb complication and 1 patient who had a grade IVa complication. Grade I and II complications were seen in 59 (6.9%) and 70 (8.2%) of patients, respectively. There were 4 intraoperative visceral injuries, and 14 cases required conversion to an open or purely laparoscopic procedure. Overall, robotic-assisted surgery in pediatric urology seems to offer similar outcomes and complication rates than its laparoscopic or open counterparts with improved cosmesis, shorter lengths of stay, and with reduced postoperative pain. However, at this time, data is too limited to assert superiority of robotic-assisted surgery for any particular case.

General and Thoracic Surgery

Robotic-assisted surgery in pediatric general and thoracic surgery have not yet reached the magnitude that it has in pediatric urology. Robotic procedures that have been reported in the pediatric literature include hepatectomy, excision of choledochal cysts, gastric fundoplication, colectomies, proctectomy with ileal pouch-anorectal anastomosis, mediastinal mass resections, lobectomies, diaphragmatic plications, and repair of congenital diaphragmatic hernias.[2]

Fundoplication

Fundoplication is the most widely performed and reported robotic-assisted surgery in pediatric general and thoracic surgery.[4] Hambraeus and colleagues[38] examined the published literature on pediatric studies comparing laparoscopic and robotic-assisted Nissen fundoplications and found several studies describing 174 children in total, among which 89 patients underwent robotic-assisted surgery and 85 patients underwent conventional laparoscopy. They found no difference between operating time, duration of hospital stay, or rate of conversion to open procedure. There were no differences in rates of intraoperative or postoperative complications.

Navarrete Arellano and Garibay González[13] reported their experiences with 186 robotic-assisted pediatric procedures, of which 84 (45.16%) were gastrointestinal. This review included 38 primary fundoplications and 13 redo fundoplications. Among primary fundoplications, they reported a 5.26% conversion to open procedure rate, a 5.26% complication rate, and 2 patients with partial dismantling of the fundoplication and hiatal hernia at subsequent follow-up. The 13 redo fundoplication procedures had no complications and 1 case required conversion to an open procedure.

Choledochal cyst resection

The first pediatric robotic-assisted choledochal cyst resection was reported by Woo and colleagues[39] in 2006. Since that time, several authors have reported small cohorts of pediatric patients undergoing robotic-assisted choledochal cyst resection. Chang and colleagues[40] described a series of 14 patients in 2012. Alizai and colleagues[41] reported 27 robotic-assisted cyst resections with hepaticojejunostomy. Five cases required conversion to an open procedure. One patient had 3 complications, including an omental hernia, an anastomotic stricture, and a subsequent bile leak. The median length of stay was 6 days. Kim and colleagues[42] retrospectively compared robotic-assisted with open procedures for choledochal cysts and found no difference in complication rates. However, they noted the patients in the robotic group were significantly older and larger than the open group and that operative times were longer in the robotic group. A recent published literature review by Wang and colleagues[43] analyzed 8 studies composed of 86 patients. Of the 86 cases, the average patient age was 6.3 years. Seven cases (8.1%) required conversion to open surgery. Eleven cases (12.8%) were done using robotic arm number 3 and the remaining cases used a hitch-stitch technique to suspend the stomach wall and the liver. The bowel was extracorporealized in 54.6% of these cases to complete the intestinal anastomosis, whereas the remaining 45.4% used a completely robotic intestinal anastomosis. There were 10 patients with complications, including 8 biliary fistulas, 1 anastomotic stenosis, and 1 wound dehiscence.[43]

Otolaryngology

Not surprisingly, pediatric robotic surgery has been used least frequently in otolaryngology.[44] Thus far, most robotic applications in otolaryngology seem to be transoral. Proponents of robotic surgery in otolaryngology argue that it is particularly useful for tongue base masses. Open surgery can easily provide access to the oropharyngeal region, including the tongue base, but can carry the morbidity of splitting the lip and the mandible or requires pharyngotomy.[45] As a result, transoral approaches are being used.[45] Kayhan and colleagues[45] reported a series of 8 pediatric patients undergoing transoral robotic-assisted tongue base resection. There was only 1 complication of minor bleeding in 1 patient on postoperative day 10, which resolved without intervention. Blood loss was minimal and hospital length of stay was an average of 2.25 days. The average overall surgery time was 47 minutes and the average robotic surgery time was 8.8 minutes. Erkul and colleagues[46] reviewed published cases of pediatric transoral robotic-assisted surgery and described 41 patients undergoing procedures including lingual and base of tongue tonsillectomy, resections of malignant disease in the oropharynx, tongue base thyroglossal duct cyst resections, repair of laryngeal cleft cysts, posterior glottic stenosis, and congenital vocal cord paralysis. Of the 41 cases, there was only 1 intraoperative complication, which was a minor buccal mucosa laceration. Of these cases, 90.2% were able to be completed robotically. Four cases were converted to an open procedure owing to inadequate visualization. Zdanski and colleagues[47] reported a series of 16 pediatric transoral robotic-assisted upper airway surgeries. They were able to complete all of the procedures robotically and recommend a 2 robotic surgeon team with a bedside surgeon to monitor the airway and assist with standard laryngeal and pharyngeal instruments.

Oncologic Operations

Minimally invasive surgery is now largely accepted in many pediatric oncologic operations. A minimally invasive approach has the standard advantages of decreasing need for narcotic analgesia, shortens time to postoperative full mobilization, and typically carries less risk of wound infection and incisional hernias.[2] Most important, it shortens the time of postoperative recovery and decreases time to adjuvant therapy.[2]

It is important to note that data from the adult literature regarding minimally invasive surgery for oncologic operations should not be extrapolated to the pediatric population, because the tumor biology, treatment, and prognosis are different.[2] Contraindications for minimally invasive surgery, including robotic surgery, in children include large or fragile tumors that carry a high risk of tumor fracture and spillage, significant adhesions from previous operations, or significant impairment in respiratory or cardiovascular physiology. Robotic surgery can also be used in supportive care in pediatric oncology including placement of gastrostomy tubes, ovarian transposition, or cryopreservation.[2]

SAFETY

Robotic surgery on older, larger children and adolescents follows several of the same surgical and safety principles as adult patients. However, smaller children and infants require special consideration when discussing robotic surgery. Many of the considerations of robotic-assisted surgery in infants are similar to those of laparoscopic surgery for this age group. Special attention must be paid to patient positioning in infants as compared with older children, because infants are frequently more pliable and extra care must be taken to avoid hyperextension and flexion. The general considerations of comfortable positioning, adequate padding, skin protection, and securing the patient to the table apply to children of all ages.[48]

As with all robotic-assisted surgeries, there are special anesthetic considerations for pediatric robotic-assisted surgery. Access to the patient by the anesthesiologist is limited after the robot is docked. Changes to patient position or access to the patient typically requires detachment of the robot. Patients must remain entirely paralyzed when the robot is docked.[49] Robotic-assisted surgery frequently requires steeper Trendelenburg or reverse Trendelenburg positioning than traditional laparoscopic surgery, which has hemodynamic consequences and requires extra care in patient securing and positioning.[50] There are renal effects of pneumoperitoneum, which causes direct compression on both the renal parenchyma itself and on the renal vein causing decreased blood flow. This renal compression further stimulates the renin–angiotensin system and can produce transient oliguria. This situation can typically be mitigated by adequate volume expansion, but extra care needs to be taken to optimize and maintain liberal intravascular volume in patients with renal dysfunction undergoing robotic-assisted surgery.[50]

Insufflation volumes and pressures are limited in small children. Insufflation volumes in a 10-kg child are less than 1 L, which decreases the working space considerably, making robotic-assisted surgery technically more challenging and increasing the potential for surgical error.[48] In infants weighing less than 10 kg, pressures of more than 9 mm Hg have been reported to have a greater impact on pulmonary mechanics and hemodynamics than lower pressures.[48] In the same randomized trial, infants who had procedures with insufflation pressures of greater than 9 mm Hg had higher pain scores, required more pain medication, and took longer to resume enteral feedings.[48]

In addition to safety issues related to the technical limitations as listed, infants and small children have unique cardiopulmonary considerations. Insufflation results in a decrease in ventricular preload as well as an increase in vagal activity with a corresponding bradycardia. These physiologic limitations can occur with either laparoscopic or robotic-assisted surgery and can create challenges for infants and children with immature or dysfunctional cardiovascular systems.[48,50]

Infants are typically more susceptible to the respiratory effects of pneumoperitoneum than older children or adults. Abdominal insufflation decreases respiratory compliance and increases airway pressures. Furthermore, the instilled CO_2 can cause hypercapnia and acidosis.[48] Prolonged operative times seen with inexperienced robotic surgeons can exaggerate the negative physiologic effects of CO_2.[51]

Despite these concerns, numerous studies have demonstrated the safety of pediatric robotic-assisted surgery in multiple surgical disciplines, including in children weighing less than 10 kg.

LOOKING FORWARD IN PEDIATRIC ROBOTIC SURGERY

Robotic-assisted surgery is safe and effective in children and is steadily increasing in its use across pediatric surgery subspecialties. The repertoire of procedures that can be performed robotically continues to expand, including procedures in younger children, infants, and neonates. However, more robust prospective studies are needed in pediatric robotic-assisted surgery to truly assess the benefits of using this approach as opposed to conventional open or laparoscopic techniques. One of the primary limitations to the implementation of robotics in pediatric surgery specifically is the availability of appropriately sized instruments for the pediatric body habitus. As smaller robotic instruments and endoscopes become commercially available use of robotic surgery in children will undoubtedly increase.

REFERENCES

1. Meininger DD, Byhahn C, Heller K, et al. Totally endoscopic Nissen fundoplication with a robotic system in a child. Surg Endosc 2001. https://doi.org/10.1007/s00464-001-4200-3.
2. Petralia P. Pediatric robotic surgery. 1st edition. In: Mattioli G, Petralia P, editors. Pediatric Robotic Surgery. 1st ed. Cham, Switzerland: Springer International Publishing; 2017. p. 1–188.
3. Mattioli G, Pini Prato A, Razore B, et al. Da Vinci robotic surgery in a pediatric hospital. J Laparoendosc Adv Surg Tech 2017;27(5):539–45.
4. Fernandez N, Farhat WA. A comprehensive analysis of robot-assisted surgery uptake in the pediatric surgical discipline. Front Surg 2019;6:1–8.
5. Bruns NE, Soldes OS, Ponsky TA. Robotic surgery may not "make the cut" in pediatrics. Front Pediatr 2015;3. https://doi.org/10.3389/fped.2015.00010.
6. Bergholz R, Botden S, Verweij J, et al. Evaluation of a new robotic-assisted laparoscopic surgical system for procedures in small cavities. J Robot Surg 2019. https://doi.org/10.1007/s11701-019-00961-y. 0123456789.
7. Cundy TP, Harley SJD, Marcus HJ, et al. Global trends in paediatric robot-assisted urological surgery: a bibliometric and Progressive Scholarly Acceptance analysis. J Robot Surg 2018;12(1):109–15.
8. Cundy TP, Shetty K, Clark J, et al. The first decade of robotic surgery in children. J Pediatr Surg 2013;48(4):858–65.
9. Chandra V, Dutta S, Albanese C. Robot-assisted pediatric surgery. In: Saxena A, Höllwarth M, editors. Essentials of Pediatric Endoscopic Surgery. Berlin, Heidelberg: Springer; 2009. https://doi.org/10.1007/978-3-540-78387-9_11.
10. Garcia I, De Armas IAS, Pimpalwar A. Current trends in pediatric robotic surgery. Bangladesh J Endosurgery 2014;2(1):15–28.
11. van Haasteren G, Levine S, Hayes W. Pediatric robotic surgery: early assessment. Pediatrics 2009;124(6):1642–9.
12. Howe A, Kozel Z, Palmer L. Robotic surgery in pediatric urology. Asian J Urol 2017;4(1):55–67.
13. Navarrete Arellano M, Garibay González F. Robot-assisted laparoscopic and thoracoscopic surgery: prospective series of 186 pediatric surgeries. Front Pediatr 2019;7:1–9.
14. Cundy TP, Marcus HJ, Clark J, et al. Robot-assisted minimally invasive surgery for pediatric solid tumors: a systematic review of feasibility and current status. Eur J Pediatr Surg 2014;24(2):127–35.
15. Meehan JJ. Robotic surgery for pediatric tumors. Cancer J 2013;19(2):183–8.
16. Childers CP, Maggard-Gibbons M. Estimation of the acquisition and operating costs for robotic surgery. JAMA 2018. https://doi.org/10.1001/jama.2018.9219.
17. O'Kelly F, Farhat WA, Koyle MA. Cost, training and simulation models for robotic-assisted surgery in pediatric urology. World J Urol 2019. https://doi.org/10.1007/s00345-019-02822-7. 0123456789.
18. Palmer KJ, Lowe GJ, Coughlin GD, et al. Launching a successful robotic surgery program. J Endourol 2008. https://doi.org/10.1089/end.2007.9824.

19. Meehan JJ, Meehan TD, Sandler A. Robotic fundoplication in children: resident teaching and a single institutional review of our first 50 patients. J Pediatr Surg 2007;42(12):2022–5.
20. Morales-López RA, Pérez-Marchán M, Pérez Brayfield M. Current concepts in pediatric robotic assisted pyeloplasty. Front Pediatr 2019. https://doi.org/10.3389/fped.2019.00004.
21. Song SH, Lee C, Jung J, et al. A comparative study of pediatric open pyeloplasty, laparoscopy-assisted extracorporeal pyeloplasty, and robot-assisted laparoscopic pyeloplasty. PLoS One 2017. https://doi.org/10.1371/journal.pone.0175026.
22. Avery DI, Herbst KW, Lendvay TS, et al. Robot-assisted laparoscopic pyeloplasty: multi-institutional experience in infants. J Pediatr Urol 2015. https://doi.org/10.1016/j.jpurol.2014.11.025.
23. Kafka IZ, Kocherov S, Jaber J, et al. Pediatric robotic-assisted laparoscopic pyeloplasty (RALP): does weight matter? Pediatr Surg Int 2019. https://doi.org/10.1007/s00383-019-04435-y.
24. Baek M, Koh CJ. Lessons learned over a decade of pediatric robotic ureteral reimplantation. Investig Clin Urol 2017. https://doi.org/10.4111/icu.2017.58.1.3.
25. Sahadev R, Spencer K, Srinivasan AK, et al. The robot-assisted extravesical antireflux surgery: how we overcame the learning curve. Front Pediatr 2019. https://doi.org/10.3389/fped.2019.00093.
26. Boysen WR, Ellison JS, Kim C, et al. Multi-institutional review of outcomes and complications of robot-assisted laparoscopic extravesical ureteral reimplantation for treatment of primary vesicoureteral reflux in children. J Urol 2017. https://doi.org/10.1016/j.juro.2017.01.062.
27. Boysen WR, Akhavan A, Ko J, et al. Prospective multicenter study on robot-assisted laparoscopic extravesical ureteral reimplantation (RALUR-EV): outcomes and complications. J Pediatr Urol 2018. https://doi.org/10.1016/j.jpurol.2018.01.020.
28. Kurtz MP, Leow JJ, Varda BK, et al. Robotic versus open pediatric ureteral reimplantation: costs and complications from a nationwide sample. J Pediatr Urol 2016. https://doi.org/10.1016/j.jpurol.2016.06.016.
29. Brown CT, Sebastião YV, McLeod DJ. Trends in surgical management of multicystic dysplastic kidney at USA children's hospitals. J Pediatr Urol 2019. https://doi.org/10.1016/j.jpurol.2019.04.024.
30. Lee RS, Sethi AS, Passerotti CC, et al. Robot-assisted laparoscopic nephrectomy and contralateral ureteral reimplantation in children. J Endourol 2009. https://doi.org/10.1089/end.2009.0271.
31. Blanc T, Pio L, Clermidi P, et al. Robotic-assisted laparoscopic management of renal tumors in children: preliminary results. Pediatr Blood Cancer 2019;e27867. https://doi.org/10.1002/pbc.27867.
32. Wiestma AC, Cho PS, Hollis MV, et al. Robot-assisted laparoscopic lower pole partial nephrectomy in the pediatric patient. J Pediatr Urol 2016. https://doi.org/10.1016/j.jpurol.2016.09.007.
33. Neheman A, Kord E, Strine AC, et al. Pediatric partial nephrectomy for upper urinary tract duplication anomalies: a comparison between different surgical approaches and techniques. Urology 2019. https://doi.org/10.1016/j.urology.2018.11.026.
34. Malik RD, Pariser JJ, Gundeti MS. Outcomes in pediatric robot-assisted laparoscopic heminephrectomy compared with contemporary open and laparoscopic series. J Endourol 2015. https://doi.org/10.1089/end.2014.0818.

35. Bansal D, Cost NG, Bean CM, et al. Comparison of pediatric robotic-assisted laparoscopic nephroureterectomy and laparoendoscopic single-site nephroureterectomy. Urology 2014;83(2):438–42.

36. Mason MD, Anthony Herndon CD, Smith-Harrison LI, et al. Robotic-assisted partial nephrectomy in duplicated collecting systems in the pediatric population: techniques and outcomes. J Pediatr Urol 2014. https://doi.org/10.1016/j.jpurol.2013.10.014.

37. Dangle PP, Akhavan A, Odeleye M, et al. Ninety-day perioperative complications of pediatric robotic urological surgery: a multi-institutional study. J Pediatr Urol 2016. https://doi.org/10.1016/j.jpurol.2015.08.015.

38. Hambraeus M, Arnbjörnsson E, Anderberg M. A literature review of the outcomes after robot-assisted laparoscopic and conventional laparoscopic Nissen fundoplication for gastro-esophageal reflux disease in children. Int J Med Robot 2013. https://doi.org/10.1002/rcs.1517.

39. Woo R, Le D, Albanese CT, et al. Robot-assisted laparoscopic resection of a type I choledochal cyst in a child. J Laparoendosc Adv Surg Tech 2006. https://doi.org/10.1089/lap.2006.16.179.

40. Chang EY, Hong YJ, Chang HK, et al. Lessons and tips from the experience of pediatric robotic choledochal cyst resection. J Laparoendosc Adv Surg Tech 2012. https://doi.org/10.1089/lap.2011.0503.

41. Alizai NK, Dawrant MJ, Najmaldin AS. Robot-assisted resection of choledochal cysts and hepaticojejunostomy in children. Pediatr Surg Int 2014. https://doi.org/10.1007/s00383-013-3459-5.

42. Kim NY, Chang EY, Hong YJ, et al. Retrospective assessment of the validity of robotic surgery in comparison to open surgery for pediatric choledochal cyst. Yonsei Med J 2015. https://doi.org/10.3349/ymj.2015.56.3.737.

43. Wang X-Q, Xu S-J, Wang Z, et al. Robotic-assisted surgery for pediatric choledochal cyst: case report and literature review. World J Clin Cases 2018;6(7):143–9.

44. Mehta D, Duvvuri U. Robotic surgery in pediatric otolaryngology: emerging trends. Laryngoscope 2012. https://doi.org/10.1002/lary.23806.

45. Kayhan FT, Yigider AP, Koc AK, et al. Treatment of tongue base masses in children by transoral robotic surgery. Eur Arch Otorhinolaryngol 2017. https://doi.org/10.1007/s00405-017-4646-0.

46. Erkul E, Duvvuri U, Mehta D, et al. Transoral robotic surgery for the pediatric head and neck surgeries. Eur Arch Otorhinolaryngol 2017. https://doi.org/10.1007/s00405-016-4425-3.

47. Zdanski CJ, Austin GK, Walsh JM, et al. Transoral robotic surgery for upper airway pathology in the pediatric population. Laryngoscope 2017;127(1):247–51.

48. Villanueva J, Killian M, Chaudhry R. Robotic urologic surgery in the infant: a review. Curr Urol Rep 2019;20(7):1–6.

49. Lee JR. Anesthetic considerations for robotic surgery. Korean J Anesthesiol 2014. https://doi.org/10.4097/kjae.2014.66.1.3.

50. Munoz CJ, Nguyen HT, Houck CS. Robotic surgery and anesthesia for pediatric urologic procedures. Curr Opin Anaesthesiol 2016. https://doi.org/10.1097/ACO.0000000000000333.

51. Mariano ER, Furukawa L, Woo RK, et al. Anesthetic concerns for robot-assisted laparoscopy in an infant. Anesth Analg 2004. https://doi.org/10.1213/01.ANE.0000137394.99683.66.

Robotic Surgery in Gynecology

Ashley S. Moon, MD[a],*, John Garofalo, MD[b], Pratistha Koirala, MD, PhD[a], Mai-Linh T. Vu, MD[c], Linus Chuang, MD[a]

KEYWORDS

- Robotic hysterectomy • Robotic myomectomy • Robotic sacrocolpopexy
- Robotic-assisted laparoscopic gynecology

KEY POINTS

- Robotic technology has improved the ability to perform complex gynecologic surgeries.
- Robotic-assisted laparoscopic gynecologic procedures are associated with early recovery and decreased hospital length of stay.
- Prospective clinical outcomes data are continuing to expand for robotic-assisted laparoscopic gynecologic surgery.

 Video content accompanies this article at http://www.surgical.theclinics.com.

INTRODUCTION

Since conventional laparoscopy (CL) or video-assisted laparoscopy became a standard surgical approach in the 1980s, multiple benefits of minimally invasive surgery have emerged, including shorter hospital admissions, smaller incisions, and decreased surgical site infection rates. Conversely, there are multiple challenges associated with CL, including a 2-dimensional visual field, less haptic feedback, difficulty with hand–eye coordination, and amplification of physiologic tremors.[1] The introduction of robotic-assisted laparoscopy (RAL) has ameliorated some of these concerns while maintaining many of the benefits of minimally invasive surgical techniques. RAL was first developed as a US military project in conjunction with the National Aeronautics and Space Administration in the 1970s. The US Food and Drug Administration approved the robotic platform in 2000 for general surgery and in

[a] Department of Obstetrics, Gynecology and Reproductive Biology, Danbury Hospital, Nuvance Health, 24 Hospital Avenue, Danbury, CT 06810, USA; [b] Department of Obstetrics, Gynecology and Reproductive Biology, Norwalk Hospital, Nuvance Health, 30 Stevens Street, Norwalk, CT 06850, USA; [c] Complete Women Care, 3711 Long Beach Boulevard, Suite 110, Long Beach, CA 90807, USA
* Corresponding author.
E-mail address: Ashley.moon@wchn.org

Surg Clin N Am 100 (2020) 445–460
https://doi.org/10.1016/j.suc.2019.12.007
0039-6109/20/© 2019 Elsevier Inc. All rights reserved.
surgical.theclinics.com

2005 for gynecologic surgery.[2] Since its inception, robotic technology has improved dramatically and adoption of RAL has been widespread, especially in pelvic and gynecologic surgery.

The robotic surgical platform allows for 3 to 4 robotic arms, which are under the control of the surgeon who is sitting at the console away from the operating table and patient. A 3-dimensional endoscope provides improved depth perception. The surgeon uses foot pedals, finger graspers, and a clutch to control the camera and direct the instruments. RAL instruments have 7° of motion compared with 4° of motion offered by CL,[1] allowing for precise manipulation and greater dexterity. These advances have allowed surgeons to perform more complex procedures, such as anastomosis and exploration of the retroperitoneal space, as well as lysis of adhesions. There is a decreased rate of conversion of RAL to open abdominal surgery as compared with CL.[3] Additionally, compared with laparotomic surgery, RAL allows for scaling large motions to micromotions and lessens operator fatigue.

The decision to perform RAL is multifactorial. Not all patients are suited for RAL owing to longer operative times than open procedures and the steep Trendelenburg position, thereby requiring increased preoperative planning and thoughtful patient selection. Financial considerations also play a role. As an emerging technology with more maintenance and equipment, the cost of RAL is significantly higher than laparotomy or CL. The learning curve associated with RAL may be considered faster given its more intuitive motion, improved imaging and instrument control compared with CL, but this is not well-established. Surgeons should be skilled at both abdominal and laparoscopic approaches for a specific procedure before performing a robotic method. Although RAL is becoming more prevalent, clinical outcomes data are still preliminary in multiple areas and are newly emerging for certain cancers. In this article, we review operative techniques for gynecologic procedures as well as considerations in patient selection and preoperative clearance. We also discuss the current data on RAL for multiple gynecologic indications, including endometrial and cervical cancers, endometriosis, myomectomy, and other benign gynecologic cases.

PREOPERATIVE PLANNING

Preanesthesia evaluation allows for assessment of the robotic approach, such as patient body habitus, chronic comorbidities, previous anesthesia complications, and prior surgeries.

Medical History

- Age of menarche, menopause
- Menstrual bleeding patterns
- Characteristics of pain
- Changes in bowel or urinary habits
- Medical conditions
- Surgical history
- Medications
- Signs and symptoms of possible hemostatic disorder
- Family history of bleeding disorders or gynecologic malignancies
- Preventative care: Pap smears, mammogram, and colonoscopy

Physical Examination

- General physical evaluation
- External pelvic examination, speculum with Pap smear if indicated, and bimanual examination

Laboratory Tests

- Pregnancy test
- Complete blood count
- Targeted screening for bleeding disorders (when indicated)

Diagnostic and Imaging Tests

- Saline infusion ultrasound examination
- Transvaginal ultrasound examination
- Magnetic resonance imaging (MRI)
- Office endometrial biopsy to assess for hyperplasia or malignancy
- Hysteroscopy-directed endometrial sampling

Imaging studies are particularly important in minimally invasive myomectomy because the limited haptic feedback of laparoscopic procedures and the total absence of haptic feedback with robotic-assisted procedures may result in incomplete removal of myomata and a higher incidence of recurrent myoma. MRI is the most accurate and reproducible means of differentiating myoma from adenomyosis and for mapping the number and position of myoma preoperatively.[4]

ENHANCED RECOVERY AFTER SURGERY

As part of an enhanced recovery after surgery (ERAS) program, of which minimally invasive technique is a tenet, preoperative optimization contributes to improving surgical outcomes.

Patient counseling and education include setting appropriate patient expectations for surgery and postoperative care. Preoperative counseling can help to decrease stress and anxiety, especially with new concepts such as robotic-assisted surgery. Smoking and alcohol cessation should also be advised, ideally for at least 4 weeks before surgery.

Based on strong randomized controlled trials of ERAS programs in colorectal patients, patients should be permitted to drink clear fluids up to 2 hours before anesthesia induction and surgery. Aside from patients with possible delayed gastric emptying, solid foods should also be allowed up to 6 hours before induction of anesthesia.[5] Complex carbohydrate drink loading may also decrease postoperative insulin resistance, improve well-being, and mitigate nausea and vomiting.[6] Routine oral mechanical bowel preparation should be avoided, especially if there is no planned enteric resection.

IMMEDIATE PREOPERATIVE AND INTRAOPERATIVE PREPARATION

The largest operating room should be used to allow for the operating table to be in different positions depending on the type of surgery. Gynecologic cases will have two back tables: one small table for vaginal instruments and another larger table for the abdominal portion of the procedure.

Two table-side assistants are used, if possible. One will perform uterine manipulation and retrieve specimens. The other will change robotic instruments, pass sutures and retrieve needles, and troubleshoot any issues with the robotic arms.

Intravenous antibiotics should be administered 60 minutes before incision because gynecologic surgeries are classified as clean contaminated. Coverage against gram-positive and gram-negative organisms is important. Cefazolin is widely used given its broad spectrum coverage and universal availability.

Anesthesia Considerations

- A foam pad should be placed over the face to avoid trauma from the robotic camera arm.
- Orogastric tube placement decompresses the stomach and avoids gastric trauma with port placement.
- With a steep Trendelenburg position and carbon dioxide insufflation, increased intra-abdominal and airway pressures may cause some anesthetic challenges.
- Using forced warm air blanket devices during surgery are crucial for normothermia maintenance to avoid impairment of wound healing and drug metabolism.
- At least two different anti-emetic classes should be used, starting with 5-HT3 antagonists.
- Intraoperative fluid overload should be avoided.

Patient Positioning

- To avoid cephalad movement of patient in steep Trendelenburg position, the operating table should have a gel pad or foam pad to allow for friction and molding to patient's body.
- Shoulder braces may be also placed to help prevent cephalad movement. Careful attention to pad placement should be observed to avoid nerve injury.
- Patient should be placed in dorsal lithotomy position with adequate sacral support.
- Bilateral arms should be padded with foam and tucked to the side with bed sheets.
- Mechanical thromboprophylaxis methods should be used (compression stockings, sequential compression devices).

Port Placement

- The surgeon or assistant places a temporary Foley urinary catheter, cervical sutures and uterine manipulator.
- The endoscope port is placed midline and supraumbilical approximately 20 to 24 cm above the uterine fundus (if the uterus is small).
- Carbon dioxide insufflation is obtained.
- The 8-mm ports for operating arms are placed along the same plane as the endoscope port, approximately 10 cm apart and ensuring no external contact between the arms.
- A first-assistant 12-mm port may be placed in the upper right or left quadrant.
- Position patient in 30° of Trendelenburg to displace bowel from pelvis, using atraumatic graspers if needed.
- Dock the robotic arms to the ports and place robotic instruments.
- Attach monopolar cautery scissors in one operating arm and bipolar cautery grasper in the opposite arm. A grasping forceps may be placed in a third operating port.
- The table-side assistant may use suction irrigator, atraumatic grasper, or needle grasper through the assistant port when indicated.

SURGICAL TECHNIQUE
Robotic Hysterectomy with or Without Salpingo-Oophorectomy

1. The retroperitoneum is dissected bilaterally to identify the ureters. Some surgeons may begin by transecting the round ligaments.

2. If performing a salpingo-oophorectomy, the infundibulopelvic ligament is sealed with coagulation and transected.
3. If the ovaries are to be preserved, the mesosalpinx and utero-ovarian ligaments are sealed with coagulation and transected.
4. At the plane of the round ligaments, the anterior and posterior leaves of the broad ligament are separated. The avascular plane of the broad ligament is developed while progressing caudally.
5. The anterior peritoneum and bladder are dissected off the uterus and cervix to develop the bladder reflection bilaterally.
6. The uterine arteries are skeletonized, sealed with coagulation, and transected at the level of the colpotomy ring.
7. The cardinal ligaments are sealed with coagulation and divided to the level of the cervical–vaginal junction.
8. Colpotomy is performed circumferentially and the cervical–vaginal junction is incised with careful uterine manipulation by the assistant.
9. The specimen is removed through the vagina followed by placement of either a sterile glove or balloon in the vagina to maintain pneumoperitoneum.
10. A 0 polyglactin suture in running fashion is used to close the vaginal cuff. The uterosacral ligaments and cardinal ligaments are incorporated in the angles of the vaginal cuff to help with pelvic support.
11. Bimanual examination is performed to ensure an intact vaginal cuff.
12. Once hemostasis is confirmed, the instruments are removed and the robot is undocked.
13. Larger fascial port sites are closed under direct visualization with a suture closure device.
14. Carbon dioxide is removed through open ports while observing for hemostasis.
15. Ports are removed under direct visualization.
16. Port incisions are injected with 0.25% bupivacaine for postoperative analgesia and closed with skin adhesive.

Lymphadenectomy for Endometrial Cancer

1. With dissection of the retroperitoneum, the paravesical and pararectal spaces are identified.[7]
2. The medial leaf of the broad ligament serves as a barrier between the pelvic lymph node-bearing tissue and the rectosigmoid colon.
3. Pelvic lymph node dissection includes the distal common iliac nodes, external iliac artery and vein nodes, and obturator nodes.
4. Nodal tissue is placed in a specimen bag for retrieval through the assistant port.
5. For para-aortic lymph nodes, the peritoneum above the right common iliac artery is incised to the level of the lower aorta and inferior mesenteric artery.
6. Nodal tissue overlying the lower aorta and distal vena cava is dissected carefully off the great vessels while the right ureter is retracted laterally.
7. The left para-aortic lymph node dissection is similarly performed without the presence of the vena cava.
8. Each unilateral nodal tissue is placed in a specimen bag and removed through the assistant port.

Sentinel Lymph Node Mapping and Biopsy for Endometrial Cancer

1. Before the uterine manipulator is placed, indocyanine green dye is prepared as 1.25 mg/mL (a 25-mg vial of indocyanine green powder diluted in 20 mL aqueous sterile water).[8]

2. At the 3 and 9 o'clock positions of the cervix, 1 mL is injected deeply into the cervical stroma. Another 1 mL is injected superficially into the cervical submucosa.[8]
3. Uterine manipulator and port placement as well as docking of robot are performed as described elsewhere in this article.
4. The retroperitoneum is dissected bilaterally to create paravesical and pararectal spaces.
5. The near-infrared fluorescence imaging is activated on the robotic platform.
6. The sentinel lymph nodes are identified and biopsied.
7. If there is no mapping, side-specific lymphadenectomy is performed as described elsewhere in this article.

Robotic Myomectomy

Myomectomy is indicated for a woman with the following conditions who desires uterine retention:

- Abnormal uterine bleeding owing to leiomyoma refractory to medical management or causing severe anemia.
- Urinary frequency or ureteral obstruction.
- Pelvic pain or pressure that compromises quality of life.
- Infertility secondary to myomas distorting the uterine cavity that cannot be removed by hysteroscopy,[9–11] large (>5 cm) intramural myomas with a history of prior adverse pregnancy outcome or failed in vitro fertilization.[12] The quality of evidence to support a benefit for improved fertility or improved pregnancy outcome from removal of myomas not distorting the uterine cavity is mixed at best.[11,13]
- Patients desiring myomectomy for infertility should have alternative etiologies investigated by an infertility evaluation, and concurrence on procedural plans from a reproductive endocrinologist.[11]
- Large myomas causing distortion of the abdominal wall that are of concern to the patient.[14]

Port placement

- Depending on the overall size of myomatous uterus, 8-mm port sites may be placed more laterally or cephalad for adequate visualization of large leiomyomas.
- Both accessory ports and laparoscopic ports should be at least 15 cm above uterus.
- This procedure may require two ports on each side of the abdomen and an epigastric port for the endoscope.
- A third robotic operating arm is useful for retraction and countertraction, especially with a robotic single-tooth tenaculum.

Steps before enucleation

1. All pelvic structures and the abdominal cavity are inspected. The number, site, and location of myomas are noted. If other pathologies are seen, they are usually treated before myomectomy.
2. For broad ligament and cervical myomas, the ureter is dissected from the pelvic brim to the cardinal ligament.[15]
3. Vasopressin is injected with a spinal needle directly into myometrium through the abdominal wall for hemostasis (see the gynecologic vasopressin protocol).[16,17]
4. The uterine arteries are temporarily occluded (if indicated by large myoma size or cervical myoma).[18]

Enucleation

1. Ideally, a transverse uterine incision is made near the base of the myoma using either unmodulated unipolar energy or harmonic energy. An anterior uterine incision is preferred, if feasible[19,20].
2. Extend the uterine incision into the pearly white myomatous tissue to avoid dissection in the vascular capsule.[21]
3. Grasp the myoma with a tenaculum to manipulate and apply traction.[22]
4. For large myomas with restricted upper abdominal space, enucleation should not be accomplished by pushing the capsule off the myoma (like peeling a glove off a hand). Traction on the myoma should not be the primary force responsible for enucleation.[23]
5. The myoma does not have to be separated completely from the capsule, which can be excised with the myoma.[23,24]
6. In situ morcellation is an option if upper abdominal space is not adequate to contain the enucleated myoma.[24]
7. Brisk bleeding during enucleation can be controlled with judicious application of bipolar energy or by loop ligation of the myoma capsule.
8. Limit the number of uterine incisions by enucleating additional myomas through the same incision if possible.[20]
9. Laparoscopic ultrasound examination is an available adjunct for multiple myomectomy to ensure removal of all myoma.[25,26]
10. Enucleated leiomyomas are placed in the posterior cul-de-sac and accounted for by stringing them on a suture and removing them from the pelvis through a mini-laparotomy after uterine reconstruction. Alternatively, a 12-mm trocar and port are used to enter the posterior cul-de-sac. A specimen bag is used to retrieve leiomyomas by vaginal extraction (Video 1).

Uterine reconstruction

1. After enucleation of all myomas through the uterine incision, fill the uterus with methylene blue-normal saline solution to check for the integrity of the endometrial lining.
2. If entered, the endometrial cavity should be repaired with rapidly absorbed 4-0 monofilament suture that is excluded from the endometrial cavity.
3. The presence of multiple defects in the endometrial cavity is an indication for placement of a uterine stent.
4. The myometrial defect should be closed in multiple layers using delayed absorbable, running barbed suture in a baseball stitch fashion to decrease dead space.[27]

Prevention of adhesions

- After hemostasis is obtained, apply an absorbable adhesion barrier over the uterine incision(s) and wet with normal saline.[28]

Pregnancy after myomectomy

- Patients should be advised to use a contraceptive method for at least 3 months after myomectomy to ensure full healing of the myometrium.[29]
- Patients should be advised that uterine rupture occurs in approximately 1% of pregnancies after myomectomy. The indication for cesarean section after myomectomy is unclear.[30]

Robotic Sacrocolpopexy

Initially reported as an open abdominal procedure for management of vaginal vault prolapse after hysterectomy by Lane in 1962, indications for sacrocolpopexy (SC) have been widened to include management of pelvic organ prolapse that has a significant degree (stage ≥2) of apical descent.[31,32] The expansion of SC to include primary procedures has been facilitated by the application of RAL SC, an effective surgical treatment of apical prolapse with high anatomic cure rate and low complication rate.[33]

Apical descent or prolapse refers to loss of pelvic support at the level of the cervical ring, where the uterosacral–cardinal ligament complex provides suspension of the apex of the vagina by broad attachment to the pelvic sidewalls and presacral ligaments. Injury to the pericervical ring results in a change in the vaginal axis to a vertical position directly over the genital hiatus. When the vagina is in a more vertical position, it is no longer compressed against the levator muscles so increases in intra-abdominal pressure are directly transmitted to the vaginal apex in a downward direction toward the genital hiatus. Because of its high rate of anatomic success (approaching 95%) and high durability, SC is the gold standard for surgical management of apical prolapse. SC can be performed by laparotomy, CL, or RAL. SC can be extended posteriorly to the perineum for rectocele repair and can be combined with anterior rectopexy for concurrent management of rectal prolapse.[34] SC can be performed for post-hysterectomy vaginal prolapse or combined with supracervical hysterectomy for uterine or uterovaginal prolapse. Perhaps the only disadvantage of SC is its longer operating time and higher cost as compared with other operations for prolapse.

Surgical technique

1. Perform supracervical hysterectomy if the patient has a uterus.[35]
2. Develop the vesicovaginal space approximately 6 to 7 cm below the level of the external cervical os, taking care to avoid the bladder trigone.
3. Develop the rectovaginal space beginning 5 to 10 mm above the rectal dissection and extending down to the level of the perineum if a distal rectocele is present or if concurrent anterior rectopexy is planned.
4. Fixation of type 1 polypropylene Y mesh to the anterior and posterior vagina can be done with permanent suture; however, monofilament delayed absorbable suture, for example, PDS or V-lock 180, seems to decrease the risk of graft and suture erosion without increasing the surgical failure rate.[36,37]
5. If using interrupted stiches, 6 to 8 sutures per side are adequate.
6. Expose a 1 × 1 cm^2 area of the anterior longitudinal ligament immediately adjacent and to the right of midline and below the L5–S1 interdisk space. This step is critical in the procedure because it is important to avoid the major vasculature, presacral veins, and right ureter.[38–40]
7. Create a tunnel in the right pararectal space by incising the peritoneum midway between the right ureter and the rectosigmoid colon.
8. Attach the sacral leg of the Y mesh to the anterior longitudinal ligament using permanent suture. A minimum of 2 stitches should be placed transversely with care to avoid puncturing the left common iliac vein upon exiting the anterior longitudinal ligament.[38] The suture should not be placed no more than 2 mm into the ligament so as to minimize the risk of L5–S1 diskitis.
9. The final step of the SC is closure of the peritoneal incision over the mesh.

REHABILITATION AND RECOVERY

One of the most significant benefits of robotic gynecologic surgery is expedited recovery and therefore early discharge from the hospital. Given no complications and significant medical conditions, patients undergoing robotic hysterectomy should be able to be discharged on the day of surgery. Otherwise, a 24-hour extended recovery admission is also practiced.

An ERAS program should be implemented after minimally invasive gynecologic surgery. The benefits of ERAS protocols have been well-studied in strong randomized trials in colorectal patients: reduced hospital stay, decreased postoperative complications, cost savings, and increased patient satisfaction.[41] There have also been multiple reports of similar benefits in gynecologic patients.[5,42–49]

Postoperative Recovery

- One dose of intravenous ketorolac 15 or 30 mg is given in the operating room if the procedure is hemostatic and the patient has adequate renal function.
- Transition to oral ibuprofen 800 mg every 6 hours and oral acetaminophen 975 mg every 8 hours as first-line analgesic treatment. If breakthrough pain occurs, oral narcotics (oxycodone, hydromorphone) may be considered sparingly.
- The Foley catheter is removed at the end of the procedure in the operating room.
- A regular diet is encouraged on the day of surgery.
- Intravenous fluids are minimized and discontinued when tolerating clear liquids.
- Early mobilization is encouraged within 24 hours.

If patients are tolerating a regular diet, voiding without difficulty, and have adequate pain control, they are discharged on the day of surgery. Instructions are given to avoid heavy lifting of more than 10 pounds and to place nothing in the vagina for at least 6 to 8 weeks. Routine outpatient postoperative visit is 2 weeks after surgery when a pelvic examination is performed to evaluate the integrity of the vaginal cuff.

CLINICAL RESULTS

The RAL surgical approach has improved gynecologic surgeries. It has the advantages of excellent visualization through the high-resolution 3-dimensional view, a wrist-like motion of the robotic arms and improved ergonomics.[50] Similar to CL, it is associated with a decrease in long-term surgical morbidity, early recovery and return to work, and improved aesthetics. However, both approaches are more likely to cause injuries than open surgeries related to trocar placement, delayed thermal gastrointestinal and urologic injuries, and vaginal cuff dehiscence.[51] Complications that are associated with the RAL approach may be a result of the use of excessive force or erroneous activation of cautery and mechanical breakdown. Results from the clinical research are detailed elsewhere in this article.

Robotic-Assisted Laparoscopic Hysterectomy

In benign gynecologic surgeries, RAL procedures have not been shown to be superior to CL or laparotomy. In the 2013 American Association of Gynecologic Laparoscopists Position Statement, it is stated that RAL approach should not replace CL or vaginal approaches.[52] The underlying rationale may include the lack of significant differences between RAL and CL approaches in intraoperative and postoperative complications, surgical bleeding, infection, and 30-day mortality rates[53] (**Table 1**). Furthermore, operative time has been reported to be longer for RAL versus CL with a mean difference of 41.18 minutes, although it did not reach statistical significance. Studies on RAL in gynecologic malignancies reported longer operative time than CL approaches; the mean difference in operative time was 46 minutes in the RASHEC 2013 trial.[54,55] It is, however, noteworthy that in this study, the RAL was performed by one surgeon, whereas the data for CL

Table 1
Clinical comparison of RAL and CL in gynecologic surgery

	Intraoperative Complications	Postoperative Complications	Operative Time (Benign Cases)	Blood Transfusions	Hospital Stay (Benign Cases)
RAL	57/1000	172/1000	75–102.7 min	20/1000	1.4–3.6 d
CL	44/1000	140/1000	68.73–191.23 min	40/1000	0.87–3.53 d
Outcomes	No differences	No differences	No differences	No differences	No differences

were collected from five other surgeons. This factor presents a potential bias in their findings.

Robotic-Assisted Laparoscopic Radical Hysterectomy for Cervical Cancer

In a recent noninferiority study published in *The New England Journal of Medicine* by Pedro Ramirez and colleagues,[56] 631 women with stage IA1 (with lymphovascular invasion), IA2, and IB1 cervical cancers were randomized to undergo radical hysterectomy by minimally invasive surgery (319 patients) or radical abdominal hysterectomy (312 patients) approaches. In the minimally invasive group, 84.4% underwent CL and 15.6% underwent RAL radical hysterectomy. The study was closed prematurely in 4.5 years when the interim analysis demonstrated an inferior disease-free survival in the minimally invasive approach group. The radical abdominal hysterectomy group had a slightly more than 10% advantage in 4.5 years disease-free survival over minimally invasive surgery radical hysterectomy (96.5% vs 80.6%). Similarly, a 5% overall survival advantage at 3 years (99.0% vs 93.8%) was observed in the radical abdominal hysterectomy group.[56] Clinicians should be cautious when choosing a minimally invasive surgical approach to manage patients with early cervical cancer. Additional studies or refinement of surgical techniques are needed to assure us of the safety of continuing to perform minimally invasive radical hysterectomy.

Robotic-Assisted Surgery in Endometrial Cancer

In a randomized study comparing RAL with CL among 96 enrolled patients, the authors found lower mean pelvic node count with RAL (22 ± 8 vs 28 ± 10; $P<.001$) than CL; however, the numbers of para-aortic lymph node count were not inferior in the RAL than CL arms (mean, 20.9 ± 9.6 vs mean, 22 ± 11). Perioperative complications and readmission rates were no different between the two groups. The robotic-assisted group had longer operative time but less blood loss and shorter length of stay.[57] A retrospective study that reviewed 102 RAL versus 115 CL versus 79 open hysterectomies for endometrial cancer found longer operating time but shorter hospital stay and decreased wound infections in the minimally invasive groups. Furthermore, there were more blood transfusions for the open hysterectomy group than CL and RAL, respectively (19% vs 3% vs 2%).[58] In another large retrospective study including 432 patients, of whom 187 underwent RAL and 245 underwent CL, intraoperative complications were similar (1.6% vs 2.9%; $P = .525$), but the rate of urinary tract injuries was statistically higher in the CL than RAL group (2.9% vs 0%; $P = .02$). The operative time was longer (218 minutes vs 161 minutes; $P = .0001$), but the length of stay was shorter (1.96 days vs 2.45 days; $P = .016$) in the RAL group. There were no significant differences in transfusions, number of lymph nodes retrieved, readmission, or reoperations.[59]

Robotic-Assisted Laparoscopic Surgery for Endometriosis

There are few studies evaluating RAL versus CL for endometriosis. In the recent multicenter, randomized, controlled Laparoscopy vs. Robotic Surgery for Endometriosis

(LAROSE) trial, the mean operative time for robotic versus laparoscopic surgery was 106.6 ± 48.4 minutes versus 101.6 ± 63.2 minutes. There were no differences in blood loss, complications, and conversion rates to laparotomy. Quality-of-life analysis reported significant improvement at 6 weeks and 6 months in both RA and CL.[60] An earlier randomized study of 78 patients reported that the mean operative time with robotic approach was 191 minutes (range, 135–295 minutes) compared with 159 minutes (range, 85–320 minutes) with CL. They did not find any differences in blood loss, length of stay, complications, or conversion rates.[61] The same authors conducted a larger trial treating 273 patients with advanced stages of endometriosis and found that both techniques were excellent. Mean operative times were not significantly different, with 196 minutes (range, 185–209 minutes) in the RAL group, and 135 minutes (range, 115–156 minutes) in the CL group, nor were there statistically significant differences in blood loss and complications. However, there were more patients in the CL group who were discharged home on the day of surgery.[62] A review of six comparative retrospective studies showed longer operative time in five of the six studies, although there were no significant differences in complications. Although one study reported a decrease in pain score for RAL, the author concluded that RAL did not provide significantly more benefits than CL.

Robotic-Assisted Laparoscopic Myomectomy

Minimally invasive myomectomy, including robotic or laparoscopic assisted approach, is superior to abdominal myomectomy, as typified by smaller incisions, shorter hospitalizations, and less postoperative pain.[63] In a 2011 study of 575 myomectomies, RAL myomectomy was associated with decreased blood loss and length of hospital stay compared with CL and abdominal myomectomy.[64] A follow-up retrospective study reviewing 374 cases of myomectomy performed at the same institution between 1995 and 2009 demonstrated no differences in long-term bleeding or fertility outcomes between RAL, CL, or abdominal approaches.[65] RAL approach should be considered when myomectomy is planned.

Robotic-Assisted Laparoscopic Versus Conventional Laparoscopic Sacrocolpopexy

Both RAL and CL SC are used to treat women with pelvic organ prolapse. In two published, randomized trials comparing RAL and CL SC, there were no differences in intraoperative and postoperative complications, although operating time was longer in the RAL arm by 40.53 minutes.[66,67] In the trial randomizing 78 women with symptomatic and significant apical support loss, the RAL group had longer operating times (202.8 minutes vs 178.4 minutes; $P = .03$) and higher pain scores one week after surgery (3.5 ± 2.1 vs 2.6 ± 2.2; $P = .044$), although there were no differences in the cost and rate of adverse events.[67] In a single-center, blinded, randomized trial for women with stage 2 to 4 post-hysterectomy vaginal prolapse, longer operating time and increased pain and cost were reported in the RAL arm.[66]

Robotic Single-Site Gynecologic Surgery

Robotic single-site surgery in gynecology was first reported in 2010.[68] The single-site robotic platform using the gel port and curved trocars facilitate the performance of a variety of gynecologic surgeries. Robotic single-site hysterectomy has been compared with laparoscopic single-site hysterectomy in several retrospective studies. Robotic-assisted single-site hysterectomy has a longer mean operating time in all studies compared with a laparoscopic approach.[69–71] Decreased time in vaginal closure and blood loss was noted in robotic-assisted single-site hysterectomy. Two retrospective studies on myomectomy reported the removal of myomas up to the size of 12.8 cm.

The mean operative time was 135 ± 59.62 minutes (range, 60–295 minutes), the mean blood loss was 182.00 ± 153.02 mL (range, 10–600 mL), and the mean skin incision length was 2.70 ± 0.19 cm (range, 2.40–3.10 cm).[72,73] Two patients needed blood transfusions. There were no other intraoperative or postoperative complications. Robotic-assisted single-site hysterectomy was found to be safe and feasible for hysterectomy. The robotic-assisted approach seems to help the surgeons overcome the technical barriers of a CL approach. Robotic-assisted single-site laparoscopic surgeries have also been performed in gynecologic cancers. The two retrospective studies that compared robotic-assisted versus laparoscopic single-site surgeries demonstrated similar operative time (102 vs 100 minutes) with less blood loss and length of stay in the robotic-assisted single-site approach. There were no intraoperative complications reported in either group.[74,75] Additional randomized studies are needed to prospectively evaluate the role of single-site surgery in gynecology.

SUMMARY

The robotic surgical platform in gynecology has allowed clinicians to adopt minimally invasive surgery by learning to perform these procedures from a RAL approach. This technique has improved our abilities in laparoscopic suturing, knot-tying, lysis of adhesions, and retroperitoneal explorations, especially in patients with large uteri. The technology has enabled general gynecologists to overcome challenges that are associated with laparoscopic surgery, and gynecologic oncologists to perform more complex surgeries, including dissections in retroperitoneal spaces. The major barriers to performing robotic surgeries are cost, training of practitioners, and lack of long-term outcomes data. Based on the existing literature, RAL surgery is considered potentially beneficial in RAL hysterectomy, and in procedures for endometrial cancer, leiomyoma, and endometriosis. Because of its potential negative impact on progression-free survival when RAL radical hysterectomy is performed on women with early-stage cervical cancer, clinicians should be cautious in its use and consider the exploratory laparotomy approach. There is a need for additional research on what measures can be taken to contain cervical cancer and to perform the procedure without the use of a uterine manipulator. There is a limited role in the use of the robotic-assisted approach in sacrocolpexy if the practitioner is able to perform the procedure with CL. The single-site RAL approach is compelling and has the potential to gain popularity with further refinement of robotic surgical tools.

DISCLOSURE

There are no commercial or financial conflicts of interest or funding sources for all authors.

SUPPLEMENTARY DATA

Supplementary data to this article can be found online at https://doi.org/10.1016/j.suc.2019.12.007.

REFERENCES

1. Lanfranco AR, Castellanos AE, Desai JP, et al. Robotic surgery: a current perspective. Ann Surg 2004;239(1):14–21.
2. Bouquet de Joliniere J, Librino A, Dubuisson JB, et al. Robotic surgery in gynecology. Front Surg 2016;3:26.

3. Sinha R, Sanjay M, Rupa B, et al. Robotic surgery in gynecology. J Minim Access Surg 2015;11(1):50–9.
4. Parker WH. The utility of MRI for the surgical treatment of women with uterine fibroid tumors. Am J Obstet Gynecol 2012;206(1):31–6.
5. de Groot JJ, Ament SM, Maessen JM, et al. Enhanced recovery pathways in abdominal gynecologic surgery: a systematic review and meta-analysis. Acta Obstet Gynecol Scand 2016;95(4):382–95.
6. Hausel J, Nygren J, Thorell A, et al. Randomized clinical trial of the effects of oral preoperative carbohydrates on postoperative nausea and vomiting after laparoscopic cholecystectomy. Br J Surg 2005;92(4):415–21.
7. Jones HW, Rock JA. Te Linde's operative gynecology. Wolters Kluwer Health; 2015.
8. Jewell EL, Huang JJ, Abu-Rustum NR, et al. Detection of sentinel lymph nodes in minimally invasive surgery using indocyanine green and near-infrared fluorescence imaging for uterine and cervical malignancies. Gynecol Oncol 2014; 133(2):274–7.
9. Seracchioli R, Rossi S, Govoni F, et al. Fertility and obstetric outcome after laparoscopic myomectomy of large myomata: a randomized comparison with abdominal myomectomy. Hum Reprod 2000;15(12):2663–8.
10. Somigliana E, Vercellini P, Daguati R, et al. Fibroids and female reproduction: a critical analysis of the evidence. Hum Reprod Update 2007;13(5):465–76.
11. Pritts EA, Parker WH, Olive DL. Fibroids and infertility: an updated systematic review of the evidence. Fertil Steril 2009;91(4):1215–23.
12. Casini ML, Rossi F, Agostini R, et al. Effects of the position of fibroids on fertility. Gynecol Endocrinol 2006;22(2):106–9.
13. Sunkara SK, Khairy M, El-Toukhy T, et al. The effect of intramural fibroids without uterine cavity involvement on the outcome of IVF treatment: a systematic review and meta-analysis. Hum Reprod 2010;25(2):418–29.
14. Sinha R, Hegde A, Warty N, et al. Laparoscopic myomectomy: enucleation of the myoma by morcellation while it is attached to the uterus. J Minim Invasive Gynecol 2005;12(3):284–9.
15. Chang WC, Chen SY, Huang SC, et al. Strategy of cervical myomectomy under laparoscopy. Fertil Steril 2010;94(7):2710–5.
16. Frederick J, Fletcher H, Simeon D, et al. Intramyometrial vasopressin as a haemostatic agent during myomectomy. Br J Obstet Gynaecol 1994;101(5):435–7.
17. Ginsburg ES, Benson CB, Garfield JM, et al. The effect of operative technique and uterine size on blood loss during myomectomy: a prospective randomized study. Fertil Steril 1993;60(6):956–62.
18. Sinha R, Sundaram M, Lakhotia S, et al. Cervical myomectomy with uterine artery ligation at its origin. J Minim Invasive Gynecol 2009;16(5):604–8.
19. Diamond MP. Reduction of adhesions after uterine myomectomy by Seprafilm membrane (HAL-F): a blinded, prospective, randomized, multicenter clinical study. Seprafilm Adhesion Study Group. Fertil Steril 1996;66(6):904–10.
20. Guarnaccia MM, Rein MS. Traditional surgical approaches to uterine fibroids: abdominal myomectomy and hysterectomy. Clin Obstet Gynecol 2001;44(2): 385–400.
21. Discepola F, Valenti DA, Reinhold C, et al. Analysis of arterial blood vessels surrounding the myoma: relevance to myomectomy. Obstet Gynecol 2007;110(6): 1301–3.
22. Hasson HM, Rotman C, Rana N, et al. Laparoscopic myomectomy. Obstet Gynecol 1992;80(5):884–8.

23. Sinha R, Hegde A, Warty N, et al. Laparoscopic excision of very large myomas. J Am Assoc Gynecol Laparosc 2003;10(4):461–8.

24. Chang WC, Huang PS, Wang PH, et al. Comparison of laparoscopic myomectomy using in situ morcellation with and without uterine artery ligation for treatment of symptomatic myomas. J Minim Invasive Gynecol 2012;19(6):715–21.

25. Angioli R, Battista C, Terranova C, et al. Intraoperative contact ultrasonography during open myomectomy for uterine fibroids. Fertil Steril 2010;94(4):1487–90.

26. Lin PC, Thyer A, Soules MR. Intraoperative ultrasound during a laparoscopic myomectomy. Fertil Steril 2004;81(6):1671–4.

27. Seinera P, Farina C, Todros T. Laparoscopic myomectomy and subsequent pregnancy: results in 54 patients. Hum Reprod 2000;15(9):1993–6.

28. Farquhar C, Vandekerckhove P, Watson A, et al. Barrier agents for preventing adhesions after surgery for subfertility. Cochrane Database Syst Rev 2000;(2):CD000475.

29. Tsuji S, Takahashi K, Imaoka I, et al. MRI evaluation of the uterine structure after myomectomy. Gynecol Obstet Invest 2006;61(2):106–10.

30. Hurst BS, Matthews ML, Marshburn PB. Laparoscopic myomectomy for symptomatic uterine myomas. Fertil Steril 2005;83(1):1–23.

31. Lane FE. Repair of posthysterectomy vaginal-vault prolapse. Obstet Gynecol 1962;20:72–7.

32. Parkes IL, Shveiky D. Sacrocolpopexy for treatment of vaginal apical prolapse: evidence-based surgery. J Minim Invasive Gynecol 2014;21(4):546–57.

33. Hudson CO, Northington GM, Lyles RH, et al. Outcomes of robotic sacrocolpopexy: a systematic review and meta-analysis. Female Pelvic Med Reconstr Surg 2014;20(5):252–60.

34. Jallad K, Barber MD, Ridgeway B, et al. The effect of surgical start time in patients undergoing minimally invasive sacrocolpopexy. Int Urogynecol J 2016; 27(10):1535–9.

35. Meriwether KV, Antosh DD, Olivera CK, et al. Uterine preservation vs hysterectomy in pelvic organ prolapse surgery: a systematic review with meta-analysis and clinical practice guidelines. Am J Obstet Gynecol 2018;219(2):129–46.e2.

36. Shepherd JP, Higdon HL 3rd, Stanford EJ, et al. Effect of suture selection on the rate of suture or mesh erosion and surgery failure in abdominal sacrocolpopexy. Female Pelvic Med Reconstr Surg 2010;16(4):229–33.

37. Tan-Kim J, Nager CW, Grimes CL, et al. A randomized trial of vaginal mesh attachment techniques for minimally invasive sacrocolpopexy. Int Urogynecol J 2015;26(5):649–56.

38. Abernethy M, Vasquez E, Kenton K, et al. Where do we place the sacrocolpopexy stitch? A magnetic resonance imaging investigation. Female Pelvic Med Reconstr Surg 2013;19(1):31–3.

39. Flynn MK, Romero AA, Amundsen CL, et al. Vascular anatomy of the presacral space: a fresh tissue cadaver dissection. Am J Obstet Gynecol 2005;192(5): 1501–5.

40. Wieslander CK, Rahn DD, McIntire DD, et al. Vascular anatomy of the presacral space in unembalmed female cadavers. Am J Obstet Gynecol 2006;195(6): 1736–41.

41. Greco M, Capretti G, Beretta L, et al. Enhanced recovery program in colorectal surgery: a meta-analysis of randomized controlled trials. World J Surg 2014; 38(6):1531–41.

42. Carter J. Enhanced recovery in gynecologic surgery. Obstet Gynecol 2013; 122(6):1305.

43. Dowdy SC, Nelson G. Enhanced recovery in gynecologic oncology - a sea change in perioperative management. Gynecol Oncol 2017;146(2):225–7.

44. Kalogera E, Dowdy SC. Enhanced recovery pathway in gynecologic surgery: improving outcomes through evidence-based medicine. Obstet Gynecol Clin North Am 2016;43(3):551–73.

45. Lindemann K, Kok PS, Stockler M, et al. Enhanced recovery after surgery for advanced ovarian cancer: a systematic review of interventions trialed. Int J Gynecol Cancer 2017;27(6):1274–82.

46. Miralpeix E, Nick AM, Meyer LA, et al. A call for new standard of care in perioperative gynecologic oncology practice: impact of enhanced recovery after surgery (ERAS) programs. Gynecol Oncol 2016;141(2):371–8.

47. Modesitt SC, Sarosiek BM, Trowbridge ER, et al. Enhanced recovery implementation in major gynecologic surgeries: effect of care standardization. Obstet Gynecol 2016;128(3):457–66.

48. Myriokefalitaki E, Smith M, Ahmed AS. Implementation of enhanced recovery after surgery (ERAS) in gynaecological oncology. Arch Gynecol Obstet 2016; 294(1):137–43.

49. Nelson G, Kalogera E, Dowdy SC. Enhanced recovery pathways in gynecologic oncology. Gynecol Oncol 2014;135(3):586–94.

50. Soto E, Lo Y, Friedman K, et al. Total laparoscopic hysterectomy versus Da Vinci robotic hysterectomy: is using the robot beneficial? J Gynecol Oncol 2011;22(4): 253–9.

51. Kho RM, Hilger WS, Hentz JG, et al. Robotic hysterectomy: technique and initial outcomes. Am J Obstet Gynecol 2007;197(1):113.e1–4.

52. AAGL Advancing Minimally Invasive Gynecology Worldwide. AAGL position statement: robotic-assisted laparoscopic surgery in benign gynecology. J Minim Invasive Gynecol 2013;20(1):2–9.

53. Lawrie TA, Liu H, Lu D, et al. Robot-assisted surgery in gynaecology. Cochrane Database Syst Rev 2019;(4):CD01142.

54. Salehi S, Åvall-Lundqvist E, Brandberg Y, et al. Lymphedema, serious adverse events, and imaging 1 year after comprehensive staging for endometrial cancer: results from the RASHEC trial. Int J Gynecol Cancer 2019;29(1):86–93.

55. Soto E, Lo Y, Friedman K, et al. Total laparoscopic hysterectomy versus Da Vinci Robotic hysterectomy: is using the robot beneficial? J Gynecol Oncol 2011;22(4): 253–9.

56. Ramirez PT, Frumovitz M, Pareja R, et al. Minimally invasive versus abdominal radical hysterectomy for cervical cancer. N Engl J Med 2018;379(20):1895–904.

57. Salehi S, Åvall-Lundqvist E, Legerstam B, et al. Robot-assisted laparoscopy versus laparotomy for infrarenal paraaortic lymphadenectomy in women with high-risk endometrial cancer: a randomised controlled trial. Eur J Cancer 2017; 79:81–9.

58. Nicole N, Rachel C, Michael M, et al. Robotic assisted, total laparoscopic, and total abdominal hysterectomy for management of uterine cancer. J Cancer Ther 2012;3(2):162–6.

59. Cardenas-Goicoechea J, Soto E, Chuang L, et al. Integration of robotics into two established programs of minimally invasive surgery for endometrial cancer appears to decrease surgical complications. J Gynecol Oncol 2013;24(1):21–8.

60. Soto E, Luu TH, Liu X, et al. Laparoscopy vs. robotic surgery for endometriosis (LAROSE): a multicenter, randomized, controlled trial. Fertil Steril 2017;107(4): 996–1002.e3.

61. Nezhat C, Lewis M, Kotikela S, et al. Robotic versus standard laparoscopy for the treatment of endometriosis. Fertil Steril 2010;94(7):2758–60.

62. Nezhat CR, Stevens A, Balassiano E, et al. Robotic-assisted laparoscopy vs conventional laparoscopy for the treatment of advanced stage endometriosis. J Minim Invasive Gynecol 2015;22(1):40–4.

63. Falcone T, Bedaiwy MA. Minimally invasive management of uterine fibroids. Curr Opin Obstet Gynecol 2002;14(4):401–7.

64. Barakat EE, Bedaiwy MA, Zimberg S, et al. Robotic-assisted, laparoscopic, and abdominal myomectomy: a comparison of surgical outcomes. Obstet Gynecol 2011;117(2 Pt 1):256–65.

65. Soto E, Flyckt R, Falcone T. Endoscopic management of uterine fibroids: an update. Minerva Ginecol 2012;64(6):507–20.

66. Paraiso MF, Jelovsek JE, Frick A, et al. Laparoscopic compared with robotic sacrocolpopexy for vaginal prolapse: a randomized controlled trial. Obstet Gynecol 2011;118(5):1005–13.

67. Anger JT, Mueller ER, Tarnay C, et al. Robotic compared with laparoscopic sacrocolpopexy: a randomized controlled trial. Obstet Gynecol 2014;123(1):5–12.

68. Kane S, Stepp KJ. Laparo-endoscopic single-site surgery hysterectomy using robotic lightweight endoscope assistants. J Robot Surg 2010;3(4):253–5.

69. Akdemir A, Yildirim N, Zeybek B, et al. Single incision trans-umbilical total hysterectomy: robotic or laparoscopic? Gynecol Obstet Invest 2015;80(2):93–8.

70. Lopez S, Mulla ZD, Hernandez L, et al. A comparison of outcomes between robotic-assisted, single-site laparoscopy versus laparoendoscopic single site for benign hysterectomy. J Minim Invasive Gynecol 2016;23(1):84–8.

71. Paek J, Lee JD, Kong TW, et al. Robotic single-site versus laparoendoscopic single-site hysterectomy: a propensity score matching study. Surg Endosc 2016;30(3):1043–50.

72. Gargiulo AR, Bailey AP, Srouji SS. Robot-assisted single-incision laparoscopic myomectomy: initial report and technique. J Robot Surg 2013;7(2):137–42.

73. Choi EJ, Rho AM, Lee SR, et al. Robotic single-site myomectomy: clinical analysis of 61 consecutive cases. J Minim Invasive Gynecol 2017;24(4):632–9.

74. Moukarzel LA, Sinno AK, Fader AN, et al. Comparing single-site and multiport robotic hysterectomy with sentinel lymph node mapping for endometrial cancer: surgical outcomes and cost analysis. J Minim Invasive Gynecol 2017;24(6):977–83.

75. Corrado G, Mereu L, Bogliolo S, et al. Robotic single site staging in endometrial cancer: a multi-institution study. Eur J Surg Oncol 2016;42(10):1506–11.

Complications of Robotic Surgery

Ramón Díaz Jara, MD, Alfredo D. Guerrón, MD, Dana Portenier, MD*

KEYWORDS

- Complications robotic surgery • Robotic malfunction • Intraoperative complications
- Robotic disadvantages • Patient positioning

KEY POINTS

- Increasing numbers of procedures are being perform using robotic-assisted platforms.
- Despite its benefits, complications occur in all aspects and stages of surgery including the preoperative, intraoperative, and postoperative periods.
- Robotic surgery has no specific surgery-related complications, but equipment malfunction and poor surgeons' training might be associated with impaired patient safety.
- Optimal equipment maintenance and troubleshooting and continuous surgeon and robotic team training, are essential to obtain the maximum benefit of using robotic devices and avoid complications.
- Complications and equipment malfunctioning should be reported promptly to improve patient outcomes.

INTRODUCTION

Without a doubt, robotic-assisted surgery has represented a revolution for surgical practice and minimally invasive surgery. Currently, several platforms are being used to perform a wide variety of procedures with different degrees of success and applications. Surgeons and industry reported better outcomes compared with conventional laparoscopy owing to several technological improvements, such as enhanced visualization owing to the 3-dimensional interface, tremor filtration, improved wrist motion freedom, motion scaling, and improved ergonomics owing to a more comfortable user interface.[1] Nowadays, robotic surgical systems are being used in a wide variety of procedures and specialties including cardiothoracic, urology, endocrine surgery, metabolic and bariatric surgery, head and neck surgery, and all the intra-abdominal surgery subspecialties. The case volume is increasing exponentially and the numbers continue to grow particularly owing to urology and general surgery

Division of Metabolic and Weight Loss Surgery, Department of Surgery, Duke University Health System, 407 Crutchfield Street, Durham, NC 27704, USA
* Corresponding author.
E-mail address: dana.portenier@duke.edu

Surg Clin N Am 100 (2020) 461–468
https://doi.org/10.1016/j.suc.2019.12.008
0039-6109/20/© 2019 Elsevier Inc. All rights reserved.

subspecialties. In 2017, approximately 877,000 robotic procedures were performed worldwide with the da Vinci Surgical System (Intuitive Surgical Systems, Sunnyvale, CA). This showed an increment compared with the 753,000 and 652,000 procedures performed in 2016 and 2015, respectively.[2]

Nonetheless, robotic surgery is not exempt from complications. It is not the intention of this article to go over complications inherent to particular procedures or specialties, but rather to categorize the complications to better understand the clinical implications and develop strategies for prevention. Like any other surgical intervention, complications can occur during the preoperative, intraoperative, and postoperative periods. Owing to the use of a platform that is controlled at a distance from the patient, it is worth reviewing issues in the aforementioned periods but also issues related to patient preparation, team dynamics, equipment failure, complications related to the surgical act, and surgical outcomes. In this article, we address the different obstacles presented by the use of this new technology.

BENEFITS OF ROBOTIC SURGERY

The benefits of robotic surgery have been reported in a variety of reports and publications. It has been postulated that robotic platforms properly integrate the surgeon into the surgical field and overcomes the disadvantages of laparoscopic surgery. Reports generated from the most widely used robotic platform suggest a smooth transition from open to minimal access techniques as a result of the technology, which improves visualization, provides enhanced manipulation of tissue by virtue of the wrist-like movement adapted to almost all the instruments, and less dependence on the surgical assistants for exposure and manipulation of the camera.

Several publications have reported that robotic surgery equals or even improves outcomes obtained by laparoscopic surgery in different specialties.[3–5] Such reports suggest that the benefits are not limited to patients, but are for surgeons as well.

Ergonomics must be specially addressed during surgery, particularly given the aging surgical workforce. Laparoscopic surgery has been associated with ergonomic issues owing to prolonged operative times, unnatural body postures, and positioning of trocars.[6,7] The robotic platforms offer the option to decrease some of these issues by providing a comfortable seating or neutral posture position, avoiding forced unnatural movements and delegating the torqueing forces to the robotic arms, decreasing the burden on surgeon's muscles in the sensitive areas like the neck, shoulders, and upper back. The ergonomic benefits can potentially help surgeon career longevity. Data have shown that, during laparoscopic procedures, a greater number of muscle groups are activated compared with robotic surgery, which implies ergonomic benefits of robotic surgery over traditional laparoscopic approach.[8] In addition, the robotic interface provides the opportunity to enhance training and education with the use of dual consoles.

ROBOT DISADVANTAGES

Robotic surgery presents several disadvantages. The robot platform requires larger operating room (OR) suites to accommodate the robotic arms, consoles, and computer towers. In some institutions, the limited OR space is creating issues with patients, staff, and equipment mobilization. The robotic platforms require the manipulation of their mechanical arms to access the surgical field and have not completely eliminated the need for assistance. A trained bedside assistant is required to perform a variety of tasks, including docking and undocking, instrument exchange, introduction and retrieval of surgical supplies (sutures, needles, staples, clips, gauze pads, etc), and in some situations provide additional exposure.

Another primary concern for surgeons is the absence of haptic sensation. Haptics is defined as the tactile feedback from the console to the surgeon's hand. Loss of touch sensation combined with the strength of robotic arms might lead to technical errors, increased operative times, and learning curves.[9] Lacking touch sensation feedback might lead to excessive use of force when handling tissues and cause inadvertent damage.

Like any device that implies an advanced technology, the robotic platform has shown higher costs when compared with other approaches.[10,11] The implementation of robotic surgery in an institution requires the maintenance and purchase of robotic supplies, both of which carry a significant economic burden for institutions. A systematic review showed that the robot results in higher costs of purchase and maintenance, as well as longer operative times. However, when a high number of robotic surgeries are performed, the procedure can be cost effective.[12]

COMPLICATIONS RELATED TO THE PATIENT POSITIONING

Injuries owing to incorrect patient positioning can be an issue. As in laparoscopic surgery, the surgery team must be aware of the possibility of having nerve injuries owing to patient's positioning,[13] as they have also been described in robotic surgery.[14] Trendelenburg's position requires special consideration because it has been related to operative complications and certain limitations particularly in older models of the Intuitive platform. Prior models were limited to single quadrant operations owing to the inability to alter the position in the OR table and move the table to accommodate the surgical field. This obstacle has been overcome with the newer version of the DaVinci platform. Prolonged operative times have been described in robotic procedures compared with laparoscopic, incurring in visual complications, cardiopulmonary complications, endotracheal tube displacement, and nerve injuries.[15] Facial protection must also be addressed and, for this purpose, there are now available commercial devices to manage this issue. Other surgical positions can result in nerve and soft tissue injuries, particularly during procedures that require bending of the operating table to create space between bony structures, such as robotic ventral hernia, in which the table has to be bent at the patient's hips to increase the distance from the subcostal margin and the pelvis and to avoid collision of the robotic arms with the patient's thighs.

Special attention must be paid with the positioning of trocars to avoid internal or external collisions of arms.[16] The latter is important because robotic arms may hit the bedside assistant or the patient. Obtaining an optimal position during the procedure is essential for the team. A newer version of the Davinci platform offers digital assistance for port placement based on target anatomy.

COMPLICATIONS RELATED TO ROBOT MALFUNCTION

We should not expect specific complications related to robotic surgery because it is the same approach as with laparoscopic surgery. Likewise, most of the risk factors reported are similar to those described for laparoscopic or open procedures.[17,18] Multiquadrant surgery has been described as a specific risk factor for complications in robotic surgery.[17,19] However, the latest da Vinci Xi, given its design, might overcome this disadvantage allowing single-dock multiquadrant surgery.[20] Hitherto, the da Vinci platform has shown not only feasibility and reproducibility, but safety, reliability, and advantages in some complex procedures.[21,22]

Nevertheless, the robotic platforms are complex equipment, integrated by different mechanical parts. The equipment and software might be defective during surgeries, which can change the surgeon's plan and compromise the safety of the surgery.

Robot malfunctions have been reported between 0.4% and 4.6%.[23,24] Borden and colleagues[25] described a robotic failure during 350 robotic-assisted radical prostatectomies. Nine procedures (2.6%) were not completed robotically owing to robotic failure. Six malfunctions were identified before the procedure began; thus, the surgeries were canceled and rescheduled. The 3 remaining malfunctions occurred while surgery was being performed, and the procedure was converted to either laparoscopic (n = 1) or open surgery (n = 2). The most common defects were setup joint malfunction (n = 2) and arm malfunction (n = 2). Kozlowski[24] described a series of 130 robotic-assisted prostatectomies where they had 6 robotic failures (4.6%). The most common malfunction was also set up joint malfunction (n = 2). Other series have described that the robotic instruments may be the most common cause of failure.[26,27]

The US Food and Drug Administration registers all the national robotic adverse events through the Manufacturer and User Facility Device Experience (MAUDE) database. United States health institutions can anonymously and voluntarily report adverse events, and the manufactures can offer a response. These complete reports are regularly monitored to detect and correct robot-related safety issues promptly.

In 2007, Andonian and colleagues[28] published a comprehensive review of the MAUDE database from 2000 to 2007. The authors found a failure rate of 0.38%, and the da Vinci robotic system was the cause of 168 robotic failures during that period. They also noted that the adverse events increased each year, but this was likely related to the increase in the number of robotic procedures. Recently, Alemzadeh and colleagues[29] performed a comprehensive MAUDE database analysis finding 10,624 adverse events related to robotic systems and instruments between 2000 and 2013. In this same period, it was expected that in the United States, 1,745,000 robotic procedures were performed and the number of adverse events per procedure was approximately 0.6%. Gynecology and urology reported the highest numbers of adverse events (86% of all robotic procedures). However, this incidence can be explained because of the greater number of procedures done by these 2 specialties. Broken pieces that fell into the surgical field (14.7%) and electrical issues (10.5%) (electrical arcing, sparking, or charring) were the most common described problems. The authors reported 410 injuries related to robotic procedures, most of the time owing to device malfunctions.

Moreover, 86 reports informed about deaths in robotic procedures; 50% of these deaths were owing to the inherent risks and complications of the performed procedure.[29] None of the reports indicated that the robotic malfunctions were the cause of deaths during the procedure, although 31.4% of the reports do not have the specific cause of death. The MAUDE database has shown that conversions to laparoscopic or open surgery and procedure abortion are rarely seen.[30] However, the limitation of these studies is that the reports to the MAUDE database are voluntary and therefore it is likely that not all the platform malfunctions are being appropriately reported.

COMPLICATIONS RELATED TO THE SURGERY AND IN THE POSTOPERATIVE PERIOD

In colorectal and esophageal surgeries, the robotic platform has not shown any specific disadvantage; it has even been shown to be more beneficial in surgeries in smaller spaces such as the male pelvis in rectal cancer.[31,32] In bariatric surgery, recently, Rogula and colleagues[33] study did not describe any clinical advantage of robotic surgery over conventional laparoscopic gastric bypass, and robotic gastric bypass actually increased the operative time. A meta-analysis comparing robotic and laparoscopic approach for gastric bypass did not find differences in 30-day mortality and readmission, but robotic surgery showed longer operative times as well.[34]

A Metabolic and Bariatric Surgery Accreditation and Quality Improvement Program database revision of robotic and laparoscopic sleeve gastrectomies found that leaks, surgical site infections, and operative time are higher in robotic surgery.[35] Longer operative times have also been found when gastric resections using robotic surgery are done owing to gastric cancer.[36] Recently, a group from the University of Virginia published a propensity-matched analysis comparing robotic and laparoscopic cholecystectomy. The authors found that the robotic approach had longer operative times and higher hospital costs compared with laparoscopic cholecystectomy.[37]

ROBOTIC TEAMS

This concept should be added to our surgical practice. Like other surgical procedures, robotic surgery is best performed when surgeons are exposed to a significant number of cases. The benefits of robotic surgery can be increased when they are performed in high-volume centers.[38] As more robotic procedures are performed, a lower incidence of complications is observed.[14,39] It is not clear how many surgeries trainees must do, but it varies by surgical procedures. Surgeons who aim to begin their robotic training must be under the supervision of experienced robotic surgeons and assisted by an appropriate operation room team as well. Every person inside the OR who is involved in the robotic surgery must be familiar with the platform and be prepared to face any challenge. Concentrating the number of cases in designated experienced personnel will optimize time and costs, which is one the most concerning issues for health institutions. Besides, the institutions that invest and support the programs of robotic surgery will have the opportunity of increasing the number of patients who, owing to the knowledge of the benefits of robotic surgery, look for hospitals that have a robot.[40]

ROBOTIC TRAINING

Currently, there is no standard curriculum for training in robotic surgery. Without a doubt, surgeons need a simulation experience before they start live cases. Live robot simulators with skill exercises (tower transfer, suture, etc) are available for training purposes.[41] Nevertheless, training on these live modules can be challenging because sometimes consoles could be in use all day, and scheduling a training session could be challenging. To overcome this issue, a virtual robot simulator can be an option for skills training.[42] It is also very important that trainees be taught to solve the most common robotic hardware and software malfunctions to avoid unnecessary conversions or surgery cancellations. It is not clear yet how robotic skills deteriorate over time, so surgeons who are not being involved in an adequate number of surgeries should be prepared and willing to practice in the simulator again.

SUMMARY

Robotic surgery represents a significant advance for surgical procedures. Despite the benefits that it entails, its practice is not exempt from complications that range from delay or cancellation of the surgeries to those that severely compromise the patient's outcomes. Once a robotic program is launched in a hospital, appropriate training for surgeons and other personnel who are going to be involved in robotic procedures must be provided to avoid incorrect use of the robot. Likewise, thorough maintenance must be carried out on all the components that make up the robot, as well as the instruments that will be used during the surgeries. The report of the robotic failures or instruments and their results must be correctly reported to the manufacturer to provide a quick and efficient solution by them. Although robotic surgery is expensive, if the cases are concentrated in centralized hospitals, a properly trained team is involved, and general maintenance is given to the robot, the surgery can be cost effective and represent a real advantage over other minimally invasive surgery modalities.

DISCLOSURE

R.D. Jara has nothing to disclose. A.D. Guerron – speaker for GORE and Medtronic, consultant Biom'up, Levita, Phenomix. D. Portenier - Educational grant from Levita Magnetics. Consultant for Intuitive and Medtronic.

REFERENCES

1. Peters BS, Armijo PR, Krause C, et al. Review of emerging surgical robotic technology. Surg Endosc 2018;32(4):1636–55.
2. Intuitive surgical 2017 annual report. Sunnyvale (CA): 2017. p. 44–5.
3. Porpiglia F, Fiori C, Bertolo R, et al. Five-year outcomes for a prospective randomised controlled trial comparing laparoscopic and robot-assisted radical prostatectomy. Eur Urol Focus 2018;4(1):80–6.
4. Prete FP, Pezzolla A, Prete F, et al. Robotic versus laparoscopic minimally invasive surgery for rectal cancer: a systematic review and meta-analysis of randomized controlled trials. Ann Surg 2018;267(6):1034–46.
5. Tsung A, Geller DA, Sukato DC, et al. Robotic versus laparoscopic hepatectomy: a matched comparison. Ann Surg 2014;259(3):549–55.
6. Berguer R, Forkey DL, Smith WD. Ergonomic problems associated with laparoscopic surgery. Surg Endosc 1999;13(5):466–8.
7. Janki S, Mulder EEAP, IJzermans JNM, et al. Ergonomics in the operating room. Surg Endosc 2017;31(6):2457–66.
8. Zarate Rodriguez JG, Zihni AM, Ohu I, et al. Ergonomic analysis of laparoscopic and robotic surgical task performance at various experience levels. Surg Endosc 2019;33(6):1938–43.
9. Toledo L, Gossot D, Fritsch S, et al. Study of sustained forces and the working space of endoscopic surgery instruments. Ann Chir 1999;53(7):587–97 [in French].
10. Finkelstein J, Eckersberger E, Sadri H, et al. Open versus laparoscopic versus robot-assisted laparoscopic prostatectomy: the European and US experience. Rev Urol 2010;12(1):35–43.
11. Steinberg PL, Merguerian PA, Bihrle W 3rd, et al. A da Vinci robot system can make sense for a mature laparoscopic prostatectomy program. JSLS 2008; 12(1):9–12.
12. Turchetti G, Palla I, Pierotti F, et al. Economic evaluation of da Vinci-assisted robotic surgery: a systematic review. Surg Endosc 2012;26(3):598–606.
13. Codd RJ, Evans MD, Sagar PM, et al. A systematic review of peripheral nerve injury following laparoscopic colorectal surgery. Colorectal Dis 2013;15(3): 278–82.
14. Ahmed F, Rhee J, Sutherland D, et al. Surgical complications after robot-assisted laparoscopic radical prostatectomy: the initial 1000 cases stratified by the Clavien classification system. J Endourol 2012;26(2):135–9.
15. Kaye AD, Vadivelu N, Ahuja N, et al. Anesthetic considerations in robotic-assisted gynecologic surgery. Ochsner J 2013;13(4):517–24.
16. Chang C, Steinberg Z, Shah A, et al. Patient positioning and port placement for robot-assisted surgery. J Endourol 2014;28(6):631–8.

17. Buchs NC, Addeo P, Bianco FM, et al. Perioperative risk assessment in robotic general surgery: lessons learned from 884 cases at a single institution. Arch Surg 2012;147(8):701–8.
18. Haga Y, Ikei S, Wada Y, et al. Evaluation of an Estimation of Physiologic Ability and Surgical Stress (E-PASS) scoring system to predict postoperative risk: a multicenter prospective study. Surg Today 2001;31(7):569–74.
19. Fantola G, Brunaud L, Nguyen-Thi P-L, et al. Risk factors for postoperative complications in robotic general surgery. Updates Surg 2017;69(1):45–54.
20. Protyniak B, Jorden J, Farmer R. Multiquadrant robotic colorectal surgery: the da Vinci Xi vs Si comparison. J Robot Surg 2018;12(1):67–74.
21. Strijker M, van Santvoort HC, Besselink MG, et al. Robot-assisted pancreatic surgery: a systematic review of the literature. HPB (Oxford) 2013;15(1):1–10.
22. Fahrner R, Rauchfuß F, Bauschke A, et al. Robotic hepatic surgery in malignancy: review of the current literature. J Robot Surg 2019;13(4):533–8.
23. Lavery HJ, Thaly R, Albala D, et al. Robotic equipment malfunction during robotic prostatectomy: a multi-institutional study. J Endourol 2008;22(9):2165–8.
24. Kozlowski PM. Mechanical failure rate of da Vinci(!R) robotic system: implantations for pre-op patient counseling. J Urol 2006;175:s372–3.
25. Borden LS Jr, Kozlowski PM, Porter CR, et al. Mechanical failure rate of da Vinci robotic system. Can J Urol 2007;14(2):3499–501.
26. Nayyar R, Gupta NP. Critical appraisal of technical problems with robotic urological surgery. BJU Int 2010;105(12):1710–3.
27. Kim WT, Ham WS, Jeong W, et al. Failure and malfunction of da Vinci Surgical systems during various robotic surgeries: experience from six departments at a single institute. Urology 2009;74(6):1234–7.
28. Andonian S, Okeke Z, Okeke DA, et al. Device failures associated with patient injuries during robot-assisted laparoscopic surgeries: a comprehensive review of FDA MAUDE database. Can J Urol 2008;15(1):3912–6.
29. Alemzadeh H, Raman J, Leveson N, et al. Adverse events in robotic surgery: a retrospective study of 14 years of FDA Data. PLoS One 2016;11(4):e0151470.
30. Lucas SM, Pattison EA, Sundaram CP. Global robotic experience and the type of surgical system impact the types of robotic malfunctions and their clinical consequences: an FDA MAUDE review. BJU Int 2012;109(8):1222–7 [discussion: 1227].
31. Matsuyama T, Kinugasa Y, Nakajima Y, et al. Robotic-assisted surgery for rectal cancer: current state and future perspective. Ann Gastroenterol Surg 2018;2(6):406–12.
32. Washington K, Watkins JR, Jay J, et al. Oncologic resection in laparoscopic versus robotic transhiatal esophagectomy. JSLS 2019;23(2).
33. Rogula T, Koprivanac M, Janik MR, et al. Does robotic Roux-en-Y gastric bypass provide outcome advantages over standard laparoscopic approaches? Obes Surg 2018;28(9):2589–96.
34. Wang L, Yao L, Yan P, et al. Robotic versus laparoscopic Roux-en-Y gastric bypass for morbid obesity: a systematic review and meta-analysis. Obes Surg 2018;28(11):3691–700.
35. Fazl Alizadeh R, Li S, Inaba CS, et al. Robotic versus laparoscopic sleeve gastrectomy: a MBSAQIP analysis. Surg Endosc 2019;33(3):917–22.
36. Alhossaini RM, Altamran AA, Seo WJ, et al. Robotic gastrectomy for gastric cancer: current evidence. Ann Gastroenterol Surg 2017;1(2):82–9.
37. Kane WJ, Charles EJ, Mehaffey JH, et al. Robotic compared with laparoscopic cholecystectomy: a propensity matched analysis. Surgery 2019;167(2):432–5.

38. Stitzenberg KB, Wong Y-N, Nielsen ME, et al. Trends in radical prostatectomy: centralization, robotics, and access to urologic cancer care. Cancer 2012; 118(1):54–62.
39. Kornaropoulos M, Moris D, Beal EW, et al. Total robotic pancreaticoduodenectomy: a systematic review of the literature. Surg Endosc 2017;31(11):4382–92.
40. Barbash GI, Friedman B, Glied SA, et al. Factors associated with adoption of robotic surgical technology in US hospitals and relationship to radical prostatectomy procedure volume. Ann Surg 2014;259(1):1–6.
41. Siddiqui NY, Galloway ML, Geller EJ, et al. Validity and reliability of the robotic objective structured assessment of technical skills. Obstet Gynecol 2014; 123(6):1193–9.
42. Newcomb LK, Bradley MS, Truong T, et al. Correlation of virtual reality simulation and dry lab robotic technical skills. J Minim Invasive Gynecol 2018;25(4):689–96.

Moving?

Make sure your subscription moves with you!

To notify us of your new address, find your **Clinics Account Number** (located on your mailing label above your name), and contact customer service at:

Email: journalscustomerservice-usa@elsevier.com

800-654-2452 (subscribers in the U.S. & Canada)
314-447-8871 (subscribers outside of the U.S. & Canada)

Fax number: 314-447-8029

Elsevier Health Sciences Division
Subscription Customer Service
3251 Riverport Lane
Maryland Heights, MO 63043

*To ensure uninterrupted delivery of your subscription, please notify us at least 4 weeks in advance of move.

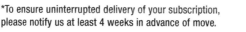

Printed and bound by CPI Group (UK) Ltd, Croydon, CR0 4YY

03/10/2024

01040478-0010